# Pain Medicine Manual
Second Edition

Commissioning Editor: *Paul Fam, Alison Ashmore*
Project Development Manager: *Belinda Henry*
Project Manager: *Rory MacDonald*
Designer: *Andy Chapman*

# Pain Medicine
# Manual Second Edition

**Edited by**

# Simon J Dolin FRCA PhD

Consultant in Pain Relief
St Richard's Hospital
Chichester, UK

# Nicholas L Padfield MBBS FRCA

Consultant in Anaesthesia and Pain Management
Pain Management Centre
St Thomas' Hospital
London, UK

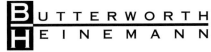

An imprint of Elsevier

Edinburgh • London • New York • Oxford • Philadelphia • St Louis • Sydney • Toronto • 2004

BUTTERWORTH-HEINEMANN
An imprint of Elsevier Limited

First edition 1996
Second edition 2004

ISBN 0750656174

**British Library Cataloguing in Publication Data**
A catalogue record for this book is available from the British Library

**Library of Congress Cataloging in Publication Data**
A catalog record for this book is available from the Library of Congress

**Notice**
Medical knowledge is constantly changing. Standard safety precautions must be followed, but as new research and clinical experience broaden our knowledge, changes in treatment and drug therapy may become necessary or appropriate. Readers are advised to check the most current product information provided by the manufacturer of each drug to be administered to verify the recommended dose, the method and duration of administration, and contraindications. It is the responsibility of the practitioner, relying on experience and knowledge of the patient, to determine dosages and the best treatment for each individual patient. Neither the Publisher nor the editors/contributors assume any liability for any injury and/or damage to persons or property arising from this publication.
**The Publisher**

 ELSEVIER SCIENCE    your source for books, journals and multimedia in the health sciences
**www.elsevierhealth.com**

Printed in China

The
publisher's
policy is to use
paper manufactured
from sustainable forests

# Contents

Contents

# List of Contributors

**Brendan Amesbury MB CHb MRCGP**
Consultant in Palliative Medicine
St Wilfrid's Hospice
Chichester, UK

**Caroline Bradbeer MBBS MRCP FRCP**
Consultant Genitourinary Physician
St Thomas' Hospital
London, UK

**Beverly J Collett MBBS FRCA**
Consultant in Pain Management and Anaesthesia
Pain Management Service
University Hospitals of Leicester
Leicester Royal Infirmary
Leicester, UK

**John Coppin MCSP SRP**
Orthopaedic Physiotherapy Specialist
Physiotherapy Department
St Richard's Hospital
Chichester, UK

**Anthony H Dickenson PhD**
Professor of Neuropharmacology
Department of Pharmacology
University College London
London, UK

**Simon J Dolin FRCA PhD**
Consultant in Pain Relief
St Richard's Hospital
Chichester, UK

**Jane M Green BSc AfBPsS**
Consultant Chartered Clinical Psychologist
Pain Clinic
St Richard's Hospital
Chichester, UK

**Richard Haigh MRCP**
Consultant Rheumatologist
Department of Rheumatology
Royal Devon & Exeter Hospital
Exeter, UK

**Jane Hazelgrove BSc(Hons) MBBS FRCA MSc**
Consultant in Anaesthesia
Department of Anaesthesia
Southampton General Hospital
Southampton, UK

**Robin S Howard PhD FRCP**
Consultant Neurologist
Department of Neurology
Guys and St Thomas' Hospital
London, UK

**John Hughes MBBS FRCA**
Consultant in Anaesthetics and Pain Management
The James Cook University Hospital
Middlesborough, UK

**Elizabeth A Matthews PhD**
Postdoctoral Research Fellow
Department of Pharmacology
University College London
London, UK

**Toby Newton-John BA(Hons) MPsychol PhD**
Consultant Clinical Psychologist
Behavioural Sciences and Dentistry
Eastman Dental Hospital
London, UK

**John K O'Dowd MR RS FRCS FRIS ORTH**
Consultant Spinal Surgeon
Department of Orthopaedics
Guy's and St Thomas' Hospital
London, UK

**Nicholas L Padfield MBBS FRCA**
Consultant in Anaesthesia and Pain Management
Pain Management Centre
St Thomas' Hospital
London, UK

**Jonathan Richardson MD FRCP FRCA**
Consultant Anaesthetist, Specialist in Pain
Department of Anaesthesia
Bradford Royal Infirmary
Bradford, UK

**Martin G Ridley MB FRCP**
Consultant Physician and Rheumatologist
Department of Rheumatology
St Richard's Hospital
Chichester, UK

**Peter Rogers MBBS FRCA**
Consultant in Pain Medicine
Pain Relief Clinic
St Mary's Hospital
Portsmouth, UK

**Anthony G Rudd FRCP**
Consultant in Stroke Medicine
Department of Elderly Care
St Thomas' Hospital
London, UK

**Karen H Simpson FRCA**
Consultant in Pain Medicine
Pain Management Service
St. James's University Hospital
Leeds, UK

**Jay R Skidmore PhD**
Professor and Director of Clinical Training
Department of Graduate Psychology
Seattle Pacific University, USA
Formerly, Consultant Clinical Psychologist
Programme Director for Pain Management
Surrey and Sussex, UK

**Catherine F Stannard MB ChB FRCA**
Consultant in Pain Medicine
The Pain Clinic
Frenchay Hospital
Bristol, UK

**Stephen P Ward FRCA**
Consultant in Pain Relief
Pain Management Unit
The Princess Royal Hospital
Haywards Heath, UK

**Stephan H Weber MD FRCA**
Consultant Anaesthetist
Department of Anaesthetics
Worthing and Southland's Hospitals
Worthing, UK

**Joanna M Zakrzewska MD FDSRCS FFDRCSI**
Senior Lecturer, Honorary Consultant
Department of Oral Medicine
St Bartholomew's and the Royal London School of
Medicine and Dentistry
London, UK

# Foreword

The burden of unrelieved chronic pain is a major problem for health services throughout the world. Epidemiological surveys reveal the large number of patients who suffer, and the major socioeconomic impact that unrelieved chronic pain has upon these individual patients, healthcare providers, social services and employers. In the UK the provision of services is patchy and sometimes inadequate, although there are centres of excellence.

In many cases patients continue to suffer because the treatments they receive fail. Treatments fail for a number of reasons. A key reason is adherence to the traditional medical model (the sequence of symptoms, signs, investigation, leading to a curative treatment). Single modality treatments, especially interventions, are prone to fail because they do not address the multidimensional biopsychosocial components of chronic pain including associated psychological or physical disability.

A major dilemma for pain services is the wide variation in the treatments employed by different practitioners for patients with ostensibly the same pain problem. This inconsistency is readily apparent to outside observers and undermines attempts to have pain medicine acknowledged as a legitimate specialty, and in addition, is in stark contrast to the strength of the basic science base. Treatments come and go in all fields of medicine and this appears to be especially so in chronic pain. Whenever possible it is essential for practitioners to employ therapies for which there is evidence of effectiveness and evidence of absence of major adverse effects. In addition there is the issue of appropriateness. It is wasteful of scarce resources and potentially harmful for patients to be subjected to inappropriate treatment. It is salutary to consider that the very long established drugs morphine and amitriptyline remain the gold standards for pharmacological pain therapies.

Education is an important factor in ensuring that healthcare practitioners are able to prescribe effective, safe and appropriate treatments for patients with chronic pain. Textbooks such as the *Pain Medicine Manual* play an important role in delivering up-to-date information and the second edition provides an opportunity to recruit new authors and to revise chapters. A multidisciplinary, team-based approach is recognized as the most effective way to deliver care for patients with chronic pain, so education must be aimed at all members of the team. The authorship of this volume reflects this multidisciplinary approach as well as the massive contribution made by basic scientists to our understanding of the pathophysiology and pharmacology of pain. Training in pain medicine is now an established component of the training programme for anaesthetists in the UK. Other countries have established separate training programmes with specific qualifications in pain medicine. This represents a major advance and should ensure that there is a supply of well-trained persons in the future.

Whatever your background, if you are interested in pain medicine and you have not done so already, you should join the International Association for the Study of Pain. The IASP and its associated national chapters work to advance the cause of pain and to alert governments and other agencies as to the magnitude of the problem.

This book provides a wide-ranging introduction to chronic pain and will allow practitioners to improve the care of their patients by utilizing effective, safe and appropriate treatments.

**Douglas Justins MB BS FRCA**
Consultant in Pain Management and Anaesthesia
Pain Management Centre
St Thomas' Hospital
London, UK

# Preface

There are now more and more physical interventions available for treating patients suffering from chronic pain. On the other hand cognitive behavioural programmes have an important place and are complementary to interventional techniques – as interventional techniques are complementary to them. Cognitive behavioural programmes are not the opposite end of the pain treatment spectrum and they are most definitely not an alternative. However they do not necessarily suit the patients who are well-adjusted, have good coping strategies and appropriate beliefs about their pain, but would simply like there to be less of it.

Every pain specialist must decide where the treatment 'philosophy' lies. But whatever they decide, the patient must come first. They, after all, are the ones suffering from the pain which we as pain specialists are enjoined to try and palliate. They are not impressed when told there is no evidence that anything works in their particular case so they will have to go and live with it – good-bye! Neither political correctness, nor the desire to use patients as experimental material for some new technique should motivate our management decisions. We are all responsible and hopefully moral practitioners who should only want the best for our patients. If we firmly believe in a procedure that has minimal risk but the potential for benefit, provided we fully inform the patient what we hope to achieve, how we hope to achieve it and the risks they face by doing it, we are not acting irresponsibly. We do have a duty to audit our results and to engage in research. We should pool our results, where practicable, and engage in multicentre collaborations, we must own up to our failures. This is all clinical governance. But if we take the easy path, and never put our professional status on the line by trying our best to palliate our patients' pain by engaging in new technologies and new procedures, we may ultimately fail our patients.

**Simon J Dolin**
**Nicholas L Padfield**

# | Pain Clinic

*Simon J Dolin*

## Reasons for existence

Pain is usually a symptom of an underlying condition that needs diagnosis and treatment. This statement is generally true with conditions of recent onset (acute) or conditions that are progressive. However in many patients pain may continue once a diagnosis has been made and treatment of the underlying condition completed. Also there are some conditions where a diagnosis has been made but treatment is only palliative rather than curative. Further there are a number of patients who continue to experience pain even though no diagnosis can be made. These patients suffer from chronic pain, i.e. pain lasting a long time ($\chi\rho o\nu o\sigma$ = period of time). Chronic pain is no longer giving useful information, in contrast to acute pain, and it is deemed reasonable to treat this pain on a symptomatic basis. Because chronic pain patients cover most medical specialties there arose a need to establish a team who had a special interest in treating the most difficult cases of chronic pain. This development has been widely welcomed by other medical specialties.

Although Bonica[1] advocated the establishment of multidisciplinary pain clinics in the 1950s, it was only in 1961 that the first modern pain treatment centre was set up at the University of Washington. In the 1970s pain clinics became more widely established with further input from the ideas of Fordyce[2] and Sternbach.[3] They established the principle of pain treatment using a multidisciplinary approach. This approach allows simultaneous treatment of physical, emotional, behavioural, vocational and social aspects of pain in a more effective way, ideally at less expense. Since then pain clinics have spread throughout the world, and they are now in the mainstream of health care delivery. Pain clinics have grown up in parallel with palliative care services for the terminally ill, and there is much common ground between them. The growth of pain clinics has also paralleled the growth of anaesthesia as a speciality and the interest amongst groups of anaesthetists in clinical areas outside the operating theatre. The involvement of anaesthetists was an extension of their role in postoperative pain relief and regional anaesthesia. Anaesthesia was not the only speciality with an early interest in chronic pain, but the majority of specialists willing to devote time to this clinical area have been anaesthetists and this trend still persists.

## Role of pain clinics

The role of the pain clinic can be summed up as follows:

- to decrease subjective pain experience
- to increase general level of activity
- to decrease drug consumption
- to return to employment or full quality of life
- to decrease further use of health care resources.

An important additional function of pain clinics is education. Patients should be taught about the difference between acute and chronic pain. Misconceptions about the nature of the pain and its significance may need to be dispelled. Patients may arrive in the pain clinic having had many opinions from doctors and other health professionals. They may have been given variable information and much disinformation on the way. The message from the pain clinic should be that, while the pain may not be curable, it should be treatable and that there are many ways in which patients can take responsibility for their pain and learn to live with it.

Much of the aim of pain clinics is to do with reducing disability and maladaptive coping styles. The primary goal is to improve the patient's level of functioning while decreasing, as much as possible, the frequency and intensity of pain. It is important that the educational message should be consistent within the team, and it is helpful if the message is reinforced at every turn. Education not only applies to patients but also to other staff within the hospital and to referring doctors. It does take considerable time and effort to communicate with colleagues about what the pain clinic is capable of and also what the operating philosophy is within the clinic. One of the important functions of the pain clinic is to terminate the cycle of perpetual specialist referral.

Teaching is also an important role of pain clinics. Undergraduates do not tend to spend time in pain clinics or, indeed, in acute pain control, and there has been criticism of this. Some medical schools have now started to address this problem. Most teaching is postgraduate, and pain therapy is now seen as an important part of anaesthetists' training. Teaching at any level by other disciplines remains unstructured at present.

There is a great need for research in the field of chronic pain. The need is for controlled clinical trials to assess the different modes of therapy. This is as true in the field of pharmacology as it is in physiotherapy and nerve blocks. Much of the currently accepted activity within the pain clinic is only partly supported by definitive clinical trials,[4] but there have been many quality clinical trials supporting the role of both interventional[5] and psychological based treatments.[6]

## Referral patterns

Referral numbers and patterns will vary enormously between pain clinics. The question is whether pain clinics should take patients on a primary, secondary or even tertiary referral basis. This will be determined in part by the nature of the pain condition and in part by the expertise available within the clinic. Some conditions such as post-herpetic neuralgia will be readily diagnosed by the general practitioner and will be suitable for primary referral. For many conditions an initial diagnostic work-up is essential. Given the wide spectrum of medical conditions the initial diagnostic work-up may need to be done by orthopaedic surgeons, rheumatologists, neurologists, gynaecologists, general physicians, general surgeons, neurosurgeons, thoracic surgeons or maxillofacial surgeons, to name a few. While some of these may work closely or be integral to the pain clinic, it is likely that most referrals will need to go through the diagnostic work-up in other clinics and then come to the pain clinic as a secondary referral.

There is a need for regional referral centres that take tertiary referral from other pain clinics, especially when techniques that are sophisticated (e.g. cordotomy) or invasive (e.g. spinal cord stimulator) are being considered. It may be that some centres with neurology and neurosurgery services will offer expertise unavailable elsewhere. It may also be appropriate to have expensive facilities, such as residential pain management programmes, concentrated at one centre rather than trying to reproduce such facilities on a smaller scale.

There will also be referrals from the local hospice or terminal care facility if this is not part of an integrated service. These referrals will tend to be at short notice and will need prompt assessment and intervention. While it will only be a small minority of patients whose pain cannot be controlled by the palliative care physicians, the techniques available within the pain clinic are usually highly effective at gaining rapid pain control in this situation.

## Staff required[7-9]

Current management of chronic pain embodies the concept that patients with complex pain problems are best served by a team of specialists with different health care backgrounds. Many different practice styles are used in achieving the coordination of services and specialists. Solo practitioners may use referrals to other specialists in their area. Larger practices may permit several specialists to work in the same premises. Pain clinics in larger hospitals may have extensive programmes involving specialists with every possible interest as well as in-patient services. The broad expertise available in a multidisciplinary team allows consideration of emotional, psychological, familial and occupational consequences of patients' pain.

The specialities involved in pain management are psychology, psychiatry, neurology, neuro-surgery, anaesthesia, rehabilitation medicine, palliative care, rheumatology and physiotherapy. There will need to be a director of the pain clinic, and this is most often but not necessarily an anaesthetist. Input from occupational therapy, dietary specialists and vocational rehabilitation will also be useful. Dedicated nursing staff are essential to the running of an effective pain clinic. Office support personnel such as a business manager, receptionist and secretarial staff, as well as good access to medical records, are essential contributors to the team. The actual mix of personnel will vary between pain clinics depending on patient demand and available funding.

The International Association for the study of pain[10] has published guidelines called *Desirable Characteristics for Pain Treatment Facilities*. Pain treatment facilities have been categorized as follows:

- Multidisciplinary pain centres, to include representatives of two medical specialties together with a psychiatrist or psychologist and offer full diagnostic and therapeutic services for outpatient, inpatient and emergency care. The centre should be part of a major health science education or research organization and should be actively engaged in research and education.
- Multidisciplinary pain clinics which will have identical facilities to the multidisciplinary pain centre but need not teach or research or be part of a major health science education or research organization.
- The pain clinic must interact with at least three physicians or different specialities, one of whom must be a psychiatrist or psychologist. It must have both diagnostic and therapeutic facilities and provide emergency care.
- Modality-oriented clinics use only one treatment modality such as nerve blocks or acupuncture.

Actual staffing levels vary enormously between pain clinics. It is not clear what constitutes the ideal staffing ratio per head of population. Proposals for two consultant sessions (one outpatient, one procedure-based) for every 250 000 head of population have been made.[11] This was upgraded to one whole-time equivalent consultant for each 100 000 population.[12] However, those who work on this basis still find themselves overwhelmed with referrals and develop waiting lists. These figures also do not take account of other specialists, therapists, nurses and administrative staff needed within the pain clinic.

## Facilities required

Just as dedicated staff are essential to the continuity of patient care and to building up team-work, so a dedicated facility is essential. The biggest challenge for pain clinics is often acquiring enough space to allow for efficient handling of the flow of patients through the clinic. A fixed locus of operation is ideal for outpatient visits, medical consultations, transcutaneous nerve stimulation (TENS) clinics, group sessions for education, psychological or physical therapies, and in-patient stay.

A conference room for regular meetings is helpful, as is a staff lounge area. There must be sufficient space for reception and secretarial services as well as storage space for equipment. The treatment area must allow access to X-ray screening when needed and have adequate monitoring devices, oxygen, suction and ready access to resuscitation facilities. The ability to do some procedures under general anaesthesia is essential . A biplane fluoroscope with a C-arm and memory is generally sufficient for imaging purposes, although some more sophisti-cated facilities include carbon fibre floating tables. A well-staffed recovery area is also essential.

In-patient services are expensive in time and resources, and so they must be limited to rel-atively few patients. In-patient care can be an excellent option for those requiring drug detox-ification to more appropriate medications, extensive psychological or behavioural therapy, or therapies involving extended administration of drugs via complex routes, e.g. epidural or intrathecal. In-patient care may also be essential when out-patient care has failed and for those who may need temporary removal from a detrimental home environment to enable therapies to be more effective.

## Funding

Sources of funding are various. In publicly funded hospitals pain clinics will have an annual contract to treat a certain number of patients and be given an agreed budget to achieve this contract. The size of the contract and the staff and facilities provided will need to be agreed on an annual basis with the purchasers of the health service. Additional contracts for further work may be obtained if the pain clinic can provide a service at a price that is attractive to other purchasers outside the local hospital. More recently, a number of general practitioners now hold their own budgets and they are free to purchase pain clinic services as needed. However, not all of the pain clinic services may be on the list from which general practitioners can pur-chase, so this avenue of funding may be limited. Specialized units such as residential pain man-agement programmes or those with special expertise may get referral from other pain clinics on an extra-contractual referral basis. The funding for these referrals will generally come from the purchasers of the referring hospital. National tertiary referral centres may need to depend largely on such referrals.

Private insurance companies are generally willing to cover patients for some, but not all, pain clinic treatments.

## Value of pain clinics

With the increasing cost of health care it is essential that pain clinics justify the money spent on them. The benefits of pain clinic treatment are not simply limited to the subjective per-ception of patients but also extend to objective behavioural variables such as return to work and decreased use of the health care system.

Pain clinic patients often try a series of different therapies (medication, both analgesic and psychotropic, TENS, acupuncture, nerve blocks, physical and psychological intervention) until relief is achieved or further attempts are discontinued. In an intriguing study Davies *et al*[13] looked at the effect of sequential therapy and were able to demonstrate good improve-ment using this approach, suggesting that allowing patients to access multiple sequential pain therapies may well be an appropriate management strategy.

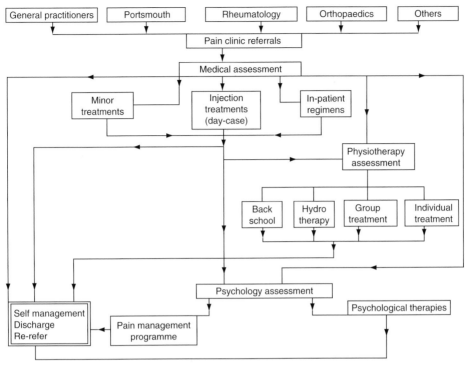

**Figure 1.1** Algorithm of possible routes through the pain clinic at St Richard's Hospital, Chichester. Decisions need to be made at a number of points about the most appropriate next step.

The role of large scale audits will become increasingly important. In the UK a national audit tool (PACS) is now in use, with annual reports being published.[14] Reports from the first year demonstrate that over 30% of patients achieved greater than one standard deviation of change in pain intensity and interference on discharge from pain clinics, with 27% of patients reporting either mild or no pain. Overall, patients reported pain relief was 34%. These figures reflect the activity of many pain clinics and indicate good effectiveness.

## Pain organizations

Many regional pain organizations have regular meetings, and most countries now have their own pain societies that have annual meetings where all disciplines involved in pain management can exchange ideas. National pain societies frequently advise their government departments of health and various speciality governing bodies. The International Association of the Study of Pain (IASP) has become the international body to which all national pain societies are affiliated. The IASP promotes the field at an international level, and it is also involved in publishing consensus guidelines and terminology for pain conditions. There is a world meeting held under the auspices of the IASP every 3 years.

The main international journal is *Pain*. There has recently been a proliferation of other journals in the field, including *Journal of Pain and Symptom Management, Journal of Palliative Care, Pain Clinics* and *Clinical Journal of Pain*. Some chronic pain literature is published in the anaesthetic journals and some important articles may be published in the mainstream medical literature, such as *The Lancet* or *New England Journal of Medicine*.

# References

1. Bonica JJ. Organisation and function of a pain clinic. *Adv Neurol* **4**: 433–443, 1974
2. Fordyce WE. *Behavioural Methods for Chronic Pain and Illness.* St Louis: CV Mosby, 1976
3. Sternbach RA. *Pain Patients: Tracts and Treatments.* New York: Academic Press, 1974
4. McQuay H, Moore A. *An evidence-based resource for pain relief.* Oxford University Press, 1998
5. Geurts JW, Van Wijk RM, Stolker RJ, Groen GJ. Efficacy of radiofrequency procedures for the treatment of spinal pain: A systematic review of randomized clinical trials. Reg Anesth Pain Med 26: 394–400, 2001
6. Flor H, Fydich T, Turk DC. Efficacy of multidisciplinary pain treatment centres: a meta-analytic review. *Pain* **49**: 221–230, 1992
7. Rowlinson JC, Hamill RJ. Organisation of a multidisciplinary pain centre. *Mt Sinai Med* **58**: 267–272, 1991
8. Hannenburg AA, McArthur JD. Establishing a pain clinic. *Intl Anesthesiol Clin Boston* **21**: 1–10, 1983
9. Bullingham RES, McQuay HJ, Budd K. Pain control centres: problem of organisation and operation in the UK. *Clin Anaesthesiol Lond* **3**: 211–221, 1985
10. International Association for the Study of Pain. *Desirable Characteristics for Pain Facilities.* Seattle: IASP, 1990
11. Mushin WW, Swerdlow M, Lipton S, Mehta MD. The pain centre. *Practitioner* **218**: 439, 1977
12. *Aneasthetists and Non-acute Pain Management.* Association of Anaesthetists of Great Britian and Ireland, Royal College of Anaesthetists and the Pain Society, 1993
13. Davies HT, Crombie TK, Brown JH, Martin C. Diminishing returns or appropriate treatment strategy? An analysis of short term outcomes after pain clinic treatment. *Pain* **70**: 203–208, 1997
14. Griffiths P, Noon J, Campbell F, Price C. Clinical governance, towards a practical solution. *Anaesthesia* **58**: 243–248, 2003

# 2 Pain Patient

*Simon J Dolin*

## Epidemiology of chronic pain

Chronic pain is a common experience and is costly both for the individual and for health care provision. A number of epidemiological studies have examined the extent of the problem. Chronic pain prevalence studies have considerable heterogeneity depending on populations chosen, chronicity definitions and the type of measure used (period or lifetime prevalence). Most studies were conducted in North America and Western Europe. Period prevalence was median 15% (range 2–40%).[1] In older patients chronic pain prevalence was in excess of 50%, rising slowly with the decades.[2]

In a randomly selected sample, chronic pain (every day for 3 months) was experienced by 17% of males and 20% of females.[3] Most of those with chronic pain reported some degree of interference with daily activities, but the impact was greatest in younger patients. Chronic pain was associated with older age, female gender, lower socio-economic status, poor education, poor health, increased levels of psychological distress and employment disadvantage. Interference was associated with younger age, female gender, lower socio-economic status, receipt of government pensions or benefits and being unemployed for health reasons. The literature on unemployment and health indicates a complex interdependence.[4] There is extensive literature on gender and pain, which indicates that females have a greater overall life experience of pain and suffer greater disability due to pain.[5]

Racial and ethnic differences have been reported. For example, non-Caucasian patients reported more severe low-back pain, and reported higher levels of pain and disability compared with Caucasian patients seen at a multidisciplinary pain centre.[6] The basis for these differences, whether biological, social or psychological remains unclear. The meaning of pain can be influenced by sociocultural factors related to ethnic background. Pain meaning can have a major influence on pain-related emotional responses (e.g. depression, guilt, anxiety) and behavioural responses (e.g. the decision to seek treatment, adherence to treatment regimens).

Chronic pain is a common complaint in childhood and adolescence. In a survey of 1300 children, 25% of respondents reported recurrent or continuous pain for more than 3 months. In girls, a marked increase occurred in chronic pain between 12 and 14 years of age. The most common types of pain in children were limb pain, headache and abdominal pain, and often multiple pain sites were reported.[7]

## Clinical presentation

Patients referred to pain clinics are most likely to present with musculoskeletal pains, in particular low-back, neck and shoulder pain. Neuropathic pain was less common, followed by facial pain/headache and visceral pain.[8] The referral pattern will, of course, vary with local special interests and expertise. Pain clinics now tend to see less cancer-related pain, as

Palliative Care teams have become more widespread and more effective. On presentation to pain clinics, mean pain intensity is on average severe with high levels of pain interference.[9] Sleep disturbance due to pain is common. Patients may have been seen by a number of physicians prior to referral (average 4.8)[10] who will have done appropriate diagnostic work-up. Patients may or may not have a meaningful diagnosis, and it is helpful for them to understand that pain clinics aim to control symptoms and not to arrive at a new or different diagnosis. Patients will have had symptoms for variable periods of time, often in excess of 1 year, and they will often have experienced failed therapies, including surgery, prior to referral.[9]

Although patients may persist in their desire to find a diagnosis in spite of multiple previous investigations, it is an important role of pain clinics to terminate further rounds of referral and to consider ways of limiting the patient's ongoing medical care. Chronic pain patients otherwise become substantial users of the health care system,[9] and once appropriate diagnosis has been completed further referrals and investigation may be counter-productive or even dangerous.

Chronic pain patients will present on a variety of analgesic medications, but most patients will be on multiple medications, often reporting at best modest benefit from these. A number of patients will present with high intake of opioid medications. Some of these patients may need to be detoxified, which can present a complex challenge to pain clinics. Patients may also present on antidepressants and, occasionally, benzodiazepines. While antidepressants may be useful in treating chronic pain the role of the benzodiazepines remains unclear.

## Psychological profile

There is a strong association between having chronic pain and having high levels of psychological distress. For example, chronic musculoskeletal pain is associated with major depressive symptoms.[11] Significant associations have been found between somatisation, anxiety, and depression scale scores and site-specific pain conditions.[12] This relationship has been demonstrated across different populations using different measures of psychological distress. There is a strong association between experiencing interference with daily activities due to chronic pain and increased levels of psychological distress.

Chronic pain and depression have a particularly close relationship. In chronic pain patients there is a high prevalence of depressive disorders; conversely, in patients with major depression pain is a frequent complaint. Importantly, pain improves with treatment of depression, and depression improves with treatment of pain.[13]

Post-traumatic stress disorder (PTSD) is commonly associated with chronic pain after injuries caused by trauma. It is characterized by dreaming and intrusive thoughts. Patients often find it painful to talk about, and it may not become apparent other than by direct questioning.[14] It is worth inquiring about because it is generally amenable to therapy.

Patient's beliefs about the meaning of their pain may be important. They may have fears that they do not readily express, such as fears about cancer or that they will end up in a wheelchair. Patient's beliefs are associated with physical disability and depression.[15]

The role of the patient within the family setting may also be important, as spouses or partners of chronic pain patients may play an important role in reinforcing pain behaviour.[16] The role of childhood victimization in the development of chronic pain in adulthood remains unclear. Various studies have cited higher incidences of reported abuse in chronic pain patients, especially for chronic pelvic pain, compared with other medical conditions and non-pain controls.[17] However, prospective studies have not confirmed the association.[18]

# Physical profile

Many chronic pain patients have become inactive, often not participating in regular exercise or employment. Much of their day may be spent resting in order to avoid pain. In addition to a loss of general fitness there may be reduction in use and range of movement of painful sites. Some patients may alternate periods of rest with excessive activity, the so-called boom–bust activity cycle. Recognition that fear of pain leads to avoidance of activity is an important observation, and it may influence treatment strategies.

# Litigation and compensation

Many chronic pain patients are actively involved in litigation when referred to the pain clinic. The relationship between litigation, compensation and clinical outcome is complex. There is a lack of prospective studies to clarify their contributions, but such studies as exist are retrospective and conclusions are contradictory.

# References

1. Verhaak PF, Kerssens JJ, Dekker J, Sorbi MJ, Bensing JM. Prevalence of chronic benign pain disorder among adults: a review of the literature. *Pain* 77: 231–239, 1998
2. Helme RD, Gibson SJ. Pain in the elderly. In: Jensen TS, Turner JA, Wiesenfeld-Hallin Z, eds. *Proceedings of 8th World Congress on Pain*. Seattle: IASP Press, 1997, pp. 919–944
3. Blyth F, March L, Brnabic J, Jorm L, Williamson M, Cousins M. Chronic pain in Australia: a prevalence study. *Pain* **89:** 127–134, 2001
4. Bartley M. Unemployment and health selection. *Lancet* **348:** 904, 1996
5. Unruh AM. Gender variations in clinical pain experience. *Pain* **65:** 123–167, 1996
6. Edwards CL, Fillingham RB, Keefe F. Race, ethnicity and pain. *Pain* **94:** 133–137, 2001
7. Perquin CW, Hazebroek-Kampschreur A, Hunfeld J, et al. Pain in children and adolescents: a common experience. *Pain* **87:** 51–58, 2000
8. Griffiths P, Noon J, Campbell F, Price C. Clinical governance: towards a practical solution. *Anaesthesia.* **58:** 243–248, 2003
9. Becker N, Bondegaard Thomsen A, et al. Pain epidemiology and health related quality of life in chronic non-malignant pain patients referred to a Danish multidisiplinary pain centre. *Pain* **73:** 393–400, 1997
10. Allen G, Galer B, Schwartz L. Epidemiology of complex regional pain syndrome: a retrospective chart review of 134 patients. *Pain* **80:** 539–544, 1999
11. Magni G, Marchetti M, Moreschi C, Merskey H, Luchini SR. Chronic musculoskeletal pain and depressive symptoms in the National Health and Nutrition Examination. I. Epidemiological follow-up study. *Pain* **53:** 163–168, 1993
12. Von Korff M, Dworkin SF, Le Resche L. An epidemiological comparison of pain complaints. *Pain* **32:** 173–183, 1988
13. Smith GR. The epidemiology and treatment of depression when it coexists with somatoform disorders, somatisation, or pain. *Gen Hosp Psychiatry* **14:** 265–272, 1992
14. Kulich R, Mencher P, Bertrand C, Maciewicz R. Comorbidity of post-traumatic stress disorder and chronic pain: implications for clinical and forensic assessment. *Curr Rev Pain* **4:** 36–48, 2000
15. Turner JA, Jensen M, Romano J. Do beliefs, coping and catastrophizing independently predict functioning in patients with chronic pain. *Pain* **85:** 115–125, 2000
16. Romano J, Turner J, Jensen M, et al. Chronic pain patient-spouse behavioural interactions predict patient disability. *Pain* **63:** 353–360, 1995
17. Walling MK, Reiter RC, O'Hara MW, Milburn AK, Liliy G, Vincnet SD. Abuse history and chronic pain in women: prevalence of sexual and physical abuse. *Obstet Gynecol* **84:** 193–199, 1994
18. Raphael KG, Widom KS, Lange G. Childhood victimization and pain in adulthood: a prospective investigation. *Pain* **92:** 283–293, 2001

# 3 Pain Pathophysiology

*Elizabeth A Matthews and Anthony H Dickenson*

Clinically significant pain has distinct neurophysiology and pharmacology to pain evoked by acute noxious stimuli. This is due to injury-evoked dysfunction and plasticity in the pain pathways. Exploitation of continually developing pharmacological, immunohistochemical, molecular and genomic techniques, furthers the knowledge of molecular and cellular mechanisms that underlie the pain systems, along with the pathophysiological changes. Much of the understanding surrounding pain transmission comes from the extensive study into cutaneous sensory input. Whereas many pains arise from damage to tissue, chronic neuropathic pains can arise from injury to both the peripheral nervous system and the central nervous system (CNS) from causes such as diabetes mellitus, herpes zoster and lesions. Characteristic symptoms experienced with chronic or persistent pain, resulting from inflammatory tissue damage or nerve injury, include expanded receptive fields, increased amplitude of response to a given stimulus (hyperalgesia), pain elicited by normally innocuous stimuli (allodynia) and spontaneous pain in the absence of external stimuli. Sensory deficits can also exist in neuropathic pain.[1]

## Primary afferent fibres

Primary somatosensory afferents are classified into Aβ, Aδ and C fibres (Table 3.1), which are differentially sensitive to noxious and non-noxious stimuli. Heavily myelinated and thus large diameter, rapidly conducting, Aβ fibres normally transmit modes of non-noxious, low intensity mechanical stimuli, from specialized encapsulated receptors on their peripheral endings. Thinly myelinated, intermediately sized and conducting Aδ fibres convey both innocuous and noxious information. C fibres lack myelination, and they are the smallest and slowest conducting afferents specialised for polymodal transmission of noxious stimuli from their free peripheral nerve endings. 'Sleeping' nociceptors, unresponsive to mechanical stimuli under normal circumstances, are only chemosensitive.

Histochemically, C fibre afferent neurones are further divided into IB4-positive and TrkA-positive populations (IB4 is a plant-derived isolectin and TrkA is a nerve growth factor receptor). These populations display functional differences in certain facets of pain transmission and differential sensitivities to trophic factors, critical not only during development but also for maintenance of afferent phenotypes in the adult nervous system and may underlie fibre alterations in persistent pain states.[2]

### Sensitization of peripheral nociceptors in inflammation

Inflammatory mediators released from areas of tissue damage chemically activate and can sensitize nociceptor terminals to subsequent thermal and mechanical stimuli, producing hyperalgesia and allodynia. Most have the ability to produce painful sensations in humans and in animal models, and blockade of their activity either through production or receptor antagonism is generally antihyperalgesic (Figure 3.1).

**Table 3.1** Properties of the sensory cutaneous primary afferent fibre types

|  | Aβ fibre | Aδ fibre | C fibre |
|---|---|---|---|
| Conduction velocity (m/sec) | 7–75 | 2–7 | 0.5–1.5 |
| Myelination | Heavy | Light | None |
| DRG cell body diameter (μm) | 45–51 | 33–38 | 20–27 |
| Stimulus conveyed | Non-noxious | Non-noxious/ noxious | Noxious |

Bradykinin (BK) is an important proinflammatory peptide. Via the B2 BK receptor positively coupled to protein kinase C (PKC), BK directly activates capsaicin-sensitive nociceptors, and is linked to modulation of noxious heat responsiveness. The B1 receptor may have increased importance in persistent inflammation, possibly due to increased expression or receptor sensitization. Bradykinin also sensitises nociceptors to other inflammatory agents including prostaglandins (PGs), 5-hydroxytryptamine (5-HT) and histamine, and vice versa. Prostaglandins are linked to the generation of cAMP and protein kinase A, which enhance activation of tetrodotoxin-resistant (TTX-resistant) Na$^+$ channels and VR1 currents, impor-

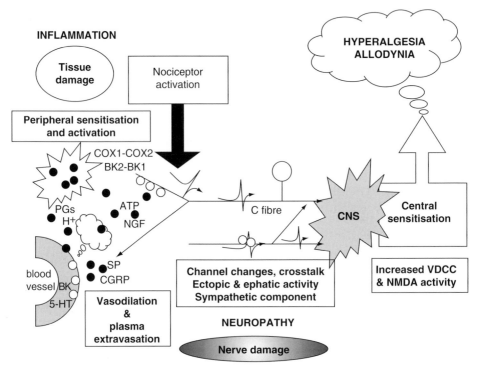

**Figure 3.1** Mechanisms of inflammatory and neuropathic pain, as described in detail in the text. Inflammatory mediators and neuropeptides (●: PGs, prostaglandins; BK, bradykinin; ATP, adenosine triphosphate; NGF, nerve growth factor; SP, substance P; CGRP, calcitonin gene-related peptide; 5-HT, 5-hydroxytryptamine) activate their peripheral receptors (o) leading to sensitization of nociceptors on primary afferent fibres. Nerve damage leads to alterations in peripheral nerves. Increased afferent barrage into the central nervous system (CNS) leads to both increased neuronal activity and central sensitization, which underlie allodynia and hyperalgesia.

tant in nociception (discussed below). Prostaglandins are produced by the cyclooxygenase (COX) enzymes. COX-1 is constitutive, whereas COX-2 is induced in the periphery by inflammation.

Some cytokines, including tumour necrosis factor-$\alpha$ (TNF-$\alpha$) and interleukin 6 (IL-6), have proinflammatory roles exerting direct effects upon sensory neurones in addition to modulatory influences upon inflammatory and immune cells. Sensitisation is mediated by cytokines through the phosphorylation and upregulation of ion channels in acute and chronic inflammatory states, respectively. Many inflammation-induced alterations to primary afferent functioning are dependent upon nerve growth factor (NGF), whose release from immune and Schwann cells is increased in inflammatory states. Nerve growth factor mediates hyperalgesia directly and indirectly by actions on nociceptors and inflammatory cells, respectively. Activation of its neuronal TrkA receptor culminates in phosphorylation of ion channels and intracellular targets to modulate expression of neuropeptide transmitters, receptors and ion channels important in nociception. Peptide neurotransmitters, predominantly released from C fibre central terminals, are also released peripherally in neurogenic inflammation. Calcitonin gene-related peptide (CGRP) and substance P mediate vasodilation and plasma extravasation, respectively.[3]

# Anatomical changes to peripheral nerves after nerve injury

Peripheral nerve damage usually results in the formation of a 'neuroma', whereby the distal end of the remaining primary afferent seals and swells. Disruption to Schwann cell distribution occurs along damaged axons and at the neuroma producing areas of demyelination that show altered conduction properties and abnormal excitability. There can also be loss of predominantly A fibre axons distal to the site of damage accompanied by sensory neuronal cell death in the dorsal root ganglia (DRG), likely a result of disrupted axonal transport of trophic factors.

## Nerve injury-induced primary afferent sprouting

Deafferentation induced by peripheral nerve damage can initiate the reinnervation of target tissue. Regeneration is not always lucrative, and success depends on fibre type and injury extent. A$\beta$ fibres are least likely to regenerate, in contrast to C fibres, and this is increasingly hindered with increasing severity of nerve injury. In some cases regeneration fails to be initiated and sensory loss in the target area results. In other situations inappropriate targeting of regenerating fibres can lead to innervation of low-threshold cutaneous receptors by nociceptive afferent neurones. Collateral sprouting can also occur, where uninjured sensory afferents of adjacent uninjured nerves, or the damaged nerve itself, expand into the deafferented area. This is mediated by all fibre types, yet smaller primary afferents appear to have the potential to expand over larger areas, which may have relevance in the development of hyperalgesia. In both axonal regeneration and collateral sprouting erroneous reinnervation of deafferented target tissue could contribute to aberrant pain sensations and abnormal central spatial representation of tactile information in neuropathic pain sufferers.[4,5]

## Ectopic activity

Ectopic activity arises when sites other than the normal transduction elements of primary afferent nerve fibres generate impulses, as a result of injury-induced alterations to their electrical transduction properties. This can be either spontaneous or stimulus-dependent in nature, and it can arise from afferent axonal sprouts innervating the neuroma, axonal areas of demyelination and DRG of A and C fibres. Spontaneous activity of primary afferent neurones occurs in the absence of stimulus. Rarely observed in an intact peripheral nervous system, this can develop after nerve injury. Clinically, positive correlations have been made between the occurrence of spontaneous firing of nociceptors innervating the painful region and neuropathic pain. In both human neuropathic pain states and animal models, stimulus-independent pain is observed and spontaneous ectopic activity seems a likely contributing factor.

Stimulus-dependent ectopic activity can arise in the injured or regenerating nerve in the neuroma or axon, whereby novel or increased sensitivity to thermal and chemical mechanical stimuli develops such that even blood vessel pulsation can evoke pain. Subsequent to nerve injury, axons become responsive to exogenous application of sensitizing inflammatory mediators, such as BK, histamine and PGs, which are normally only active at peripheral nerve terminals, and this may be important in the development of hyperalgesia. Endogenously, peripheral nerve damage has been shown to bring about a local inflammatory response involving the release of inflammatory mediators from immunocompetent cells and proliferating Schwann cells.[5]

## Pathologic interneuronal communication

Nerve injury-induced demyelination impacts upon non-synaptic modes of interneuronal communication such that abnormal interactions between different fibre types can occur. Low-threshold Aβ fibres may directly activate nociceptive C fibres, allowing innocuous stimuli to evoke painful sensations possibly contributing to allodynia. Apposition of denuded axons can allow the 'cross-excitation' of an impulse in one fibre to an adjacent fibre via 'ephatic communication'. 'Crossed-afterdischarge' involves diffusible factors, released from the activity of a group of neurones, altering the endogenous firing activity of their neighbours. Areas of demyelination and neuromas become more susceptible to such substances, and crossed-afterdischarge may enhance ectopic activity ongoing in damaged nerves as well as recruiting silent neurones.[2,4]

## Sympathetically-activated sensory system

Following peripheral nerve damage, atypical sensory-sympathetic coupling can occur. Sympathetic sprouting forms 'basket' structures that surround DRG soma, permitting close contact between sympathetic terminals, reliant upon NGF and cytokines produced by Schwann and immunocompetent cells following peripheral nerve injury. This novel sympathetic innervation allows noradrenergic modulation of DRG activity such that spontaneous or evoked firing is dramatically enhanced. Via Aβ fibres this may directly evoke allodynia, and via facilitation of a constant C fibre input into the dorsal horn it may contribute to central sensitisation. Numerous clinical and pre-clinical studies, some utilising surgical or chemical intervention, have confirmed a sympathetically-maintained component of some, but not all, types of neuropathic pain.[5]

## Abnormal dorsal horn reorganization

Primary afferent fibres terminate and make their first synapse with the CNS in the dorsal horn of the spinal cord, a site where the peripheral input undergoes anatomical convergence and neurotransmitter system modulation before projection to higher brain centres via ascending tracts (Figure 3.2). On entering the spinal cord, Aβ fibres terminate in the deep laminae of the dorsal horn where they synapse onto non-nociceptive, low-threshold second order neurones, before projection to the brain. In lamina V, Aβ fibres also terminate upon wide dynamic range (WDR) neurones, which also receive C fibre input. Aδ fibres with high-threshold

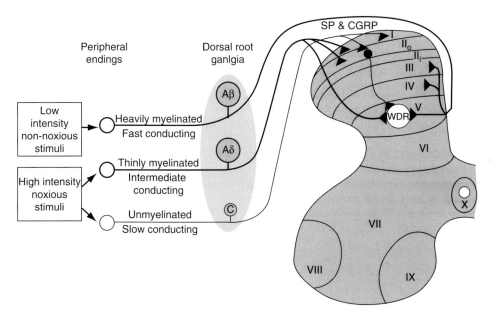

**Figure 3.2** Organization of the spinal cord laminae in lumbar segments and the termination patterns of cutaneous primary afferent fibre input. Noxious stimuli-evoked afferent input mediates the release of peptide neurotransmitters substance P (SP) and calcitonin gene-related peptide (CGRP) from C fibre terminals in the superficial laminae of the dorsal horn. Non-noxious and noxious input converges upon wide dynamic range (WDR) neurones, which then project to the brain via ascending tracts.

peripheral mechanoreceptors distribute ipsilaterally to laminae I, IIo and V, with some projections to contralateral lamina V. They terminate upon predominantly WDR and nociceptive, high-threshold second order dorsal horn neurones, which project to the brain via various ascending tracts. C fibre primary afferent fibres terminate in the superficial dorsal horn. Peptidergic TrkA-positive nociceptors distribute to laminae I and IIo, whereas the non-peptidergic IB4-positive population distribute to IIi. Lamina I contains nociceptive-specific (mechanical, heat and cold) and WDR dorsal horn neurones, the majority of which project to the brain. In contrast, the cells of lamina II only project locally to surrounding segments and serve as interneurones relaying inputs to deeper laminae, such as the WDR neurones in V.[6]

Damage to peripheral nerves can lead to alterations in the anatomical dorsal horn organization of primary afferent termination patterns that may underlie some neuropathic pain symptoms and characteristics. Peripheral nerve injury results in loss of primary afferent input, including C fibres, into the dorsal horn such that nociceptive input is reduced – a possible explanation for sensory deficits experienced by neuropathic pain patients. In contrast, deafferentation induces peripheral primary afferent regeneration. Whilst this is beneficial for restoration of original circuitry, aberrant re-wiring may underlie positive neuropathic pain symptoms such as allodynia.

Central projections of intact Aβ fibres within the deep dorsal horn conveying non-noxious information may make abnormal dorsal-oriented sprouts into lamina II after nerve injury. Alongside the induction of substance P expression in Aβ fibres, sprouting may permit innocuous input to activate nociceptive-specific spinal cord neurones. This appears a rational mechanism for touch-evoked pain; however, it is difficult to prove clinically. The existence of Aβ fibre sprouting and its functional relevance is debatable. There are discrepancies concerning Aβ fibre specificity of the tracer used for identification, and antiallodynic drugs have little impact upon Aβ fibre-evoked response electrophysiologically.[7] Furthermore, it cannot account for the induction of allodynia, since the time scale of functional reorganization of Aβ fibre terminals does not correlate with the rapidity with which allodynia can be manifest. Aβ fibre reorganization may be of importance in the maintenance of allodynia.[8]

Peripheral nerve damage can also lead to long-term changes in the CNS, contributing to the dysesthesias associated with neuropathic pain. Dorsal horn neurones display enlarged receptive fields,[9] spontaneous activity and reduced mechanical stimuli thresholds in parallel with lowered magnitudes of responses[10] alongside a loss of afferent input into the spinal cord. These observations fit well with the clinical neuropathic pain profile of both allodynia and hyperalgesia together with sensory deficits, yet how altered peripheral and central neuronal responses contribute to these symptoms still remains to be thoroughly defined. What is clear is that in the presence of dramatically reduced afferent input, dorsal horn neuronal responses manage to sustain their response magnitudes, which is indicative of central neuronal compensatory mechanisms and may explain the positive symptoms of neuropathic pain despite loss of normal sensory input.[11] The increased barrage of impulses arising from primary afferent fibres due to nerve injury is important in eliciting central sensitization and hyperexcitability of dorsal horn neurones. Ongoing peripheral activity results in sustained neurotransmitter release and activation of neurotransmitter systems within the spinal cord. Plasticity in the excitatory and inhibitory modulatory systems and functional connectivity together contribute to a persistent pain state.

# Ion channel plasticity in inflammation and neuropathy

The flow of ions through ligand-gated or voltage-dependent channels in neuronal membranes is critical for normal peripheral nerve function, controlling excitability and the propagation of action potentials. Modifications in expression and distribution of ion channels subsequent to peripheral nerve damage alters electrical properties and excitability of primary afferent fibres.

## Ligand-gated ion channels

VR1 is a ligand-gated, non-selective cation channel found predominantly on C fibre afferents. It is activated by capsaicin, heat (threshold 43°C) and H+ (pH 5.5). VR1 is, therefore, responsive to painful stimuli such as noxious heat and potentially the acidity associated with tissue inflammation. However, its role, if any, in pathophysiological pain is not yet clearly defined.

Acid-sensing ion channels (ASICs) are a family of ligand-gated cation channels, activated by H+, such that they respond to low pH. They are found throughout the nervous system, however, the dorsal root acid sensing ion channel (DRASIC) is sensory neurone-specific. Acidic conditions are associated with inflamed tissue, arthritic joints and ischaemia, producing pain and underlying hyperalgesia to both mechanical and thermal stimuli.

P2X receptors are another family of ligand-gated cation channels that respond to adenosine triphosphate (ATP). ATP is released from damaged tissues and can elicit painful sensations in humans. In particular P2X3 is only found in non-peptidergic IB4-positive C fibres. In inflammatory conditions, responses to ATP are increased and P2X3 knockout mice display altered pain processing, with preserved acute nociception.[2]

## Voltage-dependent ion channels

In the adult, non-pathological situation, DRG express at least seven types of Na+ channels. Of these, the TTX-resistant (high threshold of activation; slow activation/inactivation) the sensory neurone specific (SNS) and the neuronal sodium channel (NaN) channels are specifically expressed upon nociceptive neurones. After peripheral nerve damage their gene expression is reduced, yet translocation of SNS to the site of injury is enhanced. The lack of myelin surrounding the neuroma allows insertion of translocated $Na^+$ channels into the axonal membrane, in correlation with the materialization of ectopic spontaneous discharge. The expression of a silent TTX-sensitive $\alpha$-III embryonic $Na^+$ channel emerges in C fibres, the kinetics of which (low threshold of activation; rapidly activating/inactivating) likely permit repetitive firing in injured neurones that probably contributes to ectopic activity. A similar pattern of TTX-sensitive channel increase and TTX-resistant decrease is also mirrored in damaged A$\beta$ fibres. Ectopic neuronal discharge can be reduced by systemic and topical administration of $Na^+$ channel blockers, including some anticonvulsants, antiarrhythmics and local anaesthetics. Pre-clinical and clinical data report reductions in neuropathic pain behaviours or symptoms following $Na^+$ channel blockade. During persistent inflammation SNS expression is likewise increased, and spinal SNS antisense oligonucleotide treatment reverses hyperalgesia. Furthermore, SNS sensitivity is enhanced by inflammatory mediators such as PGs, adenosine and 5-HT.[3,4,12]

Voltage-dependent $Ca^{2+}$ channels (VDCCs) are critical to the sensory pathway in various aspects. In response to membrane depolarization they mediate $Ca^{2+}$ entry into numerous cell types, and thus underlie synaptic transmission of sensory information from the periphery to the brain via the control of depolarization-coupled neurotransmitter release, neuronal excitability and intracellular changes, including gene induction. Sensory neurones express a number of classes of VDCCs (L, N, P, Q, R and T), distinguished by their electrophysiological and pharmacological profiles. N- and P/Q-type VDCCs, sensitive to block by $\omega$-conotoxin-GVIA and $\omega$-agatoxin IVA, respectively, are widely expressed throughout the brain and spinal cord. The N-type channel is concentrated in laminae I and II of the superficial dorsal horn, where nociceptive primary afferents synapse. Upon substantial membrane depolarization, N- and P/Q-type are the VDCCs responsible for release of excitatory neurotransmitters, critical for wind-up and central sensitization. There is an established role for VDCCs in nociception, and the contribution of the different channel subtypes appears to alter depending on the nature of the pain. A predominant nociceptive role for N-type VDCCs has been established, which is enhanced after neuropathy and inflammation. P/Q-type channels appear to play a modest role in sensory transmission. They are implicated in the initiation of a facilitated pain state, especially inflammation, with little influence in the maintenance of neuropathy. L- and T-type channels appear to have a limited role in sensory transmission. T-type VDCC activation occurs close to resting potential; they allow $Ca^{2+}$ influx when cells are at rest, thus regulating cell excitability and most likely the depolarization required to activate high-voltage activated N- and P/Q-type channels necessary for neurotransmission.[13–15] It is noteworthy that SNX-111 and gabapentin (GBP), with analgesic efficacy in patients, may exert their effects via binding to VDCCs. Gabapentin has been demonstrated to bind to the auxillary $\alpha_2\delta$ subunit of VDCCs, where it is assumed to act as an antagonist, and it may highlight the importance of VDCCs as targets in pain control.[7,15]

# Neurochemical changes of primary afferent fibres

Neurotransmission between nociceptive primary afferent neurones and secondary neurones in the dorsal horn is dependent on neurotransmitters that are produced in the DRG-located cell bodies of primary afferent neurones and stored in presynaptic vesicles of central terminals awaiting depolarization-coupled release. Translocation of neurotransmitters to peripheral terminals is relevant to neurogenic inflammation. Neurotransmitters comprise excitatory amino acids (EAAs), such as glutamate and aspartate, associated with fast excitatory neurotransmission, and neuropeptides, such as calcitonin gene-related peptide (CGRP) and substance P, which can exert longer-lasting actions. Chronic pain can mediate alterations to the different primary afferent neurochemical phenotypes.

## Neurochemical downregulation

In rat and monkey DRG approximately 45% and 75%, respectively, of neurones are CGRP-immunoreactive, and these are primarily nociceptive primary afferents. Likewise, 40% of monkey DRG neurones synthesise substance P mRNA and this is nociceptive fibre specific. Following nerve injury, there is a marked reduction in the expression of both these peptides in the DRG, explained by the transient loss of TrkA receptors on the peripheral terminals of TrkA-positive, peptidergic primary afferents, and disrupted axonal transport of NGF to the DRG. Furthermore, nerve injury-induced spontaneous activity within the DRG may result in a depletion of presynaptic terminal stores of peptide due to increased activity-dependent vesicular release.[2,16]

## Neurochemical upregulation

Other peptides are upregulated in sensory neurones following peripheral nerve damage in a manner serving to predominantly enhance pain transmission. Although overall levels of substance P mRNA are downregulated, in contrast to nociceptive fibre substance P decrease, the previously quiescent expression of substance P in Aβ fibres is induced after nerve injury. This fibre switch to a nociceptive mode from a previously tactile-specific function may have relevance to touch-evoked pain.

Vasoactive intestinal polypeptide (VIP), not normally expressed in lumbar ganglia, is also upregulated in DRG after nerve injury. Nerve growth factor may act to prevent expression of VIP, the inhibitory effect of which would be removed on the decrease of NGF after nerve injury. Vasoactive intestinal polypeptide is important in glycogenolysis and, therefore, its upregulation may reflect active processes of nerve regeneration. However, it appears to mediate a central excitatory role in pain transmission.

Galanin is normally expressed in a limited number of small diameter DRG neurones. Although its role is somewhat unclear, galanin generally enhances nociception. Following peripheral nerve damage, its expression is upregulated in small diameter neurones and induced in larger cells and can exert inhibitory actions in the dorsal horn.

Neuropeptide Y, not normally expressed in sensory neurones, is also induced after nerve injury in large diameter neurones. This is paralleled by an increase of corresponding $Y_2$ receptors on peripheral afferents and central Aβ fibre terminals. Centrally, it may produce antinociceptive effects, yet peripherally it may be pro-nociceptive.

Nitric oxide (NO) is a neuronal modulator found throughout the CNS, produced on demand from L-arginine by nitric oxide synthase (NOS). NO may be linked to events downstream of N-methyl-D-aspartate (NMDA) receptor activation, underlying central sensitization as well as exerting peripheral actions. It is possibly important in chronic pain states. Following peripheral nerve damage, small DRG neurones show an increase in NOS mRNA. Nitric oxide synthase inhibitors have antinociceptive effects, although changes in NOS do not parallel behavioural allodynia[2].

Nerve injury and inflammation induce a complex pattern of anatomical, neurochemical and receptor alterations in primary afferent fibres, often in a fibre type-specific manner. Some of the changes observed are purely targeted to the development of persistent pain, but some of those apparently associated with regeneration of damaged nerves may also contribute to enhanced nociception. Although a general consensus prevails, the extent and specifics of such changes may be subject to slight variation in different pre-clinical models, and not all changes are permanent. There is substantial progress in the understanding of the relationship these nervous system alterations have to the onset and nature of pathological pain behaviours and their clinical relevance.

# References

1. Greenspan JD. Quantitative assessment of neuropathic pain. *Curr Pain Headache Rep* **5**: 107–113 2001
2. Millan MJ. The induction of pain: an integrative review. *Prog Neurobiol* **57**: 1–164, 1999
3. Kidd BL, Urban LA. Mechanisms of inflammatory pain. *Br J Anaesth* **87**: 3–11, 2001
4. Suzuki R, Dickenson AH. Neuropathic pain: nerves bursting with excitement. *Neuroreport* **11**: R17–21, 2000
5. Taylor BK. Pathophysiologic mechanisms of neuropathic pain. *Curr Pain Headache Rep* **5**: 151–61, 2001
6. Sorkin LS, Carlton SM. Spinal Anatomy and Pharmacology of Afferent Processing. In: Yaksh TL, Lynch III C, Zapol WM, Maze M, Biebuyck JF, Saidman LJ, eds. *Anesthesia: Biologic Foundations.* Philadelphia: Lippincott-Raven, 1997, pp. 577–609
7. Matthews EA, Dickenson AH. A combination of gabapentin and morphine mediates enhanced inhibitory effects on dorsal horn neuronal responses in a rat model of neuropathy. *Anesthesiology* **96**: 633–640, 2002
8. Blomqvist A, Craig AD. Is neuropathic pain caused by the activation of nociceptive-specific neurons due to anatomic sprouting in the dorsal horn? *J Comp Neurol* **428**: 1–4, 2000
9. Suzuki R, Kontinen VK, Matthews E, et al. Enlargement of the receptive field size to low intensity mechanical stimulation in the rat spinal nerve ligation model of neuropathy. *Exp Neurol* **163**: 408–413, 2000
10. Chapman V, Suzuki R, Dickenson AH. Electrophysiological characterization of spinal neuronal response properties in anaesthetized rats after ligation of spinal nerves L5-L6. *J Physiol* **507**: 881–894, 1998
11. Dickenson AH, Matthews EA, Suzuki R. Central nervous system mechanisms of pain in peripheral neuropathy. In: Hansson PT, Fields HL, Hill RG, Marchettini P, eds. *Progress in Pain Research and Management. Neuropathic pain: pathophysiology and treatment.* Seattle: IASP Press, 2001, pp. 185–106
12. Baker MD, Wood JN. Involvement of Na+ channels in pain pathways. *Trends Pharmacol Sci* **22**: 27–31, 2001
13. Matthews EA, Dickenson AH. Effects of spinally delivered N- and P-type voltage-dependent calcium channel antagonists on dorsal horn neuronal responses in a rat model of neuropathy. *Pain* **92**: 235–246, 2001
14. Matthews EA, Dickenson AH. Effects of ethosuximide, a T-type Ca(2+) channel blocker, on dorsal horn neuronal responses in rats. *Eur J Pharmacol* **415**: 141–149, 2001
15. Vanegas H, Schaible H. Effects of antagonists to high-threshold calcium channels upon spinal mechanisms of pain, hyperalgesia and allodynia. *Pain* **85**: 9–18, 2000
16. Wilcox GL, Seybold V. Pharmacology of Spinal Afferent Processing. In: Yaksh TL, Lynch III C, Zapol WM, Maze M, Biebuyck JF, Saidman LJ, eds. *Anesthesia: Biologic Foundations.* Philadelphia: Lippincott-Raven, 1997

# 4 Pain Pharmacology

*Elizabeth A Matthews and Anthony H Dickenson*

Acute pain can be successfully controlled by a variety of pharmacological agents, yet clinically significant chronic pain, resulting from inflammation or nerve injury, is fundamentally distinct, and it often responds poorly to traditional therapeutic approaches. Knowledge of the pharmacologically defined peripheral, spinal and brain systems involved in pain transmission has arisen from extensive study into sensory input in the clinical and pre-clinical settings. In response to a noxious stimulus, the central terminals of nociceptive primary afferent fibres, located in the dorsal horn of the spinal cord, release a diverse array of products, including amino acids, neuropeptides and neuromodulators. Activation of their respective receptor systems at postsynaptic sites predominantly results in excitation of dorsal horn neurones. However, within the spinal cord there are both excitatory and inhibitory systems, and the overall central excitability and degree of transmission of pain here is established by the interplay between the two.

## Excitatory receptor systems

### Neuropeptides

Substance P (a member of the neurokinin (NK) family) is the predominant nociceptive excitatory neurotransmitter peptide. It acts at the NK1 receptor to mediate slow depolarizations and sustained excitatory postsynaptic potentials (EPSPs) important for the recruitment of $N$-methyl-D-aspartate (NMDA) receptors for activation. Substance P is only released in response to noxious and persistent peripheral stimulation, since it is normally only expressed by C fibres, and, therefore, in nerve injury and inflammatory states. In the spinal cord, substance P-containing neurones are localized to the superficial dorsal horn, half arising from nociceptive primary afferent fibres and half from intrinsic dorsal horn neurones.[1] NK1 receptors are found on spinal cord neurones in the superficial laminae and on deeper cells with dendrites located superficially.[2]

The actions of substance P may be enhanced in persistent pain states. Under inflammatory and neuropathic conditions upregulation of NK-1 receptors occurs in the superficial dorsal horn, NK antagonists attenuate spinal sensitization after sciatic nerve section, and Aβ fibres phenotypically transform, allowing them to synthesise substance P[3]. In contrast, a decrease in spinal substance P itself is observed after nerve injury. In the presence of peripheral inflammation, substance P responsive dorsal horn neurones are necessary for spinal hyperexcitability and behavioural hyperalgesia but not normal acute noxious transmission and NK1 receptor knockout mice selectively show reduced hyperalgesia. Expression of substance P and its mRNA is increased in primary afferent neurones in the presence of peripheral inflammation. Destruction of the substance P containing cells in the spinal cord leads to noxious deficits in animals, but antagonists of the receptor have not been analgesic in patients, perhaps reflecting the need for a better understanding of this peptide.[4]

Calcitonin gene-related peptide (CGRP) is another important excitatory peptide, although CGRP-containing terminals are less abundant than those for substance P. It is found in laminae I, II, V and X, arising predominantly from nociceptive primary afferents. Activation of CGRP dorsal horn receptors serves to enhance the actions of substance P, but its role is comparatively less well defined due to a lack of useful antagonists. Calcitonin gene-related peptide mediates slow membrane depolarizations and increased intracellular $Ca^{2+}$ levels by both $Ca^{2+}$ influx and release from internal stores. Like substance P, the expression of CGRP and its mRNA is increased in primary afferents during peripheral inflammation.[5]

## Excitatory amino acids

The excitatory amino acids (EAAs) comprise glutamate and aspartate, found in both small and large primary afferent fibres.[6] Within the spinal cord, glutamate-containing fibres and terminals are found in laminae I–IV, the majority arising from primary afferent neurones although some are intrinsic. Aspartate-containing terminals are found in laminae I–III and separate from the glutamate population. The EAAs are considered to be fast neurotransmitters and their superficial dorsal horn localization implies an important role in pain transmission. Glutamate is predominantly found co-localized with substance P, probably ensuring that both are released from nociceptive afferents upon noxious stimulation.[3]

Glutamate receptors are subdivided into slow G-protein-coupled metabotropic receptors and fast ligand-gated ionotropic receptors. The ionotropic receptors are further characterized by synthetic agonists into AMPA (α-amino-3-hydroxy-5-methyl-4-isoxazolepropionic acid, which contribute to fast transmission of acute innocuous and noxious stimuli), kainate and NMDA receptors.[7] All three receptors are prominently localized to the superficial dorsal horn, with some located in deeper laminae probably expressed on wide dynamic range (WDR) neurones. The NMDA receptor has been the most extensively studied glutamate receptor owing to its ubiquitous central nervous system (CNS) expression. It is an ionotropic receptor coupled to a cation channel, which is quiescent under resting conditions due to intra-channel $Mg^{2+}$ block. Only upon the binding of glutamate, in addition to the co-agonist glycine, and sufficient membrane depolarization to relieve the $Mg^{2+}$ block, is the complex activated and $Ca^{2+}$ influx occurs. Ketamine, at analgesic doses, is an NMDA-receptor/channel blocker.

Prolonged peripheral input into the spinal cord via nociceptive C fibres is known to enhance dorsal horn neuronal responses to subsequent afferent input – an experimental phenomenon known as 'wind-up' used to study central sensitization and spinal cord hyperexcitability. The NMDA receptor is critical for wind-up, and consequently it is important in events that enhance and prolong sensory transmission[7]. Central sensitization is characterised by reduced thresholds and exaggerated responses to stimuli, and enlarged receptive fields; at the level of the spinal cord, NMDA receptor activity is heavily implicated.[8] The inherent properties of the NMDA receptor/channel complex described permit its role in the development of wind-up and central sensitization. Repetitive nociceptive afferent input mediates a sustained release of glutamate, substance P and CGRP, which activate AMPA and neuropeptide receptors. These actions combine to relieve $Mg^{2+}$ block, thus recruiting NMDA receptors into glutamatergic transmission. $Ca^{2+}$ influx through the NMDA receptor itself mediates further membrane depolarizations recruiting more NMDA receptors ... and so on. These convergent events result in amplified activation of the NMDA receptor. Increased and sustained $Ca^{2+}$ influx results, which sets in motion signal transduction cascades culminating in secondary modifications of ionic currents via receptor/ion channel phosphorylation, as well as long term alterations in receptor/neurotransmitter expression via gene transcription processes. Central sensitization is normally kept under control by inhibitory controls, yet in neuropathic and inflammatory pain central sensitization can persist and become pathological.

After nerve injury, there is evidence to show an ipsilateral enhancement of glutamate release and an upregulation of glutamate receptors. Administration of NMDA receptor antagonists in models of neuropathic pain and inflammation have proved effective in reducing hyperalgesic and allodynic behaviours, as well as dorsal horn neuronal responses[9]. Likewise, the hypothesized roles for NMDA receptors in central sensitization and its link to the development of neuropathic pain have been proven in clinical neuropathic pain states with the use of antagonists, but with limiting side-effects.[10]

## Other neuromodulators

As mentioned, elevated intracellular $Ca^{2+}$ levels arises from sustained afferent input due to its influx through activated voltage-dependent $Ca^{2+}$ channels (VDCCs) and ionotropic receptors, such as the NMDA receptor complex, in addition to its release from intracellular $Ca^{2+}$ stores by activation of G-protein-linked receptors, such as NK1. Downstream events leading to increased intracellular $Ca^{2+}$ include activation of enzymes such as cyclooxygenase 2 (COX-2) and nitric oxide synthase (NOS) required for the synthesis of prostaglandins (PGs) and nitric oxide (NO), respectively, as well as protein kinase C (PKC) activation. Prostaglandins and NO are released in the spinal cord following prolonged nociceptive transmission involving NMDA-receptor activation. Through prostanoid receptors in the dorsal horn, PGs cause increased spinal neurotransmitter release from primary afferents, yet spinal COX-2 inhibitors appear only to be effective as antihyperalgesics in persistent pain states, not in the acute situation. It is proposed that NO also increases presynaptic neurotransmitter release, acting as a retrograde transmitter, and its synthesis is implicated in the pro-nociceptive actions of substance P on dorsal horn neurones. Indeed, NOS inhibitors are antinociceptive in animal models of neuropathy and inflammation. Protein kinase C comprises a family of phosphorylating enzymes that, in particular, are known to phosphorylate the NMDA receptor priming it for further activation. Spinally administered PKC inhibitors have been demonstrated to be antihyperalgesic in animal models of facilitated nociception.[11]

Cholecystokinin (CCK) functions as an anti-opioid peptide, although its mechanism is not fully understood. There are two identified receptors for the peptide CCK, named CCKA and CCKB, the latter being the predominant type in the spinal cord of rats, whereas it is CCKA in primates. Its effect is not due to direct hyperalgesia, since CCK does not alter non-pathological pain thresholds, nor is it mediated via binding to opioid receptors. Cholecystokinin receptor antagonists have been found to be antinociceptive against neuropathic pain administered alone, and they are able to re-establish the effect of morphine lost after neuropathy.[12] It is proposed that nerve injury increases activity of the CCK system, through either changes in the peptide or its receptors, and this in turn reduces the efficacy of opioids in neuropathic pain, which can possibly be overcome by dose escalation.

Effective analgesia has the potential to be mediated by the selective inhibition of some of the afore mentioned excitatory spinal cord systems, reducing pain transmission before the information is conveyed up to higher brain centres. In addition to blocking excitatory events, the inhibitory spinal cord receptor systems can be exploited. In general these systems involve G-protein-coupled receptors that increase $K^+$ conductance and hyperpolarize neuronal membranes. Agonists that act on such receptors at a presynaptic location, particularly on C fibre terminals, will in effect reduce neurotransmitter release and pain transmission as it enters the spinal cord. In parallel, hyperpolarization mediated by activation of inhibitory receptors at postsynaptic sites serves to prevent dorsal horn neuronal depolarization in response to any excitatory neurotransmitters.

# Inhibitory Receptor Systems

## Opioids

The endogenous inhibitory opioid system has been manipulated to provide pain relief since the discovery of opium, of which morphine is the main active component. There are three classical opioid receptor types, namely mu, delta and kappa, plus the recently defined opioid-like receptor (ORL-1).[13] They are G-protein-coupled receptors, which upon activation inhibit cAMP formation and subsequently open $K^+$ channels (mu, delta and ORL-1 receptors). The resultant neuronal hyperpolarization decreases VDCC opening and $Ca^{2+}$ influx. In the case of kappa opioid receptor activation this reduction of $Ca^{2+}$ influx is direct. Endogenously, mu, delta and kappa receptors are activated by endorphin, enkephalin and dynorphin peptides, respectively, and exogenous agonists are potentially valuable analgesics (Table 4.1). Under normal conditions the spinal opioid system is not tonically active. ORL-1 is a recent addition to the opioid receptor family and is endogenously activated by the peptide nociceptin (or orphanin FQ), yet it only displays a low affinity for the universal opioid receptor antagonist, naloxone. Its physiological function and pain modulation role are as yet not thoroughly defined.[14]

Within the spinal cord, opioid receptors are mostly located in the superficial dorsal horn (laminae I and II), with a smaller population in deeper layers. The contribution of mu, delta and kappa receptors to the total opiate binding throughout the spinal cord is estimated at 70%, 24% and 6%, respectively, at a predominantly (>70%) presynaptic location that relates to C fibre afferent terminals. The main mechanism of spinal opioid analgesia is, therefore, via activation of presynaptic opioid receptors, which act to selectively decrease transmitter release from C fibre afferents and thus selectively inhibit nociceptive transmission. The remaining 30% of opioid receptors are located postsynaptically on interneurones, and the dendrites of projection cells. Here, any opioid-mediated cell hyperpolarization will not exert nociceptive-specific effects.[13]

The opioid system displays a substantial amount of plasticity in persistent pain states. Whilst such changes are beneficial in the presence of inflammation, neuropathic pain due to peripheral nerve damage more often than not displays reduced sensitivity to opioids. This is evident both pre-clinically and clinically, and is surrounded by much controversy.[15] Mechanisms by which opioid sensitivity may be reduced after nerve injury include a reduction of spinal opioid receptors, non-opioid receptor-expressing Aβ fibre-mediated allodynia, increased CCK antagonism and NMDA-mediated dorsal horn neuronal hyperexcitability, likely requiring a greater opioid inhibitory counteraction.[16]

Opioid receptors are distributed throughout the CNS, especially in areas other than the spinal cord also concerned with nociceptive processing such as the thalamus and supraspinal

| Table 4.1 | Agonists and antagonists of the opioid receptors | | | |
|---|---|---|---|---|
| | mu | delta | kappa | ORL-1 |
| Endogenous agonist | Endorphins | Enkephalins | Dynorphins | Nociceptin/OFQ |
| Synthetic agonist | Morphine DAMGO | DPDPE | Enadoline | None |
| Antagonist | Naloxone CTAP | Naloxone Naltrindole | Naloxone Nor-BNI | Pheψ |

DAMGO, [D-Ala$^2$,N-Me-Phe$^4$,Gly-ol$^5$]-enkephalin; DPDPE, [D-Pen$^2$, D-Pen$^5$]-enkephalin; CTAP, D-Phe-Cys-Tyr-D-Trp-Arg-Thr-Pen-Thr-NH$_2$; OFQ, orphanin FQ; Pheψ, [Phe$^1$ψ (CH$_2$NH)Gly$^2$]NC$_{(1-13)}$NH$_2$

midbrain and brainstem structures – the periaquaductal gray and the rostroventromedial medulla. Exogenous application of morphine into these sites elicits antinociceptive effects by increasing the activity of inhibitory descending controls that terminate in the dorsal horn.[17] The pathway that descends from the rostroventromedial medulla contains mostly enkephalin, 5-hydroxytryptamine (5-HT, or serotonin), γ-aminobutyric acid (GABA) and glycine containing fibre.

Opioid receptors are also found in the periphery and their expression is increased in nociceptive primary afferents during inflammation. Endogenously opiates are released from immune cells and exogenous agonists developed for peripheral application have been shown to be antinociceptive in inflammatory states.[18]

## Inhibitory amino acids

GABA is the major inhibitory neurotransmitter in the CNS, and its extensive distribution permits it to tonically control spinal cord excitability. The majority of GABA terminals arise from interneurones, though some are from descending tracts, and are mostly concentrated in the superficial dorsal horn (laminae I–III). GABA-ergic terminals can also contain other substances, such as glycine, galanin, enkephalin and neuropeptide Y in different populations, and they contact mainly nociceptive Aδ and C fibre terminals. There are two receptors for GABA in the spinal cord, $GABA_A$ and $GABA_B$, both of which are found pre-and postsynaptically on nociceptive afferents. $GABA_A$ is a ligand-gated $Cl^-$ channel, modulated by barbiturates and benzodiazepines. $GABA_B$ is a G-protein-coupled receptor linked to the inhibition of $Ca^{2+}$ influx via $K^+$ and $Ca^{2+}$ channel mediated actions.

Under normal conditions the GABA-ergic control of nociceptive transmission is near maximally activated, so loss of GABA-ergic control favours the generation of hyperexcitability. Plasticity within this system is implicated in pathophysiological pain states. $GABA_B$ agonists have been shown to be more effective than $GABA_A$ agonists in ischaemia-induced rat spinal cord injury, yet electrophysiologically midazolam, a positive allosteric modulator of $GABA_A$ receptor function, was shown to be more effective in inhibiting nociceptive activity after spinal nerve ligation (SNL).[19]

Glycine is another inhibitory amino acid and is found in dorsal horn neurones localized superficially, mostly in coexistence with GABA. It acts via a strychnine-sensitive receptor that is a ligand-gated $Cl^-$ channel to inhibit dorsal horn neurones, and spinal strychnine mediates allodynia and nociceptive behaviour in rats, so its role in nociceptive transmission appears similar to that of GABA. Little is known regarding changes to the glycinergic system after nerve injury, but increased glycine levels have been reported. In contrast glycine is a co-agonist at the NMDA receptor, but spinal levels are such that this affects its activation.[3]

## Monoamines

The majority of nociceptive pathways (including the spinoreticular and spinothalamic tracts) are under the control of bulbospinal projections originating in brainstem nuclei. The nucleus raphe magnus gives rise to 5-HT-containing projections, the locus caeruleus and lateral tegmentum cell systems contain noradrenaline, and these are released in the spinal cord selectively in response to high-intensity stimulated afferent input.[17]

The role of descending serotonergic pathways in the modulation of pain transmission is somewhat complicated by the multiplicity of its target 5-HT receptors, activation of which exerts both pro- and antinociceptive actions dependent on the differing effector mechanisms and neuronal locations. Dense 5-HT labelling is found in laminae I and II, the majority arising from supraspinal sites, in addition to a small interneuronal population. Stimulation of the nucleus raphe magnus displays a biphasic, excitatory followed by inhibitory, influence on dorsal horn neurones. Importantly, these descending pathways display plasticity after nerve damage. Chronic pain patients show changes in spinal levels of 5-HT, and deep laminae terminating serotonergic terminals sprout into lamina II such that nociceptive transmission is enhanced. Blockade of 5-HT re-uptake by tricyclic antidepressants may account for their noted analgesic effects. In brief, $5\text{-HT}_{1B}$ and $5\text{-HT}_{1D}$ mediate selective inhibition of nociceptive neurones and are implicated in headache[20]. $5\text{-HT}_{2C}$ and $5\text{-HT}_{2A}$ are positively coupled to phospholipase C and suppress $K^+$ current. $5\text{-HT}_3$ increases intracellular $Ca^{2+}$ either directly by activation of a cation channel that triggers the opening of VDCCs or via induction of phospholipase C. The localization of $5\text{-HT}_{2A, 2C}$ and $_3$ on excitatory interneurones or primary afferent terminals mediates the pro-nociceptive actions of 5-HT or descending facilitation.[21]

Noradrenaline-containing spinal cord terminals are localized to laminae I, II and V, and arise purely from supraspinal sites. Within the spinal cord there are two $\alpha_2$-adrenergic receptors and these are G-protein-coupled. $\alpha_{2C}$ have a presynaptic location in primary afferents and $\alpha_{2A}$ are found in secondary dorsal horn neurones. They inhibit dorsal horn neurones by presynaptic inhibition of neurotransmitter release and postsynaptically by hyperpolarization, mediated by coupling to inwardly rectifying $K^+$ channels. Although modulation of nociception by $\alpha_2$-adrenergic agonists such as clonidine is proven, sedative side-effects are problematic in their clinical use.[21] Anti-depressants used in neuropathic pain act to increase synaptic levels of noradrenaline and 5-HT leading to inhibition of sensory events at spinal levels by block of reuptake of these monoamines.

## Purines

The purines, including adenosine produced by adenosine triphosphate (ATP) metabolism, alongside ATP itself, are implicated in the modulation of nociception, although centrally the role of the adenosine receptor system is more defined. Adenosine-like immunoreactivity is detected in lamina II of the dorsal horn. Three differentially G-protein-coupled receptors for adenosine have been characterized and the A1 receptor is predominant in the antinociceptive effects of spinally applied adenosine and adenosine analogues, exerted through $K^+$ channel mediated hyperpolarization. Additionally those receptors found on the terminals of primary afferent fibres inhibit $Ca^{2+}$ current and neuropeptide release. Adenosine inhibits NMDA receptor-mediated hyperexcitability[22] and adenosine analogues are effective against neuropathic pain in both clinical and pre-clinical studies, in a manner that may be enhanced after nerve injury.[23]

## Inhibitory neuropeptides

Galanin-containing dorsal horn cells are found superficially, localized to interneurones, projection neurones and primary afferent terminals, sometimes in coexistence with substance P, CGRP, CCK and NOS. There are three cloned galanin receptors, namely GalR1, 2 and 3, which are G-protein-coupled. In normal animals, galanin release seldom occurs in response to noxious and innocuous stimulation and low levels are pro-nociceptive. Nerve injury upregulates galanin synthesis, and high doses appear to be antinociceptive. Thus, the spinal administration of galanin has complex but predominantly inhibitory/antinociceptive effects, which are enhanced in models of neuropathy.[24]

The $Y_2$ receptors for neuropeptide Y normally occur in small diameter dorsal root ganglia (DRG) neurones and their activation inhibits $Ca^{2+}$ currents, probably via a $G_0$ coupling. Receptor activation can block the release of substance P from cultured neurones; spinal neuropeptide Y has been reported to exert potent analgesic effects, and the receptor system appears to display nerve injury-induced changes that are beneficial.[3]

## Cannabinoids

There are two identified cannabinoid receptors, CB1 and CB2. CB1 is found on central and peripheral neurones. In the spinal cord its mRNA has been located to medium and large DRG cell bodies and at both presynaptic and postsynaptic spinal sites. Its activation here has been demonstrated to release dynorphins and may be involved in endogenous inhibitory tone. Negatively coupled to adenylate cyclase, activation of CB1 inhibits neuronal activity. Cannabinoid agonists are also antihyperalgesic in the presence of inflammation and nerve injury, possibly mediated via actions in both the CNS and in the periphery, and activity within this system may increase in the presence of persistent pain.[25]

From this account it is clear that there are multiple excitatory and inhibitory transmitter systems that interact at many levels of the nervous system to determine the final level of pain. Analgesic strategies revolve around blocking excitation or enhancing inhibitions – improvements in our knowledge of the pharmacology of pain should lead to a better range of analgesic therapies for the clinic.

# References

1. Sorkin LS, Carlton SM. Spinal Anatomy and Pharmacology of Afferent Processing. In: Yaksh TL, Lynch III C, Zapol WM, Maze M, Biebuyck JF, Saidman LJ, eds. *Anesthesia: Biologic Foundations.* Philadelphia: Lippincott-Raven, 1997: pp. 577–609.
2. Todd AJ, McGill MM, Shehab SA. Neurokinin 1 receptor expression by neurons in laminae I, III and IV of the rat spinal dorsal horn that project to the brainstem. *Eur J Neurosci* **12**: 689–700, 2000
3. Millan MJ. The induction of pain: an integrative review. *Prog Neurobiol* **57**: 1–164, 1999
4. Hunt SP, Mantyh PW. The molecular dynamics of pain control. *Nat Rev Neurosci* **2**: 83–91, 2001
5. Wilcox GL, Seybold V. Pharmacology of Spinal Afferent Processing. In: Yaksh TL, Lynch III C, Zapol WM, Maze M, Biebuyck JF, Saidman LJ, eds. *Anesthesia: Biologic Foundations.* Philadelphia: Lippincott-Raven, 1997
6. Dickenson AH, Stanfa LC, Chapman V, et al. Response properties of dorsal horn neurons: pharmacology of the dorsal horn. In: Yaksh TL, Lynch III C, Zapol WM, Maze M, Biebuyck JF, Saidman LJ, eds. *Anesthesia: Biologic Foundations.* Philadelphia: Lippincott-Raven, 1997: pp. 611–624.
7. Dickenson AH, Chapman V, Green GM. The pharmacology of excitatory and inhibitory amino acid-mediated events in the transmission and modulation of pain in the spinal cord. *Gen Pharmacol* **28**: 633–638, 1997
8. Suzuki R, Kontinen VK, Matthews E, et al. Enlargement of the receptive field size to low intensity mechanical stimulation in the rat spinal nerve ligation model of neuropathy. *Exp Neurol* **163**: 408–413, 2000
9. Suzuki R, Matthews EA, Dickenson AH. Comparison of the effects of MK-801, ketamine and memantine on responses of spinal dorsal horn neurones in a rat model of mononeuropathy. *Pain* **91**: 101–109, 2001
10. Sang CN. NMDA-receptor antagonists in neuropathic pain: experimental methods to clinical trials. *J Pain Symptom Manage* **19**(Suppl 1): S21–25, 2000
11. Yaksh TL, Hua XY, Kalcheva I, et al. The spinal biology in humans and animals of pain states generated by persistent small afferent input. *Proc Natl Acad Sci USA* **96**: 7680–7686, 1999
12. Wiesenfeld-Hallin Z, de Arauja Lucas G, Alster P, et al. Cholecystokinin/opioid interactions. *Brain Res* **848**: 78–89, 1999
13. Dickenson AH, Suzuki R. Function and dysfunction of opioid receptors in the spinal cord. In: Kalso E, McQuay H, Wiesenfeld-Hallin Z, eds. *Progress in Pain Research and Management, vol 14.* Seattle: IASP Press, 1999, pp. 17–44
14. Darland T, Heinricher MM, Grandy DK. Orphanin FQ/nociceptin: a role in pain and analgesia, but so much more. *Trends Neurosci* **21**: 215–221, 1998
15. Rowbotham MC. Efficacy of opioids in neuropathic pain. In: Hansson PT, Fields HL, Hill RG, Marchettini P, eds. *Neuropathic pain: pathophysiology and treatment, vol 21.* Seattle: IASP Press, 2001, pp. 203–213

16. Dickenson AH. NMDA receptor antagonists: interactions with opioids. *Acta Anaesthesiol Scand* **41**: 112–115, 1997
17. Heinricher M. Organizational characteristics of supraspinally mediated responses to nociceptive input. In: Yaksh TL, Lynch III C, Zapol WM, Maze M, Biebuyck JF, Saidman LJ, eds. *Anesthesia: Biologic Foundations.* Philadelphia: Lippincott-Raven, 1997, pp. 643–661
18. Machelska H, Binder W, Stein C. Opioid receptors in the periphery. In: Kalso E, McQuay HJ, Wiesenfeld-Hallin Z, eds. *Opioid Sensitivity of Chronic Noncancer Pain. Progress in Pain Research and Management; vol 14.* Seattle: IASP, 1999, pp. 45–58
19. Kontinen VK, Dickenson AH. Effects of midazolam in the spinal nerve ligation model of neuropathic pain in rats. *Pain* 85: 425–431, 2000
20. Goadsby PJ. The pharmacology of headache. *Prog Neurobiol* **62**: 509–525, 2000
21. Millan MJ. Descending control of pain. *Prog Neurobiol* **66**: 355–474, 2002
22. Dickenson AH, Suzuki R, Reeve AJ. Adenosine as a potential analgesic target in inflammatory and neuropathic pains. *CNS Drugs* **13**: 77–85, 2000
23. Suzuki R, Gale A, Dickenson AH. Altered effects of and A$_1$ adenosine receptor agonist on the evoked responses of spinal dorsal horn neurones in a rat model of mononeuropathy. *J Pain* **1**: 99–110, 2000
24. Xu XJ, Hokfelt T, Bartfai T, et al. Galanin and spinal nociceptive mechanisms: recent advances and therapeutic implications. *Neuropeptides* **34**: 137–147, 2000
25. Iversen L, Chapman V. Cannabinoids: a real prospect for pain relief? *Curr Opin Pharmacol* **2**: 50–55, 2002

# 5 Measurement of Pain

*Toby Newton-John*

There is no doubt that modern health care provision is being influenced by the principles of evidence-based practice. It is no longer acceptable for treatments to be delivered on the basis of anecdotal evidence for their efficacy, or because of clinical 'hunches' that they are useful, or because that is the way things have always been done. In order to demonstrate the value of a given intervention, various parameters of the treatment must be assessed and then evaluated according to clearly defined criteria. The purpose of this chapter is to discuss various forms of assessment that may be used in a pain clinic setting.

The chapter is intended to be pragmatic rather than idealistic – few clinicians have an excess of time or resources to devote to a lengthy and extensive assessment process. Equally, many chronic pain sufferers experience difficulties with prolonged sitting and/or writing, and with concentration and the unfamiliarity of form-filling. Their capacity to engage in a lengthy assessment may also be compromised. Hence there is always a balance to be found between obtaining sufficient information from patients and not overloading and overwhelming them. Equally, it is important to consider the practical resources available for systematically administering and scoring questionnaires, interpreting the results, entering the data on computer and carrying out analyses of the data. There is little point in administering a long and detailed assessment battery if the information obtained is not going to be utilized.

Self-report is by far the most expedient method for obtaining information about patient functioning, and, therefore, the most popular assessment format. Although a range of other methodologies have been developed and validated, such as structured clinical interviews, protocolized physical examinations and observational coding systems of pain behaviour, the focus of this chapter will be on the application of self-report instruments in the pain clinic. Again, pragmatism is the overriding notion.

Before proceeding, it is worth noting that treatment evaluation is by no means only the reason for carrying out a standardized assessment. The measurement tools described can enhance the clinical information obtained at the assessment stage by offering insights about patient function that would otherwise be difficult to quantify. Furthermore, the measures can be used as a means of describing the population of patients attending the service in greater detail than basic throughput information. A single assessment battery may serve clinical needs as well as facilitating a research project and providing audit information.

For the reader with a particular interest in the assessment of chronic pain, there are several texts that should be consulted. In particular, the textbook by Turk and Melzack[1] and the chapter by Williams[2] are essential reading.

## Measurement of pain quality

The core element of pain assessment is the quantification of the pain itself. The three methods most commonly used are Verbal Rating Scales (VRS), Visual Analogue Scales (VAS) and Numerical Rating Scales (NRS). The VRS format offers subjects a choice between adjectives (e.g. no pain, mild, moderate, severe) which have been assigned a priority rankings of severity (e.g. 0–3). Although straightforward to complete and, therefore, associated with high levels of compliance,[3] the VRS suffers from several methodological flaws. The forced choice format means that subjects have to select an adjective that may not accurately reflect their experience of their pain. They must be able to discriminate between each adjective in the list (some scales contain 15 adjectives), which requires a considerable degree of both language ability and capacity for self-reflection. Further, the rank-scoring format assumes equal intervals between points on the scale, which is unlikely to be the case. For example, the difference between no pain and mild pain is considered to be the same as between moderate and severe pain, when in fact the subjective experience of this difference may be quite different.

The VAS involves a (usually) 10 centimetre line, anchored with *'no pain at all'* at one end and *'pain as bad as it can be'* at the other. The respondent is asked to place a mark upon the line to represent the severity of the pain. Alternatively the NRS uses a numerical parameter (e.g. 0–10, 0–20 or 0–100) and the respondent is asked to rate the pain intensity by giving it a corresponding number. Pain 'thermometers' also use visual cues to represent degrees of pain intensity by resembling a temperature gauge, but will often include word descriptors as well as numerical parameters.

These tools appear deceptively simple for measuring a construct as complex and variable as the experience of pain. Indeed, one study has exposed the individuality with which respondents with the same condition complete the same pain measure,[4] and highlighted the response biases that are an inherent part of all self-report assessment. However, there has also been a considerable amount of research to support the utility of these methods. The extensive review of this literature by Jensen and Karoly[3] found that the VAS was highly sensitive to clinical changes but more prone to scoring error, whereas the NRS was preferable for the elderly or cognitively impaired and was generally the preferred measure when working with a heterogeneous patient population.

An altogether different method for assessing the quality of pain experience is the widely used McGill Pain Questionnaire (MPQ).[5,6] In addition to a VAS and Present Pain Index giving overall pain intensity scores, the more recent short form of the scale uses 15 adjectives to describe pain (e.g. 'throbbing', 'gnawing', 'fearful'), with the respondent rating each one on a scale from 0 (none) to 3 (severe). The adjectives offer a means of assessing both the sensory and affective dimensions of pain (see below), and the wealth of empirical studies on the MPQ attests to the discriminative capacity of the measure.[7] For example, it has been shown that post-herpetic neuralgia sufferers choose reliably different pain descriptors from patients with phantom limb pain or toothache.

## Multiaxial measures of pain

One of the criticisms of the pain quality measures outlined above has been that the assessment of pain intensity alone carries the erroneous implication that pain is a unidimensional construct. A number of assessment tools have therefore been developed that attempt to measure multiple aspects of the pain experience.

The Medical Outcome Study 36-Item Short Form Health Survey[8] (SF–36) is a broad-based measure of quality of life in the context of illness. As well as assessing physical and mental health functioning across eight domains, it has a Bodily Pain scale and asks about the degree of interference due to pain over the past week. It has been widely used with different chronic illness populations, and a particular strength is its age and sex-based normative data, which have been derived from US population surveys. However, concerns have been raised as to its applicability for chronic pain patients, and whether it is sufficiently sensitive for detecting clinically significant changes following treatment. A briefer but psychometrically sound measure of general disability is the Pain Disability Index (PDI),[9] which asks about the degree of disruption to seven life areas due to pain, from recreational and occupational activity to self-care behaviours. A 0–10 Likert scale format for each item means that the PDI is rapidly completed and scored.

A multiaxial measure that has been the mainstay of much of the psychological literature on chronic pain carried out in the US is the West-Haven Yale Multidimensional Pain Inventory[10] (WHYMPI). Using 56 items and three sections, it covers many of the important aspects of chronic pain adjustment within a single measure, including perceived control over pain, interference in daily activities due to pain, a measure of the significant other's responses to pain, and an activity scale. Normative data for various pain subgroups have been generated, and a number of studies have suggested that WHYMPI scores may categorize chronic pain patients into one of three groups: dysfunctional, interpersonally distressed and adaptive coper profiles.[11,12]

In the UK, there has been a move towards using the Brief Pain Inventory (BPI)[13] as a composite measure of functioning that can be used with a wide range of chronic pain conditions. The BPI uses 0–10 numerical rating scales to assess the interference of pain with mood, walking, general activity, work, relations with others, sleep and enjoyment of life. It can be administered and scored rapidly, and has been translated into several languages. It has also become the measure on which the Pain Audit Collection System (PACS)[14] database has been developed. This computerized database was designed to be as user-friendly as possible, such that entering information for a given patient episode takes only a couple of minutes. The PACS package includes applications for both pain clinic and pain management programme formats and can be obtained free of charge by contacting the authors directly (*admin@west-onking.com*). There can be few excuses for not using a system as simple and time efficient as this one.

## Self report of functional activities

Other than improving pain intensity itself, the stated goal of chronic pain treatment is often an increase in the range and scope of activities – or conversely a decrease in the level of disability experienced by the patient. Several of the measures described above offer general measures of disability, but there are a range of tools that offer more specific information about what the patient is capable or not capable of doing.

Perhaps the most commonly used measure in back pain is the Roland–Morris disability scale,[15] with the Oswestry Low Back Pain Disability Questionnaire[16] also widely used. One limitation of these functional activity measures is their focus on back pain specifically, which renders them less useful for upper limb or facial pain patients. Self report of functional activity in the context of chronic orofacial pain (e.g. chewing, smiling, yawning) can be assessed using the Oral Health Impact Profile,[17] which is brief and straightforward to complete, whereas functional activity in upper limb pain tends to be assessed behaviourally, for example, with a loaded reach test or typing tolerance assessment.

### Pain beliefs/cognitions

The assessment of patient beliefs about pain encompasses many domains, from ideas about the aetiology of the pain (somatic only vs multifactorial cause; mysterious vs identifiable), to expectations about treatment (confident to self manage vs reliance upon medical input) to expectations of outcome (complete relief from discomfort vs improvement in quality of life despite some discomfort). The impact that pain cognitions can have upon adjustment is highlighted by the recent research examining the concept of 'catastrophizing'. This term is loosely defined as an exaggerated negative 'mental set' brought to bear during actual or antic-ipated pain experience.[18] Patients who tend to think catastrophically during a flare-up of chronic pain (e.g. 'This will overwhelm me.' 'I will never get better.' 'There is nothing that I can do that will help in this situation.') are also the most disabled, and use the most health care resources including analgesic use and number of hospitalizations.[3,18] To assess this, the Pain Catastrophising Scale (PCS)[19] was derived from the widely used Coping Strategies Questionnaire[20] and is comprised of 13 items scored on a scale from 0 (never think this when in pain) to 4 (think this all the time when in pain).

Self-efficacy is another cognitive construct to have received considerable empirical atten-tion in the pain literature. It refers to the personal conviction that one can successfully per-form certain behaviours in a specific situation. With regard to chronic pain, this means a belief that one can carry out specific tasks (e.g. socialise, do housework, cope without pain medication) in the presence of ongoing pain. The Pain Self-Efficacy Scale[21] is a 10-item questionnaire that asks about patient confidence to pursue everyday activities despite pain, and particularly low scores on this measure have been shown to predict drop-out from pain management treatment.[22]

As every clinician working in a pain management setting will be aware, there are certain patients who are very reluctant to take on a self-management approach to managing their pain. They persist in seeking a medical solution and reject any attempt to introduce a reha-bilitation model for coping with their pain. One way of understanding this reluctance is to consider that the patient is not yet prepared to make the necessary changes, and requires further time and/or information in order to move towards the self-management approach. The Pain Stages of Change Questionnaire[23] was developed out of the psychological litera-ture examining behavioural changes in relation to addictions, and it seeks to quantify whether the patient is ready or not to accept a pain management intervention. The evidence thus far for the predictive power of the measure is mixed; however, being able to better identify which patients are most likely to benefit from which treatments remains a useful objective.

## Mood

The assessment of mood state is a vital aspect of any pain assessment. The current International Association for the Study of Pain (IASP) definition of pain formally recognizes that both sensory and emotional factors are part of all pain experience, and consequently any attempt to isolate one from the other is artificial. Assessing the patient's mood state gives a context within which pain scores can be interpreted, which is particularly important when rat-ings are towards either extreme of the scale.

Low mood is commonly assessed in relation to chronic pain because of the high concor-dance between depressive illness and pain – as many as 50% of chronic pain patients meet cri-teria for major depressive episode.[24] The assessment of depression in chronic pain is also problematic because of the overlap in symptomatology between the two disorders (poor sleep, lack of concentration, fatigue). This can cause an inflation in depression scores, which gives a misleading profile for a pain patient.[2,3] Furthermore, none of the depression measures reported here can be used as a diagnostic tool, as that requires a formal clinical assessment. Rather, these measures indicate the degree of depressive symptomatology.

The Beck Depression Inventory (BDI)[25] is the most widely used self-report measure of depressive symptoms, and has been extensively used in the field of chronic pain research. It contains useful items relating to cognitive symptoms of depression, but does suffer from the confound described above, and scores must, therefore, be interpreted with caution. The Hospital Anxiety and Depression Scale (HADS)[26] is a useful alternative, as it was specifically developed for use with medical and surgical patients and does not contain items pertaining to somatic symptoms (unfortunately it also says very little about the actual beliefs underlying the mood problem). Two separate scales of 7 items are derived, each pertaining to anxious or depressive symptoms.

Anxiety is well recognized as a potential exacerbating factor of pain, and specific measures of pain-related anxiety have been developed. The Pain Anxiety Symptom Scale[27] is a useful tool for assessing a variety of cognitive, somatic and behavioural symptoms of anxiety in relation to pain. These are symptoms that a generic anxiety measure such as the HADS would not necessarily detect. More recently, the fear-avoidance model of chronic pain has been increasingly shown to be relevant in the development and maintenance of long-term disability,[28] and the measure specifically developed to assess fear of movement is the Tampa Scale for Kinesiophobia.[29] This is a 17-item questionnaire exploring patient anxieties about the likelihood of (re)injury from normal movement. A patient who holds grave fears about damaging themselves as a result of simple exercise is going to need considerably more clinical attention than a patient who is not avoidant of activity or movement.

## Personal preferences

From the large pool of assessment tools discussed above, I use the same battery with chronic musculoskeletal pain patients attending a multidisciplinary pain management programme as with chronic orofacial pain patients attending for individual psychological treatment. The measures are:

- 0–100 NRS – pain intensity – current and average over the past week
- 0–100 NRS – pain-related distress – current and average over the past week
- 0–100 NRS – pain-related interference in daily activities – average over the past week
- Pain Disability Index – general measure of disability
- Pain Self-Efficacy Questionnaire – confidence to carry out activity despite pain
- Pain Anxiety Symptom Scale – fears about pain and the effects of pain/Tampa Scale for Kinesiophobia – fears of (re)injury due to movement (substitute Oral Health Impact Profile for chronic orofacial pain patients)
- Beck Depression Inventory – severity of depressive symptomatology.

All assessment batteries represent a compromise between detail and expediency, and the group listed above also demonstrates this compromise. Nevertheless, all of the measures have been subject to psychometric testing and found to be both valid and reliable. The length of the assessment is within most patient's limits of concentration and sitting/writing tolerance, and all measures are sensitive to change following pain management treatment. This is not a gold standard assessment battery, but perhaps represents a useful starting point for a practitioner who is developing an assessment protocol for audit, research or purely clinical purposes.

# Definitions

In helping to interpret the results of different tests and assessments, the following definitions might prove useful. They are provided by the International Association for the Study of Pain Task Force on Taxonomy, 1994.

- Allodynia – Pain due to a stimulus which does not normally provoke pain.
- Dysaesthesia – An unpleasant abnormal sensation, whether spontaneous or evoked.
- Hyperalgesia – An increased response to a stimulus which is normally painful.

- Hyperpathia – A painful syndrome characterized by an abnormally painful reaction to a stimulus, especially a repetitive stimulus, as well as an increased threshold.
- Pain threshold – The least experience of pain which a subject can recognize.
- Pain tolerance level – The greatest level of pain which a subject is prepared to tolerate.
- Paraesthesia – An abnormal sensation, whether spontaneous or evoked.

# References

1. Turk DC, Melzack R. Handbook of Pain Assessment. 2nd edn. New York: Guilford Press, 2001
2. Williams AC de C. Pain measurement in chronic pain management. *Pain Revs* **2**: 39–63, 1995
3. Jensen MP, Karoly P. Self report scales and procedures. In: Turk DC, Melzack R, eds. *Handbook of Pain Assessment. 2nd edn.* New York: Guilford Press, 2001, pp. 15–34
4. Williams AC de C, Davies HTO, Chadhury Y. Simple pain ratings hide complex idiosyncratic meanings. *Pain* **85**: 456–463, 2000
5. Melzack R. The McGill Pain Questionnaire: major properties and scoring methods. *Pain* **1**: 277–299, 1975
6. Melzack R. The short-form McGill Pain Questionnaire. *Pain* **30**: 191–197, 1987
7. Melzack R, Katz J. The McGill Pain Questionnaire: appraisal and current status. In: Turk DC, Melzack R, eds. *Handbook of Pain Assessment. 2nd edn.* New York: Guilford Press, 2001, pp. 35–52
8. Ware JE, Sherbourne CD. The MOS 36-item Short Form Health Survey (SF–36). *Med Care* **30**: 473–483, 1992
9. Pollard A. Preliminary validity study of The Pain Disability Index. *Percept Mot Skills* **59**: 974, 1984
10. Kerns RD, Turk DC, Rudy, TE. The West Haven-Yale Multidimensional Pain Inventory (WHYMPI). *Pain* **23**: 345–356, 1985
11. Turk DC, Okifuji A, Sinclair JD, Starz TW. Pain, disability and physical functioning in subgroups of patients with fibromyalgia. *J Rheumatol* 23: 1255–1262, 1996
12. McCraken LM, Spertus IL, Janeck AS, Sinclair D, Wetzel FT. Behavioral dimensions of adjustment in persons with chronic pain: pain-related anxiety and acceptance. *Pain* **80**: 283–289, 1999
13. Cleeland C. Measurement of pain by self report. In: Chapman CR, Loeser JD, eds. *Issues in Pain Management.* New York: Raven Press; 1989, pp. 391–403
14. Weston King Associates. 2002 PACS Data Collection and Analysis Package. Unit 6, The Lookout, Packet Quays, High Street, Falmouth, Cornwall TR11 2UE
15. Roland M, Morris R. A study of the natural history of back pain. Part 1: development of a reliable and sensitive measure of disability in low back pain. *Spine* **8**: 141–144, 1983
16. Fairbank JC, Couper J, Davies JB, O'Brien JP. The Oswestry low back pain disability questionnaire. *Physiotherapy* **66**: 271–273, 1980
17. Slade GD. Derivation and validation of a short-form oral health impact profile. *Community Dent Oral Epidemiol* **25**: 284–290, 1997
18. Sullivan MJL, Thorn BT, Haythornthwaite JA, et al. Theoretical perspectives on the relation between catastrophizing and pain. *Clin J Pain* **17**: 52–64, 2001
19. Sullivan MJL, Bishop S, Pivik J. The Pain Catastrophizing Scale: development and validation. *Psychol Assess* **7**: 524–532, 1995
20. Rosensteil AK, Keefe, FJ. The use of coping strategies in low back pain patients: relationship to patient characteristics and current adjustment. *Pain* **17**: 33–40, 1983
21. Nicholas MK. An Evaluation of Treatment for Chronic Low Back Pain. Unpublished doctoral dissertation. University of Sydney, Australia, 1988.
22. Coughlan GM, Ridout KL, Williams AC de C, Richardson PH. Attrition from a pain management programme. *Br J Clin Psychol* **34**: 471–479, 1995
23. Kerns RD, Rosenberg R, Jamison RN, Caudill MA, Haythornthwaite J. Readiness to adopt a self-management approach to chronic pain: the Pain Stages of Change Questionnaire (PSOCQ). *Pain* **72**: 227–234, 1997
24. Banks SM, Kerns RD. Explaining high rates of depression in chronic pain: a diathesis-stress framework. *Psychol Bull* **119**: 95–110, 1996

25. Beck AT, Ward CH, Mendelson M, Mock N, Erbaugh J. An inventory for measuring depression. *Arch Gen Psychiatry* **4**: 561–571, 1961
26. Zigmond AS, Snaith RP. The Hospital Anxiety and Depression Scale. *Acta Psychiatr Scand* **67**: 361–370, 1983
27. McCraken LM, Zayfert C, Gross RT. The Pain Anxiety Symptoms Scale: development and validation of a scale to measure fear of pain. *Pain* **50**: 67–73, 1992
28. Vlaeyen JWS, Linton SJ. Fear-avoidance and its consequences in chronic musculoskeletal pain: a state of the art. *Pain* **85**: 317–332, 2000
29. Kori SH, Miller RP, Todd DD. Kinesiophobia: a new view of chronic pain behavior. *Pain Manage* 35–43, 1990

# 6  Neuropathic Pain

*Stephen P Ward*

Neuropathic pain has been defined by the International Association for the Study of Pain (IASP) as 'Pain initiated or caused by a primary lesion or dysfunction in the nervous system'.[1] This simple definition vastly understates a complex and fascinating spectrum of painful conditions arising as a consequence of neural injury.

The neurophysiological processes responsible for the genesis of neuropathic pain remain poorly understood, but they are certainly far more complex and unpredictable than those mechanisms responsible for nociceptive pain. Nociceptive pain is mediated by stimulation of Aδ and C fibre polymodal nociceptors the response to which usually serves a biologically useful role in localizing noxious stimuli. In contrast, nerve injury may initiate a highly complex cascade of pathophysiological events unreliant on nociceptor stimulation that may culminate in the perception of pain.

It must be emphasized that nerve injury does not always result in a painful state. Only a relatively small proportion of patients develop neuropathic pain following nerve injury and the reasons for this unpredictability (e.g. genetic or environmental influences) remain elusive.

Painful conditions with a neuropathic component are estimated to comprise 25% of referrals to pain clinics in the UK. When all categories of neuropathic pain conditions are taken into account, the population prevalence in the UK is approximately 1%.[2] Within diagnostic categories such as syringomyelia the incidence may be as high as 75%.[3] An ageing population will almost certainly see the overall incidence rise as over half of patients over 70 years of age currently attending pain clinics in the UK have a neuropathic component to their presenting condition.[2]

## Classification

The term 'neuropathic pain', when applied clinically and diagnostically, simply indicates that peripheral or central neural injury is the likely underlying mechanism and not ongoing nociceptor activation. In this sense, neuropathic pain is a symptom of neurological dysfunction and not, in itself, a disease.

Traditionally, we have grouped together patients whose neuropathic pain conditions are similar in terms of clinical features and anatomical distribution, and this has encouraged the classification of neuropathic pain into discrete syndromes and aetiological groups (Table 6.1).

Whilst this classification is simple to comprehend and easy to apply, a fundamental problem is apparent. Pain clinic treatments of neuropathic pain conditions have evolved in concert with this classification to the extent that many treatments have become almost 'syndrome specific' and empirical. For example, we may diagnose post-herpetic neuralgia based on the clinical features and anatomical distribution of the pain and treat the patient with a medication thought to be effective on the basis of a few randomized, controlled trials (eg. amitriptyline, gabapentin). We may also prescribe according to 'tradition' (eg. carbamazepine in trigeminal neuralgia).

| **Table 6.1** | Conditions with a neuropathic component |
|---|---|
| **Peripheral** | |
| Post-herpetic neuralgia | |
| Trigeminal and glossopharyngeal neuralgia | |
| Phantom limb pain | |
| Complex regional pain syndromes | |
| Painful diabetic neuropathy | |
| Traumatic nerve injury | |
| Ischaemic neuropathy | |
| Nerve compression/entrapment | |
| **Central** | |
| Post-stroke pain | |
| Multiple sclerosis | |
| Syringomyelia | |
| Spinal cord injury | |

What has become apparent over the last decade, however, is that multiple mechanisms underlie the pathogenesis of neuropathic pain and that very different mechanisms may ultimately lead to a near identical clinical presentation.[4] Conversely, different clinical syndromes may be a product of identical mechanisms.

Our patient with post-herpetic neuralgia may have, as the underlying mechanism, central sensitization. Another may demonstrate predominantly primary afferent ectopic activity. Whilst clinically the presentations may be nearly identical, the different mechanisms demand treatments specific to those mechanisms. Failure to understand and implement this concept may explain the often disappointing results from clinical trials and, more importantly, our failure to treat neuropathic pain adequately in the pain clinic.

Whilst the classification of neuropathic pain based on underlying mechanism is logical and desirable, our current inability to determine the mechanism accurately by clinical examination alone precludes this. In addition, individuals may demonstrate multiple mechanisms, and the relative importance of these mechanisms may vary with time. We are beginning to understand many of these mechanisms and the ways in which they present, but it will be many years before we see a true mechanistic classification and subsequent treatment algorithm.

## Clinical features

The great variability in the underlying mechanisms of neuropathic pain is reinforced by an equally variable clinical presentation.

Pain due to neuropathy is projected and almost always confined to the innervation territory of the injured peripheral nerve, root or central pathway. Pain may occur immediately[5] or may be delayed – often for weeks and even months after nerve injury.

Characteristic of all the neuropathic pain states is the presence of spontaneous and/or stimulus evoked pain. Spontaneous pain is often described as burning, shooting, lancinating, stinging or stabbing, and these descriptors may be offered alone or in combination and may be continuous or episodic. Many patients with nociceptive pain will also use these descriptions, and we must be cautious not to secure a diagnosis on the basis of this alone.

Stimulus-evoked pain, specifically allodynia and hyperalgesia, is more pathognomic of neuropathic pain.

- Allodynia is pain due to a stimulus that does not normally provoke pain.[1] Whilst considered almost a hallmark feature of neuropathic pain states, allodynia may also be apparent in nociceptive pain conditions (e.g. acute joint inflammation, sunburn). Allodynia is usually invoked by an innocuous mechanical stimulus that can be further classified into subgroups (dynamic, static, punctate and skin stretch). Whether the subtypes reflect a difference in the underlying mechanism is unknown.[6] Allodynia may also result from chemical and thermal (cool and warm) stimulation.
- Hyperalgesia is an increased response to a stimulus that is normally painful.[1] Hyperalgesia to pin-prick or thermal stimulus may be confined to the area of injury (primary hyperalgesia – probably reflecting C fibre sensitization) or may extend to undamaged areas adjacent to the injury (secondary hyperalgesia – probably reflecting dorsal horn or central sensitization)

Patients commonly complain of other 'positive' non-painful sensory symptoms following nerve injury such as paraesthesia and itching and 'negative' symptoms such as hypoaesthesia and hypoalgesia.

Taking a history and conducting a meticulous examination is usually sufficient to diagnose neuropathic pain. There are validated neuropathic pain scales and questionnaires available that may be useful (e.g. Neuropathic Pain Scale (NPS),[7] Leeds assessment of neuropathic symptoms and signs (LANSS) Pain Scale[8]) and a pain drawing is often helpful in documenting symptoms within an innervation territory. The examination should include careful evaluation of somatosensory function as the sensory abnormalities are often confined to a single modality.

Useful equipment for testing sensation in the pain clinic includes a camel or sable brush for the sensation of touch and for detecting allodynia, a pin for the sensation of pain and a cold and warm roller ($25°C$ and $40°C$) for temperature sensation.[9]

Other more involved methods used to evaluate neuropathic pain include electromyography, nerve conduction studies and quantitive sensory testing (QST).

## Mechanisms

Our understanding of the mechanisms underlying neuropathic pain suggests that nerve injury can provoke a highly complex cascade of reparatory processes involving both peripheral and central somatosensory systems that can result in often permanent changes in these systems. Over the last decade, improved basic scientific techniques and reliable animal models have furthered our understanding of this phenomenon.

The following mechanisms, both peripheral and central, have been described:

- Ectopic discharge – after nerve injury, spontaneous ectopic discharges are observed in primary sensory neurones – dorsal root ganglion (DRG) neurones.[10] Action potentials depend on the depolarization of voltage-gated sodium channels of which there are nine or more isoforms within the nervous system. In DRG neurones, three isoforms are preferentially expressed (PN1, SNS and NaN). It has become apparent that hyperexcitability of DRG neurones after axonal injury results, in part, from changes in the expressions of genes that encode sodium channels in these cells. These changes include the downregulation of several sodium channel genes and the upregulation of transcription of previously silent sodium channel genes.[11] Models of neuropathic pain also reveal changes in cytokine expression in injured nerves, the DRG and in the central nervous system (CNS). Interleukin 1β (IL-1β) and tumour necrosis factor (TNF) may activate or sensitize afferent neurones, and there is ample evidence that proinflammatory cytokines induce or increase neuropathic pain.[12]
- Cross-excitation – injured axons may make electrical or chemical contact with adjacent uninjured fibres resulting in cross-excitation. When Aβ fibres activate C fibres, a non-noxious stimulus may produce pain.[13]

- Nociceptor sensitization – local damaged neurones may release substance P thus sensitizing the adjacent nociceptors of both injured and uninjured axons. Additionally, nerve injury results in a dramatic increase in cellular prostaglandin synthesizing enzyme cyclooxygenase 2 (COX-2) at the injury site and adjacent region. Overproduction of prostaglandins may sensitize nociceptors and may also be involved in central plasticity and sensitization at the spinal cord level.[14]
- Central sensitization – repetitive C fibre stimulation can result in prolonged discharge of dorsal horn cells, a phenomenon known as 'wind-up'. At a cellular level, this central nervous system change appears to be associated with the NMDA receptor. C fibre stimulation can activate dorsal horn interneurones causing them to release excitatory amino acids (aspartate and glutamate), which excite wide dynamic range neurones via the NMDA receptor. NMDA receptor activation initiates a cascade of events including an increase in intracellular calcium, activation of protein kinases, phosphorylating enzymes and nitric oxide synthetase. The resultant release of neurotransmitters and inflammatory chemicals can further activate excitatory amino acid production.[15] Prolonged activation of these NMDA receptors may lead to long standing and often irreversible changes in the central nociceptive pathways.
- Spinal cord reorganization – following nerve injury, degeneration and loss of C fibre terminals in lamina II of the dorsal horn may allow the sprouting of Aβ fibres into this vacated territory. This may allow non-noxious information to be interpreted as painful.
- Spinal cord disinhibition – nerve injury may result in the degeneration and death of dorsal horn inhibitory neurones. Decreased production of inhibitory amino acids such as γ-aminobutyric acid (GABA) and a reduction in the GABA receptor population has also been reported.[16]

The list of mechanisms above is by no means exhaustive, but it serves to illustrate the complexity of neuropathic pain, the relationships between central and peripheral nervous systems and the rationale for the various treatments available.

# Management

Experience tells us that early, aggressive treatment of neuropathic pain is more likely to be successful than late intervention. Unfortunately, neuropathic pain is often a late diagnosis and patients who quite reasonably display an abnormal and exaggerated response to painful and non-painful stimuli are often dismissed as psychologically distressed malingerers.

Treatment is predominantly pharmacological, and it has emerged over the years partly as a result of the research activity directed at elucidating the mechanisms of neuropathic pain but, more often than not, through trial and error and serendipity.

# Pharmacological treatment

## Antidepressants

The analgesic properties of the tricyclic group of antidepressants were noted as early as 1960 and have become the mainstay of treatment for neuropathic pain. The analgesic effect of tricyclic antidepressants can be explained by several pharmacological mechanisms including inhibition of presynaptic reuptake of noradrenaline and 5-hydroxytryptamine (5-HT, or serotonin), postsynaptic receptor blockade, NMDA receptor antagonism, calcium channel blockade and sodium channel blockade.

Several randomized controlled trials and subsequent systematic reviews have demonstrated the efficacy of this class of drugs. Taken together, controlled trials of the tricyclics show that 60–70% of patients with neuropathic pain respond to these drugs with a number needed to treat (NNT) of approximately 2–3 (to achieve 50% pain relief).[17] The different tricyclics appear to compare favourably with each other with little intradrug variability.

Several of the commonly used tricyclics including amitriptyline, nortriptyline, imipramine and desipramine are metabolized by the enzyme CYP2D6 and exhibit genetic polymorphism. This polymorphism is responsible for the marked pharmacokinetic variability observed with these drugs, and it explains both the often disappointing results achieved with treatment and the great variability in tolerance.

The dosages used are considerably less than those used in the treatment of depression. A typical dosing regimen for amitriptyline would be 10 mg orally at bedtime with a gradual escalation in 10 mg increments over a 2–3 week period to a maximum of 50–75 mg per day.

The side-effects of the tricyclics include sedation and the anticholinergic effects of eye and mouth dryness. The sedative effect is often welcome and beneficial but, if unwanted, it may be prudent to use one of the less sedative secondary amines such as nortriptyline or desipramine.

The newer selective serotonin (5-HT) reuptake inhibitors (SSRIs) such as fluoxetine and paroxetine have not compared favourably with the tricyclics and are seldom used.

## Anticonvulsants

This group of drugs, like the antidepressants, has been used in the treatment of neuropathic pain for almost four decades with carbamazepine demonstrating its efficacy in the treatment of trigeminal neuralgia as early as 1966.[18] Only carbamazepine, phenytoin, gabapentin and lamotrigine have been subject to randomized controlled trials in neuropathic pain, but several anecdotal reports suggest that nearly all anticonvulsants demonstrate some analgesic activity.

- Carbamazepine is structurally related to the tricyclic antidepressants and the mechanisms of action are likely to be similar. Eleven randomized controlled trials in various neuropathic pain conditions (predominantly trigeminal neuralgia) have demonstrated its effectiveness with a NNT of 2–3.[19,20] The doses used in these studies varied from 300–2400 mg per day with side-effects preventing ongoing treatment in 0% to 11%. Tolerable side-effects occurred in up to 50% of patients including dizziness, sedation and ataxia.
- Gabapentin is a structural GABA analogue with no direct GABA-ergic action. The mechanism of action is thought to be related to the effect of gabapentin on the $\alpha2\delta$ calcium channel subtype. Two large randomized controlled trials of gabapentin in post-herpetic neuralgia (NNT 3.2)[21] and painful diabetic neuropathy (NNT 3.8)[22] have established its efficacy in the treatment of these conditions, and several smaller studies in various neuropathic pain conditions have yielded similar results. Study doses ranged from 900–3600 mg per day with the drug proving well tolerated and safe and demonstrating no significant interaction with other medications. The most frequent reported adverse effects were somnolence and dizziness. In the UK, the maximum recommended dosage for the treatment of neuropathic pain is 1800 mg per day, yet most clinicians would advance above this dose if the drug is well tolerated. In an attempt to minimize the side-effects, the drug is normally titrated from 300 mg to 1800 mg per day over several days or even weeks.
- Lamotrigine is one of the newer antiepileptic agents that blocks voltage dependant $Na^+$ channels and inhibits glutamate release. In doses of 50–400 mg per day lamotrigine has demonstrated efficacy in the treatment of trigeminal neuralgia with an NNT of 2.1.[23] Similar outcomes are seen in studies of lamotrigine in post stroke pain. A study of lamotrigine given to patients with various neuropathic pain conditions, however, showed the drug to be no more effective than placebo.[24]

## Local anaesthetics and anti-arrhythmics

Several studies have demonstrated the effectiveness of intravenous lignocaine in the treatment of neuropathic pain. Doses of up to 5 mg/kg have been shown to provide long lasting pain relief in painful diabetic neuropathy, post-herpetic neuralgia, complex regional pain syndrome and post-stroke pain. In an attempt to mirror this effect, which is almost certainly due to sodium channel blockade, with an oral substitute, mexiletine has been subject to five randomized controlled trials – four in painful diabetic neuropathy and one in post-stroke pain. Unfortunately, the results have proved equivocal and overall the NNT is a disappointing 10.

## Opioids

Much debate surrounds the use of opioids in neuropathic pain. Many early studies suggested that neuropathic pain is only slightly sensitive or not sensitive at all to opiates. More recent work clearly demonstrates that a subgroup of patients respond well to opiates and that opioid responsiveness is partly a matter of dosage.[25] Patients with neuropathic pain simply require higher doses to experience analgesia.

Evidence is available for the effectiveness of oxycodone in post-hepatic neuralgia (PHN), tramadol in painful diabetic neuropathy and fentanyl in patients with various neuropathic pain conditions. Methadone has been successfully used to treat neuropathic pain in cancer, possibly reflecting its considerable NMDA receptor affinity.[26]

## NMDA receptor antagonists

Ketamine non-competitively antagonises NMDA receptors and has proven benefit in the treatment of neuropathic pain. Unfortunately, the psychomimetic side-effects associated with this drug limit its usefulness clinically. Better tolerated NMDA receptor antagonists such as dextromethorphan and amantadine have demonstrated encouraging results, but still the side-effect profiles associated with all these agents preclude widespread use.

## Topical agents

Topical capsaicin cream (0.025% and 0.05%) when applied repeatedly for a prolonged period, has been shown to provide some relief in a number of neuropathic pain conditions including PHN, diabetic neuropathy, stump pain, trigeminal neuralgia and scar pain. The mechanism probably relates to substance P depletion, but there is some evidence to suggest an additional ability to trigger membrane depolarization and to open non-selective cation channels. Capsaicin cream is often a useful adjunct to treatment with side-effects limited to a mild and short lived burning sensation, which is normally well tolerated.

Topical lignocaine has shown some promise in the management of PHN. Randomized controlled trials of 5% lignocaine gel patches reveal that 30–53% of patients with PHN report at least moderate benefit with this treatment with a low incidence of side-effects.

## Drugs in development

With the huge advances in determining the mechanisms underlying neuropathic pain comes the insight necessary to develop appropriate pharmacological treatments. Several novel drugs are currently under development and investigation and are certain to impact on our treatment of neuropathic pain in the future. For example, venom obtained from the poisonous marine snail of the genus *Conus* when fractionated contains a variety of small peptides. One of these omega-peptides blocks N-type calcium channels occurring on neurones but not cardiovascular muscle. This drug, under the name ziconotide, is currently undergoing phase I trials in neuropathic pain and shows great promise.[27] Others include butyl-para-aminobesoate, an ester local anaesthetic and ABT-594, a nicotinic receptor agonist.

## Neurostimulation

Spinal cord stimulation (SCS) has been used in the treatment of neuropathic pain conditions since the 1960s. This reversible, minimally invasive and safe technique has documented efficacy in the treatment of a wide variety of neuropathic pain conditions, and it appears to be cost effective. SCS is an invaluable treatment modality in carefully selected patients resistant to conservative measures.

Transcutaneous electrical nerve stimulation (TENS) is a well tolerated and often useful adjunct to conservative therapy, and it has been used in PHN, phantom limb pain and post-stroke pain.

## Additional management strategies

We must remember that neuropathic pain is often a chronic condition and, as such, benefits from a multidisciplinary approach to treatment. In addition to pharmacological therapy and neuromodulation, other treatment modalities should be available in the pain clinic (eg. physical rehabilitation and psychological intervention). There are a number of specific interventional procedures available for the treatment of individual neuropathic pain conditions dealt with in other chapters (eg. neuro-ablative procedures and microvascular decompression for trigeminal neuralgia, sympathetic blocks for complex regional pain syndromes).

## Conclusion

Neuropathic pain conditions present us with one of the greatest challenges in our field. The presentation is often late, and the clinical features are seldom identical from one patient to the next.

Our treatment is heavily reliant on pharmacotherapy and is, for the most part, disappointing and inadequate. We rely on drugs designed to treat other medical problems, with diverse modes of action and often troublesome side-effects.

Neuromodulation is a valuable and effective treatment modality, which is currently underused, but which demands large resources both financial and in terms of manpower, training and facilities.

We are now beginning to elucidate the mechanisms of neuropathic pain and with this knowledge will come a revolution in its treatment.

Selective drugs targeting individual receptors, pathways and genes are in development and herald exciting changes in the way we manage our patients.

## References

1. Merskey H, Bogduk N. *Classification of Chronic Pain: Description of Chronic Pain Syndromes and Definition of Pain Terms.* Seattle: IASP Press, 1994.
2. Bowsher D. Neurogenic pain syndromes and their management. *Br Med Bull* **47**: 644–666, 1991
3. Boivie J. Central pain. In: Wall PD, Melzack R, eds. *Textbook of Pain.* Edinburgh: Churchill Livingstone, 1999, pp. 879–914.

4. Woolf CJ, Mannion RJ. Neuropathic pain: aetiology, symptoms, mechanisms, and management. *Lancet* **353**: 1959–1964, 1999

5. Hayes C, Molloy AR. Neuropathic pain in the perioperative period. *Intl Anaesthesiol Clin* **35**: 67–81, 1997

6. Pappagallo M, Oaklander AL, Quatrano-Piacentini AL, et al. Heterogenous patterns of sensory dysfunction in postherpetic neuralgia suggest multiple pathophysiologic mechanisms. *Anaesthesiology* **92**: 691–698, 2000

7. Galer BS, Jensen MP. Development and preliminary validation of a pain measure specific to neuropathic pain: the neuropathic pain scale. *Neurology* **48**: 332–338, 1997

8. Bennett M. The LANSS Pain Scale: the Leeds assessment of neuropathic symptoms and signs. *Pain* **92**: 147–157, 2001

9. Hansson P. Possibilities and potential pitfalls of combined bedside and quantitative somatosensory analysis in pain patients. In: Boivie J, Hansson P, Lindblom U, eds. *Touch, Temperature and Pain in Health and Disease: Mechanisms and Assessments, Progress in Pain Research and Management, vol 3.* Seattle: IASP Press, 1994, pp. 113–132

10. Zhang J-M, et al. Axotomy increases the excitability of dorsal root ganglion cells with unmyelinated axons. *J Neurophysiol* **78**: 2790–2794, 1997

11. Black J A, et al. Sodium channels as therapeutic targets in neuropathic pain. In: Hansson P, Fields H L, Hill R G, Marchettini P eds. *Neuropathic Pain: Pathophysiology and Treatment, Progress in Pain Research and Management, vol. 21.* Seattle: IASP Press, 2001, pp. 19–36

12. Sommer C. Cytokines and neuropathic pain. In: Hansson P, Fields H L, Hill R G, Marchettini P, eds. *Neuropathic Pain: Pathophysiology and Treatment, Progress in Pain Research and Management, vol. 21.* Seattle: IASP Press, 2001, pp. 37–62.

13. Amir R, Devor M. Functional cross-excitation between afferent A- and C-neurons in dorsal root ganglia. *Neuroscience* **95**:189–195, 2000

14. Ma W, Eisenach JC. Morphological and pharmacological evidence for the role of peripheral prostaglandins in the pathogenesis of neuropathic pain. *Eur J Neurosci* **15**: 1037–1047, 2002

15. Dickenson AH, Chapman V, Green GM. The pharmacology of excitatory and inhibitory amino acid-mediated events in the transmission and modulation of pain in the spinal cord. *Gen Pharmacol* **28**: 633–638, 1997

16. Castro-Lopez J, Tavares I, Coimbra A. GABA decreases in the spinal cord dorsal horn after peripheral neurectomy. *Brain Res* **620**: 287–291, 1993

17. McQuay HJ, et al. A systematic review of antidepressants in neuropathic pain. *Pain* **68**: 217–227, 1996

18. Campbell FG, Graham JG, Zilkha KJ. Clinical trial of carbazepine (tegretol) in trigeminal neuralgia. *J Neurol Neurosurg Psychiatry* **29**: 265–267, 1966

19. Killian JM, Fromm GH. Carbamazepine in the treatment of neuralgia. *Arch Neurol* **19**: 129–36, 1968

20. Nicol C. A four year double blind randomised study of Tegretol in facial pain. *Headache* **9**: 54–57, 1969

21. Rowbotham M, et al. Gabapentin for the treatment of postherpetic neuralgia: a randomized controlled trial. *JAMA* **280**: 1837–1842, 1998

22. Backonja M, et al. Gabapentin for the symptomatic treatment of painful neuropathy in patients with diabetes mellitus: a randomized controlled trial. *JAMA* **280**: 1831–1836, 1998

23. Zakrzewska JM, et al. Lamotrigine (lamictal) in refractory trigeminal neuralgia: results from a double-blind placebo controlled crossover trial. *Pain* **73**: 223–230, 1997

24. McCleane G. 200 mg daily of lamotrigine has no analgesic effect in neuropathic pain: a randomised, double-blind, placebo controlled trial. *Pain* **83**: 105–107, 1999

25. Portenoy RK, Foley KM, Inturrisi CE. The nature of opioid responsiveness and its implications for neuropathic pain: new hypotheses derived from studies of opioid infusions. *Pain* **43**: 273–286, 1990

26. Gorman AL, Elliott KJ, Inturrisi CE. The d- and l-isomers of methadone bind to the non-competitive site on the N-methyl-D-aspartate (NMDA) receptor in rat forebrain and spinal cord. *Neurosci Lett* **223**: 5–8, 1997

27. Bowersox SS, Luther R. Pharmacotherapeutic potential of omega-conotoxin MVIIA (SNX-111), an N-type neuronal calcium channel blocker found in the venom of Conus magus. *Toxicon* **36**: 1651–1658, 1998

# 7 Complex Regional Pain Syndrome

*John Hughes*

Complex regional pain syndrome (CRPS) describes chronic painful conditions predominantly involving the limbs that are characterized by burning pain, changes in skin colour, temperature, altered sweating, oedema and loss of function. They involve a variety of conditions variously described as: causalgia, Sudeck's atrophy, post-traumatic pain syndromes and minor causalgia. The French and orthopaedic literature frequently refer to algodystrophy. In 1953, Bonica suggested that these terms be included under the heading of Reflex Sympathetic Dystrophy (RSD), some suggested that causalgia remained a separate entity.

The International Association for the Study of Pain (IASP) in 1994 defined RSD and causalgia under the heading of complex regional pain syndrome.[1] These are sub-classified into CRPS type I (RSD) and CRPS type II (causalgia), the latter is defined by the signs of CRPS and a defined peripheral nerve injury.

Sympathetically maintained pain (SMP) is defined as a pain that is maintained by sympathetic efferent innervations or by circulating catecholamines.[1] It may be a feature of several painful conditions including CRPS, post-herpetic neuralgia and some cancer pains but is not an essential requirement. A pain that is relieved by sympathetic blockade may be described as SMP. This implies some involvement of the sympathetic nervous system with the modulation of that pain. Patients may have both SMP and sympathetically independent pain.

## Aetiology

The epidemiology is unknown. Most patients are adults but children may be involved.[2]

### Incidence

- Estimates of the incidence of RSD following trauma varies, many cases may be self limiting.
- Presenting causes to the pain clinic; trauma 45–65%, post-operative 10–20%, inflammatory processes 2%, cardiac 3%, others 4% and no precipitating cause in 10–20%.[2,3]
- The female to male ratio is approximately 3 to 1 with a mean age of onset at 40–50 years.[2,3]
- Data from Sweden with a population of 8.6 million only captures numbers from hospital admission lists.[4]

### Precipitating factors

The precipitating factors associated with CRPS include:

- Trauma including surgical (from inconsequential to major nerve damage)
- Neurological disturbances (CVA, Parkinsonism, epilepsy)

- Inflammatory disease
- Neoplastic disease (brain, lung, ovarian and breast most commonly)
- Myocardial infarction[3]
- Pregnancy, familial[5] and iatrogenic (isoniazid, ethambutol cyclosporin).

However, there may be no apparent precipitating cause.

Psychological states predisposing to or perpetuating CRPS remain controversial. Some consider the stress of organized sport to precipitate or perpetuate CRPS in children.[6]

It should be noted that the severity of the injury bears no relation to the severity of the CRPS.

# Pathophysiology

In 1873, Létiévant postulated a mechanism where the peripheral nerve was the point of irritation, with transmission to the spinal centres causing abnormal neural activity and, if the impulses were strong enough, to higher centres. Since then there have been advances, but there remains a discrepancy between clinicians and basic scientists as to the mechanism of CRPS. Further research is clearly required.[7]

## Peripheral and central mechanisms

Current opinion is leaning towards central mechanisms to explain CRPS.[8] This allows explanation of the distribution of clinical findings. Some workers continue to investigate the role of peripheral mechanisms.

## Psychological mechanisms

Psychological changes may be reactive or predispose to the development of CRPS. In paediatric cases there is a suggestion that anxiety, life stress and depression play a role in its development.[9]

# Diagnosis

Since the reclassification of RSD to CRPS[1] the features shown in Table 7.1 are required to make the diagnosis. Confusion in the literature exists as the criteria are applied in differing ways by different authors.

| Table 7.1   Diagnostic criteria |
| --- |
| • Regional pain (disproportionate to initiating event) |
| • Sensory changes (allodynia, hyperalgesia) |
| • Abnormalities of skin temperature |
| • Abnormal sudomotor activity |
| • Oedema |
| • Abnormal movements and weakness may exist |
| • CRPS 2 a peripheral nerve lesion must exist |
| • Other causes having first been excluded |

The diagnosis remains clinical. Few patients show all the signs and symptoms making diagnosis difficult in some. Investigations support clinical suspicion but no single test confirms the diagnosis; objective testing helps in equivocal cases. A careful history is essential and starts with the first symptoms. Patients may have more than one chronic pain, and it is the clinician's responsibility to assess what processes are active and which are causing the primary problem.

The differential diagnoses that need to be considered include: bony lesions, unrecognized sprain or fracture, arthritis, aseptic necrosis, Paget's disease, osteomas, infections, tumours (benign or malignant), diabetic osteopathy, post-trauma vasospasm, bursitis, tenosynovitis, calcification of tendons or ligaments, Raynaud's syndrome, phantom pain, frostbite, phlebitis, scleroderma, connective tissue diseases and myofascial syndromes.[10]

# Clinical findings

Onset of CRPS may be immediate or delayed (days, weeks or months). It may be insidious or fulminant. A spectrum of severity exists from the obvious to the bizarre and frequently one symptom or sign predominates almost to the exclusion of others. Patients are, therefore, at risk of misdiagnosis.

CRPS has been described as a progressive disease passing through three stages. The value of staging is limited, progression is not inevitable and specific symptoms to each stage do not exist. A discussion of the clinical findings may be more useful.

## Pain

- Pain is a diagnostic requirement, does not correspond to known peripheral or segmental distributions, may spread proximally to involve the whole limb or beyond to the ipsilateral or contralateral side of body.
- Pain is greater than that normally associated with the injury. It is said to be burning or aching in character and exacerbated with movement, dependence, physical contact or emotional stimuli. With time the pain may reduce in intensity but frequently remains the major problem.
- Allodynia, hyperalgesia, hyperaesthesia, hyperpathia and dysaesthesia are common. Hypaesthesia may also occur. (see Table 7.2 for definitions)

## Skin changes

- Trophic changes (skin, hair, nails) usually occur but tend to be late in the disease.
- The skin may be warm, dry and red due to vasodilatation or cyanotic and cold due to vasoconstriction. About 90% of patients show a colour and or temperature difference.[2]

| Table 7.2 Definitions | |
|---|---|
| Allodynia | Pain to a non-nociceptive stimulus |
| Hyperalgesia | Increased response to nociceptive stimulus |
| Hyperaesthesia | Increased sensitivity to stimuli (not special senses) |
| Hyperpathia | Excessive response to stimulus or after-sensation |
| Dysaesthesia | Unpleasant sensation to an innocuous stimulus |
| Hypaesthesia | Decreased sensitivity |

- Increased sweating may occur, with either a hot or cold limb.
- Changes in temperature and colour can occur spontaneously or be triggered by environmental temperature changes.
- Localized oedema and tenderness is common, becoming indurated and non pitting often with a glazed look.
- Nail growth may be increased or decreased, with nails becoming brittle, cracked and grooved.
- Hair growth also changes, becoming accelerated, thin or absent.
- The trophic changes seen in adults appear to occur in the most severe paediatric cases and are reversible.[11]
- Dermatological manifestations occasionally occur and include cutaneous ulceration and reticulate hyperpigmentation.[12]

## Muscles and joints

- Marked irreversible atrophic changes in muscle and subcutaneous tissue can occur.
- Movement is often reduced secondary to pain. Joints become weak with limited movement and develop ankylosis. Flexor tendon contractures similar to Dupuytren's also occur.
- Thickening of joints and muscle-wasting further limit movement, increase weakness, result in joint pain and further limitation of function.
- Muscle spasm, dystonia and tremor also occur; they may precede the pain, occur in a mirror distribution or occasionally without pain. These features can develop at any stage of the disease process. Tremor increases with movement, is an enhanced physiological tremor and does not correlate with other symptoms. Weakness and incoordination may progress to the stage where the patient is unable to move (pseudoparesis).[2]

## Psychological considerations

The psychological components of CRPS must not be overlooked.[8] Some suggest that CRPS is solely reactive or that psychological states predispose some individuals to its development,[9] others feel there is a population at higher risk of developing CRPS,[11] and a further postulate is that CRPS leads to psychological disturbance. Whichever the case, psychological changes are well documented and require attention if successful outcomes are to be achieved.

- Patients often appear anxious, withdrawn and emotionally unstable; drug addiction and suicidal tendencies sometimes occur.[2]
- Those who have had unsuccessful treatments coupled with suggestion that the problem is psychogenic often have an exacerbation of their psychological disturbance.
- In children, anxiety, stress and depression play a role in RSD.[9] These stresses range from academic to physical abuse, include family conflicts such as parental separation and life-threatening illness in a sibling.

# Investigations[8]

The role of laboratory investigations is limited and no single test is diagnostic. They serve to reinforce clinical evaluation. Negative results help refute the diagnosis in equivocal cases.

## Blood tests

The use of full blood count, erythrocyte sedimentation rate, antibody screens is to exclude other disease states. The presence of coexisting disease is common.

## Radiology

Radiological changes are not pathognomonic but aid diagnosis:

- Diffuse soft-tissue swelling occurs in up to 90% of patients.
- Osteoporosis varies from patchy to diffuse in nature. It occurs within the area of CRPS and is often in the epiphysial regions of small bones in the hand or foot.

Similar changes occur in conditions with high bone turnover such as thyrotoxicosis or following immobilization.

## Nuclear medicine

Technetium (99mTc) scanning may be of benefit in diagnosing CRPS.[10] Both increased and decreased uptake has been described. In children, decreased blood flow is more common in the early phase scan with soft tissue rather than bone uptake in the late one.[11]

## Thermography

This technique aids diagnosis, but it is of more benefit if negative to refute cases that are clinically difficult to evaluate. Differences of 1°C or more are considered significant.

Diffuse temperature changes (increased or decreased) occur between the affected and normal limb and are often evident clinically.[2] Thermographic differences may occur before cutaneous changes are evident and disappear with resolution of the syndrome.

## Pressure pain thresholds[13]

Pressure pain thresholds can be measured using a dolorimeter. The ratio between the affected and unaffected side helps diagnosis of CRPS and ratios below 0.77 are suggestive.

Formal quantitative sensory testing is time consuming and remains a research tool in the main. On occasions it is beneficial.

## Sympathetic nerve blockade

Initially a sympathetic block is performed (e.g. stellate ganglion block for the upper limb). If the pain eases along with evidence of sympathetic block (loss of sweating and increased temperature) a diagnosis of sympathetically maintained pain can be made.

Doppler flow monitoring helps confirm the effectiveness of sympathetic blockade particularly if the procedure is performed under sedation or general anaesthesia. Increases in blood flow are detected within minutes of the block.

If a sympathetic block demonstrates sympathetically independent pain an appropriate peripheral nerve block could be performed (e.g. axillary plexus block). If pain persists despite adequate blockade then a diagnosis of central pain can be made.

# Management[4,8,14]

Complex regional pain syndrome is a complex condition with both physical and psychological elements. Many treatments are available but evidence for benefit is often lacking or weak.[8] Current management tends to have a component of 'trial and error' with varying evidence for each intervention.

Others have suggested (consensus report) that management should be aimed at restoration of function, relief of pain and provide psychological support.[4] Active patient participation[15] is important and a multidisciplinary team approach often provides the best outcomes. Medical and psychological intervention is focused to achieve a level of functional restoration. Below are outlines of interventions that are used, the order is for convenience and not prioritized.

Attempting to prevent the development of CRPS is important[16] and requires: early treatment at the site of injury (including, debridement and stabilisation of fractures), adequate analgesia (including nerve blocks), early mobilization and psychological support. Good evidence is lacking but some studies have been carried out.[8]

## Physiotherapy

- Physiotherapy is aimed at maximizing mobility and may be effective on its own. It starts very gently avoiding interventions that increases pain.
- Good analgesia, improved mobility and reduced anxiety increases patient confidence.
- An exercise programme is essential and should include home activities and set goals within realistic boundaries. The ultimate aim is a return to normal function.
- Modalities include, stress-loading, active and passive movement, muscle stimulation and pool therapy.

## Transcutaneous electrical nerve stimulation[17]

Transcutaneous electrical nerve stimulation (TENS) provides analgesia of varying duration and coupled with physiotherapy provides good relief (especially in children).

It is easily taught, non-invasive, inexpensive and allows improved compliance with home exercise programmes. Occasionally TENS exacerbates pain.

## Psychological therapies

Psychological or psychiatric disturbance is often associated with chronic pain. It may have a role in the causation and maintenance of CRPS or result from it. Patients who fail standard treatment should be considered for psychological evaluation and management. This may prevent unnecessary treatments and the negative effects they have.[9]

In the early stages of CRPS there may be no significant psychological disturbance. Care is required when suggesting psychological assessments as patients may consider this as an accusation of psychiatric disease. Similarly caution is required when confronting patients as they often require an 'honourable exit' to avoid feeling trapped and having to admit to a psychological disturbance.[15] Maintaining patients motivation is important; anxiety exacerbates CRPS and measures to reduce it form part of management.[10]

## Sympathetic blockade

Sympathetic blockade provides analgesia of varying duration. A positive result demonstrates the presence of SMP. Repeat blocks often extend analgesia and help to elucidate the placebo responder. Successful blockade with good modification of pain can be used in conjunction with physiotherapy to increase mobility of the affected limb.

### Regional sympathetic blocks (stellate ganglion blocks for upper limb and lumbar sympathetic blocks for lower limb)[16]

Characteristically the effect outlasts the duration of local anaesthetic by hours or days; ideally blocks are repeated as soon as possible after the effect wears off. The onset of the block is usually rapid, with warmth of the limb (measurable temperature change) and reduction in pain, reduced oedema follows hours later and function improves more slowly.

Sensory testing allows accurate assessment of sympathetic involvement and the level of block achieved.

### Intravenous regional blockade (IVRB)

Intravenous regional blockades involve the administration of an active pharmacological agent with 0.5% prilocaine to reduce the pain of injection. The volumes used range from 40 to 60 ml depending on the extremity to be blocked. The tourniquet is kept inflated for 20 minutes after injection of agent to minimize the risk of systemic effects. These blocks may have an advantage when disease prevents nerve block or if the patent refuses nerve blocks.

IVRB with guanethidine 10–20 mg produces skin temperature changes lasting approximately 3 days and pain relief of greater duration.[18] This is, however, challenged by recent work suggesting there is no significant benefit.[19] Some evidence exists for the efficacy of guanethidine in patients with SMP but not sympathetically independent pain.[20] Side-effects may prevent or interrupt treatment; they increase with age and include orthostatic hypotension and thrombophlebitis. Other agents have been used. Bretylium (1.5 mg/kg) or reserpine (1.25 mg) have similar effects and side-effects to guanethidine. Hypertension and tachycardia occur initially with bretylium secondary to noradrenaline release. Ketorolac has also been used in conjunction with local anaesthetic.

## Drug treatment

- Antidepressants (amitriptyline, doxepin, desipramine, dothiepin) have been used with benefit for neuropathic pain over many years. The dosage is often lower than that for depression, and it has to be individually titrated to benefit or side-effects. Improvements in sleep and mood may also be seen. The newer selective serotonin (5-HT) reuptake inhibitors (SSRI) have not shown this benefit.
- Anti-convulsant drugs (carbamazepine, gabapentin, valproate) are established agents in treating neuropathic pain.
- Steroids have been used in early CRPS. There is some evidence for benefit.[14] Use in children has not shown clear benefits and they should therefore be avoided in this group.[6]
- Non-steroidal anti-inflammatory drugs (NSAIDs) may help on their own, for their opioid sparing effect or for associated joint pains.
- Opioids are of benefit in selected patients with neuropathic pain. Their use has increased over recent years but caution should be used. Epidural or intrathecal use has been beneficial in some. Controversy remains with opioid use and long term benefits need to be evaluated.
- Bisphosphonates have been explored and show some promise for managing the osteoporosis and to some extent the pain of CRPS.
- Calcitonin may have a mild effect on pain and influence osteoporosis. The long term benefits of calcitonin are unknown.
- α-adrenoreceptor antagonists (phenoxybenzamine, prazosin) have been effective in some patients. Their use is limited by side-effects.

- Clonidine may be useful for small areas of CRPS if applied topically to the area of pain. It has also been used intrathecaly and epiduraly in CRPS.
- Topical capsaicin has provided temporary analgesia to areas of CRPS.

## Neuroaugmentation

### Infusion techniques

These prolong the period of analgesia, allow intensive physiotherapy, permit desensitization of central pathways and minimize the number of injections.[6] Techniques include intrathecal, epidural, plexus, paravertebral and pleural blocks. Inpatient trials help assess the potential benefit of these techniques in individuals. The duration of percutaneous systems is limited by the risks of infection and patient acceptability. With outpatient infusions the patients, helpers and medical staff have to evaluate the benefits against the logistical difficulties such as infection and filling and maintaining pumps. Implanted pumps have advantages and become cost effective at approximately 3 months. Tolerance may develop, but it can be overcome by having a drug holiday or by rotating opioids

### Spinal cord stimulation[3,21]

This technique may help when conservative management fails to provide lasting results. Evidence is mixed with few good quality studies. Benefit is moderate and further studies need to be done. Most of the evidence is from case series. Implantation involves a two stage surgical procedure, starting with a temporary electrode to assess effectiveness. If there is satisfactory clinical relief the second stage is to implant a permanent system. Complications include electrode movement or fracture, haematoma, temporary nerve palsies and scar formation around the electrodes.

## Neuroablative procedures

Consensus suggests that neuroablative techniques be reserved for situations where conservative therapy has failed to maintain control. Good evidence for benefit is lacking. There must be a history of successful sympathetic blockade with local anaesthetic.[22] Patients need to be well motivated and to continue with the other modalities after the procedure. They must be aware that the benefit may not be permanent and that side-effects may be. Great caution is required when undertaking neuroablative procedures. Percutaneous procedures require X-ray control to ensure correct needle placement. One study suggests that only a small minority of cases required this type of therapy.[6]

- Radiofrequency sympathectomy can be performed on a day case basis and avoids the complications of open surgery. It has been shown to be safe but has not gained in popularity.
- Neurolytic sympathectomy with phenol 7–10% or alcohol 50–100% may be used. The current feeling is that phenol does not provide permanent relief; recurrence occurs in 30% of patients who benefit. Post-sympathectomy neuralgia occurs in 20–40% of cases, starts 10–14 days after the procedure and is usually self limiting. It occurs more commonly with lumbar sympathectomy.[22] Permanent damage to adjacent structures can occur.
- Surgery should be reserved for those who have only temporary relief following a significant period of intensive conservative therapy (3–6 months). The clinician must be sure of the diagnosis as most failures are due to incorrect diagnosis or inadequate sympathectomy. In one series[23] over 90% of patients had their pain reduced by 50% or more. The

best results were in those with less severe disease of shorter duration, but only 3 patients were able to return to their full time activities.

- Thoracoscopic cervical sympathectomy is a minimally invasive procedure with a patient satisfaction rates of up to 62%.[24] The evidence remains weak but in selected individuals this may have a role to play. Reactive hyperhydrosis may be a problem. Surgical ablative procedures including, dorsal root entry zone (DREZ) lesions, rhizotomy, cordotomy, thalamotomy and excision of cortical structures have not proved to be of long term benefit.
- On very rare occasions, with severe disease, limb amputation has been the only treatment available.[5] Amputation is neither standard treatment nor is it always successful in relieving pain. It may do no more than exchange a painful limb for a painful phantom limb.

## Management of motor abnormalities

The majority of patients with motor disturbances and CRPS obtain some relief with sympathetic blockade or sympathectomy. Spasms may be treated with benzodiazepines or baclofen.[25] Limitation of shoulder movement frequently accompanies upper limb CRPS,[2] and this may be helped by suprascapular nerve block.

# Outcome

- CRPS is self-limiting in many, but it can persist for years.
- Outcomes from one case series suggests that 60% have residual symptoms and only 20% of patients reached prior activity at 18 month follow-up.[3] The morbidity for non-responders to treatment may be significant.[23]
- No outcome figures are available for patient recovery in the general population.
- In paediatric populations, 94% reported their schoolwork had suffered and only 46% were symptom free at follow-up (median 3 years).[6]

# Conclusion

- CRPS causes a spectrum of disability from the self-limiting to the irreversible and permanently debilitating.
- CRPS is not rare; it is probably under-diagnosed in both adult and paediatric populations. Diagnostic criteria have been defined to aid diagnosis.
- The pathophysiology remains obscure with some debate as to a psychogenic cause.
- Management is difficult, and there is inadequate evidence for a clear strategy. No single treatment is effective.
- Current management is empirical and based on consensus or expert opinion. It involves multidisciplinary approaches including a component of functional restoration.
- Many patients will respond to treatment; not all will be cured but efforts have to be made to palliate their distress. True outcomes remain unknown.

# References

1. Merskey H, Bogduk N. *Classification of Chronic Pain*. 2nd edition. Seattle: IASP Press, 1994
2. Veldman PHM, Reynen HM, Arntz IE, et al. Signs and symptoms of reflex sympathetic dystrophy: prospective study of 829 patients. *Lancet* **342**: 1012–1016, 1993

3. Subarrao J, Stillwell GK. Reflex sympathetic dystrophy syndrome of the upper extremity: analysis of total outcome of management of 125 cases. *Arch Phys Med Rehab* **62**: 549–554, 1981

4. Stanton-Hicks M, Baron R, Boas R, et al. Complex Regional Pain Syndromes: guidelines for therapy. *Clin J Pain* **14**: 155–166, 1998

5. Erdmann MW, Wynn-Jones CH. 'Familial' reflex sympathetic dystrophy syndrome and amputation. *Br J Accident Surg* **23**: 136–138, 1992

6. Wilder RT, Berde CB, Wolohan M, et al. Reflex sympathetic dystrophy in children. Clinical characteristics and follow-up of seventy patients. *J Bone Joint Surg – Am Vol* **74**: 910–919, 1992

7. Janig W. The puzzle of (reflex sympathetic dystrophy): Mechanisms, hypothesis, open questions. In: Janig W, Stanton-Hicks M, eds. *Reflex Sympathetic Dystrophy: a Reappraisal Progress in Pain Research and Management Vol 6*. Seattle: IASP Press, 1996, pp. 1–24

8. Bogduk, N. Complex regional pain syndrome. *Curr Opin Anaesthesiol* **14**: 541–546, 2001

9. Bruehl S, Carlson CR. Predisposing psychological factors in the development of reflex sympathetic dystrophy. A review of the empirical evidence. *Clin J Pain* **8**: 287–299, 1992

10. Rothschild B. Reflex sympathetic dystrophy. *Arthritis Care Res* **3**: 144–153, 1990

11. Silber TJ, Majd M. Reflex sympathetic dystrophy syndrome in children and adolescents. Report of 18 cases and review of the literature. *Am J Dis Child* **142**: 1325–1330, 1988

12. Webster GF, Schwartzman RJ, Jacoby RA, et al. Reflex sympathetic dystrophy. Occurrence of inflammatory skin lesions in patients with stages II and III disease. *Arch Dermatol* 127: 1541–1544, 1991

13. Bryan AS, Klenerman L, Bowsher D. The diagnosis of reflex sympathetic dystrophy using an algometer. *J Bone Joint Surg – Br Vol* **73**: 644–646, 1991

14. Kingery WS. A critical review of controlled clinical trials for peripheral neuropathic pain and complex regional pain syndromes. *Pain* **73**: 123–139, 1997

15. Amadio PC. Pain dysfunction syndromes. *J Bone Joint Surg – Am Vol* **70**: 944–949, 1988

16. Bonica JJ. *The Management of Pain*, vol 1. Philadelphia: Lea & Febiger, 1990, pp. 220–243

17. Kesler RW, Saulsbury FT, Miller LT, et al. Reflex sympathetic dystrophy in children: treatment with transcutaneous electric nerve stimulation. *Pediatrics* **82**: 728–732, 1988

18. Hannington-Kiff JG. Pharmacological target blocks in hand surgery and rehabilitation. J *Hand Surg – Br Vol* **9**: 29–36, 1984

19. Livingstone JA, Atkins RM. Intravenous regional guanethidine blockade in the treatment of post-traumatic complex regional pain syndrome type 1 (algodystrophy) of the hand. *J Bone Joint Surg – Br Vol* **84**: 380–386, 2002

20. Jadad AR, Caroll D, Glynn CJ. Intravenous regional sympathetic blockade for pain relief in reflex sympathetic dystrophy: a systematic review and a randomized double-blind crossover study. *J Pain Symptom Management* **10**: 13–20, 1995

21. Kemler MA, Reulen JPH, Barende GAM, et al. Impact of spinal cord stimulation on sensory characteristics in complex regional pain syndrome type I: A randomized trial. *Anesthesiology* **95**: 72–80, 2001

22. Payne R. Neuropathic pain syndromes, with special reference to causalgia and reflex sympathetic dystrophy. *Clin J Pain* **2**: 59–73, 1986

23. Olcott C 4th, Eltherington LG, Wilcosky BR, et al. Reflex sympathetic dystrophy – the surgeon's role in management. *J Vascular Surg* **14**: 488–492; discussion 492–495, 1991

24. Robertson DP, Simpson RK, Rose JE, et al. Video-assisted endoscopic thoracic ganglionectomy. *J Neurosurg* **79**: 238–240, 1993

25. Schwartzman RJ, Kerrigan J. The movement disorder of reflex sympathetic dystrophy. *Neurology* **40**: 57–61, 1990

# 8 Muscle and Soft Tissue Pain

*Richard Haigh*

Musculoskeletal pain is very common and accounts for a large proportion of the burden of chronic pain. Epidemiological studies commonly report that up to 20% of people complain of widespread pain and around 10% suffer from regional pain. If American College of Rheumatology (ACR) diagnostic criteria (see below) are used, approximately 3–5% of females and 1% of males suffer from fibromyalgia. The prevalence of chronic musculoskeletal pain is consistent across North America, the UK and Europe.

Developments in our understanding of pain mechanisms in musculoskeletal disorders have allowed us to move away from the perception that 'pain equals damage in the periphery'. Evidence of dysfunctional pain processing and perturbations in the interaction between central sensory and motor systems have provided new explanations for chronic pain states.[1] However, the 6 Ds (Dramatization of complaints, Drug misuse, Dysfunction/disuse, Dependency, Depression and Disability) of the chronic pain syndrome still apply to the clinic setting.

## The scope of muscle and soft tissue pain syndromes

There are a host of painful conditions causing muscle and soft tissue pain. These are listed in Table 8.1 under five main groups. Joint pathology is not considered in this chapter.

The three conditions most commonly presenting to a pain clinic (and difficult to diagnose and manage) are considered in detail below. These are fibromyalgia/chronic widespread pain, myofascial pain and 'RSI'.

## Fibromyalgia: chronic pain or chronic poor coping?

Descriptions have been found in the medical literature as far back as the early 17th century of chronic widespread pain, tender points, fatigue, and multiple other somatic symptoms. Some physicians accept the fibromyalgia (FMS) construct and the ACR diagnostic criteria,[2] based on the presence of widespread pain and tender points.

These criteria have been subject to much debate and criticism, and have led some to challenge the diagnosis and construct itself, claiming that it has no scientific basis and that the diagnostic label has no practical value in management of patients with chronic pain. These sceptics refer to the unnecessary medicalization of psychosocial distress and describe a 'dustbin diagnosis', proposed when an alternative explanation of symptoms cannot be provided.

The term 'chronic widespread pain' (CWP) may be more useful – it avoids both the controversial ACR criteria and unnecessary conflict with the patient about whether you are a 'believer' or 'non-believer', but simply acknowledges the nature of the problem. An alternative definition of widespread pain has been proposed, which utilizes a more stringent definition that requires the presence of more diffuse limb pain.[3]

**Table 8.1** Muscle and soft-tissue pain syndromes (excluding arthritis)

| | |
|---|---|
| Pathology at tendon, bursa and enthesis (see Table 8.2) | Bursitis<br>Tendonosis<br>Enthesis |
| Biomechanical problems | Hypermobility (local and generalized)<br>Leg length discrepancy<br>Mechanical foot problems |
| Neurovascular aetiology | Carpal tunnel syndrome<br>Medial and ulnar nerve entrapment in forearm<br>Suprascapular nerve entrapment<br>Thoracic outlet syndrome<br>Lumbar spinal stenosis<br>Meralgia parasthetica<br>Tarsal tunnel syndrome |
| Regional pain syndromes | Temporomandibular disorders<br>Myofascial pain syndrome<br>Repetitive strain syndrome |
| Generalized pain syndromes | Fibromyalgia/chronic widespread pain<br>Multiple chemical sensitivity syndrome<br>Chronic fatigue syndrome |

There is no dispute however, that chronic widespread pain is common both in the community and in hospital populations, and patients suffering from chronic widespread pain report increased functional impairment, marked disability and consequently face barriers to participation in society, often in excess of those with chronic disease such as rheumatoid, inflammatory bowel disease and diabetes.[4] In addition, patients consult many physicians before receiving appropriate treatment and advice and some undergo unnecessary surgery.

The diagnosis of FMS is being made with increasing frequency. FMS is one of the three most common new rheumatological diagnoses made in North America,[5] and it has been suggested that it is the single most common disorder in rheumatological practice. Patients with FMS utilize hospital resources such as outpatient consultations, have more surgical interventions and complain of more comorbid medical conditions than patients with other rheumatic disorders. There are clearly significant resource and cost health care issues surrounding FMS, notwithstanding those relating to work loss, social welfare and medicolegal issues including the so-called post-traumatic FMS.

There is an overlap between patients with both widespread pain and prominent symptoms of fatigue, and patients who fulfill the criteria for chronic fatigue syndrome, and who also have

**Table 8.2** Pathology at tendon, bursa and enthesis

| | |
|---|---|
| Bursitis | Sub deltoid; olecranon; iliopsoas; greater trochanteric; prepatellar; anserine; retrocalcaneal |
| Tendonosis | Shoulder (rotator cuff, supraspinatus, biceps)<br>Wrist (deQuervain's: APL and EPB), extensor, flexor (trigger finger)<br>Achilles<br>Posterior tibial |
| Enthesis | Epicondylitis<br>Plantar fasciitis |

chronic widespread pain. The approach to the management of these two conditions does not differ a great deal, especially when considering sleep, physical therapy modalities and cognitive-behavioural therapy.

## Diagnosis

### Clinical presentation
Cardinal features:

- Widespread myalgia and arthralgia
- Axial pain
- Severe stiffness: mornings, post exercise and generalized gelling phenomena
- Deconditioning and intolerance of exercise
- Poor-quality unrefreshing sleep
- Fatigue
- Exacerbating features: weather, environmental temperature, stress, exercise
- Tender points on examination

Other complaints – there are a number that commonly present with widespread pain, implying either shared predisposing risk factors or aetiology:

- Subjective joint swelling
- Painful paraesthesia (in the absence of objective neurological abnormality)
- Chronic headaches
- Palpitations
- Irritable bowel syndrome
- Pelvic pain, dyspareunia and dysmenorrhoea
- Female urethral syndrome
- Mitral valve prolapse
- Temporomandibular joint dysfunction
- Restless legs syndrome
- Multiple allergy and multiple chemical sensitivity syndromes
- Cognitive dysfunction
- Anxiety disorders
- Depression
- Hyperventilation
- Raynaud's phenomenon
- Chronic fatigue syndrome

### Diagnostic criteria
The ACR criteria are designed for case definition and research purposes, and they need not be strictly applied in the clinic setting. The criteria are included as they are widely quoted in both clinical and research reports. The alternative 'Manchester criteria' differ in that they require more diffuse limb pain for a diagnosis of CWP, and seem to identify a group of subjects whose pain is likely to be truly 'widespread' and is associated more strongly with factors such as psychological disturbance, fatigue, sleep problems and tender points.[3]
ACR Criteria 1990[2]:

- Pain history
  - Widespread pain in all 4 quadrants of the body (i.e. both sides, above and below the waist and the axial skeleton)
  - Constant for 3 months

- At least 11 of 18 anatomically specific tender points (TPs). (Elicited by palpation to cause the examiner's nail bed to blanch, or about 4 kg force, no referred pain and referred to as 'painful' by the patient)
  - Suboccipital muscle insertions at occiput
  - Lower cervical paraspinal
  - Trapezius at midpoint of the upper border
  - Supraspinatus at its origin above medial scapular spine
  - 2nd costochondral junction
  - 2 cm distal to lateral epicondyle in forearm
  - Upper outer quadrant of buttock
  - Greater trochanter
  - Knee just proximal to the medial joint line.

All of the above sites are bilateral.

## Differential diagnosis

Diffuse muscle and joint pain has a wide differential diagnosis. It requires a thorough clinical assessment to exclude inflammatory joint and muscle disease, and systemic disease ranging from hypothyroidism to systemic lupus erythematosus to carcinomatosis.

Differential diagnosis of fibromyalgia syndrome:
- Endocrine
  - Hypothyroidism*
  - Osteomalacia/hyperparathyroidism*
  - Cushing's syndrome
- Joint disease
  - Inflammatory
  - Osteoarthritis/spondylosis
- Polymyalgia Rheumatica
- Autoimmune connective tissue disease/vasculitis, e.g. systemic lupus erythematosus
- Neuromuscular disease
  - Idiopathic inflammatory myopathy*
  - Drug induced myopathy* (including alcohol)
  - Toxic myopathy*
  - Metabolic myopathy*
  - Post-polio syndrome
  - Myasthenia
  - Infective, e.g. viral, Lyme disease*
  - Parkinsonism
- Depression
- Other pain syndromes
  - Chronic fatigue syndrome
  - Myofascial pain syndrome
- Carcinomatosis*
- Amyloid*.

(* Indicates may present with weakness in association with myalgia).

Useful investigations in patients complaining of widespread pain:
- Urinalysis and microscopy
- Acute phase reactants, e.g. erythrocyte sedimentation rate/C-reactive protein
- Full blood count

- Muscle enzymes, e.g. creatine phosphokinase
- Electrolytes and renal function
- Blood glucose
- Calcium group
- Anti-nuclear antibody/rheumatoid Factor
- Thyroid function tests[*]
- Chest X-ray.

[*] TFTs have the best yield in patients with no other suspicion of systemic disease.

## Pathophysiology: soma or psyche?

Theories concerning the generation and perpetuation of chronic widespread musculoskeletal pain in FMS are varied. These include muscle pathology, neurochemical and neuroendocrine abnormalities, sleep disorders, pain physiology and psychological and psychiatric abnormalities. There is increasing evidence that FMS/CWP may be a central pain processing disorder, with associated neuroendocrine features.

### Muscle pathology

There has been no consistent reproducible evidence that points to muscle pathology as the culprit. Skin blood flow abnormalities have revealed a local vasoconstriction, suggesting that local hypoxia may contribute to TPs. Some doubt the relevance of TPs as they can be found in normal subjects, and their number and severity are normally distributed. The presence of TPs may be related to poor sleep and psychological distress.

When pathological changes are seen in FMS muscle (these include non-specific type II fibre atrophy, an increase of lipid droplets, a slight proliferation of mitochondria and a slightly elevated incidence of ragged red fibres), it is not clear whether these physiological and anatomical abnormalities should be considered as primary pathology or the secondary effects of disuse and deconditioning. However, features such as the increased perception of effort during exercise and a time lapse between exercise and pain may be explained by enhanced muscle nociception and microrupture of muscle fibres respectively.

### Sleep

Non-restorative deep sleep, associated with reduction/absence of δ (stage 4 Non-REM) activity on the electroencephalogram, is also implicated. Moreover, by interfering with sleep patterns in normal volunteers, FMS-like symptoms can be induced.[6,7] Regular exercises improve sleep quality, and the relationship between the two may influence symptoms in FMS. Fatigue is also associated with sleep disturbance.

### Neuroendocrine

There are a host of biochemical, metabolic, and immunoregulatory abnormalities associated with fibromyalgia. These include perturbations in 5-hydroxytryptamine (5-HT, serotonin), substance P, hypothalamic-pituitary-adrenal (HPA) axis, growth hormone (GH) and cytokines, most of which are involved in sleep physiology, and in central and peripheral pain mechanisms. Whether these abnormalities are important in the pathophysiology of FMS or secondary is still unclear. Some of the reported abnormalities are:

- Abnormally low 5-HT levels and a relationship between low 5-HT levels and fibromyalgia symptoms.
- 5-HT transporter gene (5-HTT) polymorphism – SS genotype in fibromyalgia may be associated with higher levels depression and psychological distress.

**59**

- Cerebrospinal fluid (CSF) substance P levels are 2–3 times normal.
- Abnormal red blood cell ATP (involved in 5-HT metabolism)
- HPA axis dysfunction at many levels – 5-HT is involved in the circadian regulation and the stress-induced stimulation of the HPA axis.
- Growth hormone deficiency and low levels of insulin-like growth factor I (IGF-I) – disrupted sleep affects GH levels and (IGF-I) is involved in tissue repair.
- CSF nerve growth factor (involved in substance P production) higher in fibromyalgia.
- Abnormal cytokine levels – cytokines such as interleukin–2 (IL–2) are elevated in FMS patients, and, when given intravenously, it reproduces FMS-like symptoms.[8] Il–6 and Il–8 have also been found elevated in FMS (substance P influences their production)
- Autonomic dysfunction clinical reports, vasomotor irregularities, responses to ganglion blockade, muscle blood flow alterations.

## Pain processing

Considerable evidence from the pain physiology literature supports defective pain processing as being responsible for the increased pain perception in FMS.[9] This does not imply causality, but it can help our understanding of the characteristic pain complaints and signs of primary hyperalgesia, secondary hyperalgesia and allodynia, and neurogenic inflammation observed in FMS patients.

Pain processing abnormalities:

- Increased afferent nociceptive activity
- Central sensitization of receptors
- Abnormal pain thresholds
- Enhanced axon reflex and flare following capsaicin application
- CNS imaging studies of the 'pain pathway' are invariably abnormal (and differ from other pain conditions and arthritis).[10]

## Psychosocial

Psychological factors play an important role in any chronic painful condition, and FMS is no different. However, the role of personality and psychological factors in the genesis of FMS remains controversial. What is not in doubt though, is that FMS/CWP is associated with significant psychological comorbidity. There are increased rates of depression, anxiety, distress, and health-care seeking behaviours compared with control subjects without pain or other disease group populations.[11] There are also suggestions from a wide variety of sources that factors such as somatization,[12] hypervigilance, attentional factors, and coping styles (such as catastrophization) strongly influence pain and distress in FMS. There are also increased rates of depression in relatives of those with FMS.

Further evidence of psychological distress describes FMS patients self-reporting reduced Quality of Life and increased functional impairment to a greater extent than many other patients with other chronic disease.[4] Though these factors are important in chronic pain, a causal relationship cannot be confirmed or refuted. Despite some reports of increased rates of post-traumatic stress disorder and childhood sexual abuse in FMS, the association has not been shown to be causal.

## More controversies

Debate continues to rage about the role of trauma triggering FMS. Most of the evidence is retrospective and supports an association, but whether this relationship is causal has yet to be proven. There is no evidence of a link between Gulf War service and FMS. Despite silicone implants being more common in women with FMS, there is no evidence of increased rates of FMS in women following implants.

## Management

There is a paucity of controlled trial evidence to guide the treatment of FMS. There is evidence to support a trial of pain modifying antidepressant medication, a graded aerobic exercise programme[13] and cognitive-behavioural therapy[14] – though the timing of such interventions and which patients to select for a particular approach is not clear. The involvement of a multidisciplinary team is often essential when dealing with distressed, challenging patients. The team must work within defined, efficient and consistent decision making processes and with clear lines of communication within the team identified.

A pragmatic approach to FMS is outlined below:

- Baseline assessment of pain, disability, and a measure of distress/depression.
- Empathetic listening, and acknowledgment that the patient is experiencing a difficult pain problem. Frankly discuss the limits of medical knowledge and treatment in this condition.
- There is no benefit gained from challenging a patient's belief in the existence of FMS – unless you feel that there is another legitimate medical diagnosis. A compromise label of 'chronic widespread pain' may be acceptable.
- Prognosis – although all health professionals in the pain team have encountered severely distressed and disabled patients with FMS, published reports suggest that such cases are uncommon, and importantly, another more serious diagnosis is not discovered on follow-up. The majority of patients improve with advice and treatment. However, persistent pain problems are common, and an association between the report of CWP and subsequent death from cancer in the medium and long term has been reported.[15] The nature of this association is unclear.
- Identify barriers to recovery, such as pending litigation or compensation claims.
- Address possible causal or perpetuating factors – such as inflammatory or degenerative joint disease or psychosocial factors. Ongoing nociceptive pain may 'drive' the FMS pain experience.
- Avoid excessive use of physical therapy modalities, activity limitation, and prescribed work absence.

A treatment plan may include:

- Analgesia. Many patients feel that paracetamol; non-steroidal anti-inflammatory drugs (NSAIDs), compound analgesia and opiates are not helpful. However, despite the lack of evidence for 'inflammation', NSAIDs are often preferred.
- A graded paced aerobic and flexibility exercise programme.[16] (*Suggested advice: daily exercise; set attainable, realistic goals; warm up is essential; stretch all the major muscle groups on rising and before bed; start at low levels of exercise and build up slowly; afternoons and evenings are best; expect and plan for an increase in pain initially; exercise in water may be beneficial especially to start things off; group exercise is useful; once a programme is developed, there is usually no need for frequent physiotherapy review, exercise at home is as useful as in hospital*).
- Pain modifying techniques, such as transcutaneous electrical nerve stimulation (TENS), activity pacing, relaxation training, visual imagery and distraction.
- Low doses of antidepressant medication (amitriptyline: 10–25 mg) may improve sleep and decrease pain. If there is no response after 2–4 weeks, stop treatment. Patients with

FMS are very sensitive to these medications and often complain of a marked 'hangover'. A combination of evening low dose amitriptyline and morning fluoxetine may be tried.[17]
- Identify and manage depression.
- Acupuncture, dry needling and local anaesthetic/corticosteroid injections may give short-term relief from a particularly distressing TPs/trigger points. However, TPs are often widespread precluding purely local treatment, and patients may become dependent on this interventional approach at the expense of other self-management techniques.
- Construct a setback plan in collaboration with the patient.
- Cognitive-behavioural therapy[14] – this is a process in which patients reconceptualize their pain experience, are taught pain coping skills, and given opportunity for behavioural rehearsal and guided practice. The knowledge and skills obtained through the process are then applied in an effort to exert control over the FMS pain experience.

# Myofascial pain syndromes

Reports consistent with the current concept of the myofascial pain syndrome (MPS) have been written for over a century, though the construct widely accepted today derives from Travell's seminal work, later modified following her collaboration with Simons.[18,19]

In MPS, localized pain is attributed to a muscle and its surrounding fascia. Myofascial pain is a very common cause of regional pain, especially in the cervical, lumbar and temporo-mandibular regions. In fact, most people will have experienced a localized myofascial pain problem at one time or another. Trigger points (TrPs) and taut bands are characteristic of MPS. There is considerable variation between clinicians in the identification of taut bands, muscle twitch, and active TrPs, and therefore some question the reliability of this diagnosis.

A taut band:

- Is a tight palpable area within a muscle ('rope like induration')
- Produces pain when the muscle is stretched
- Restricts range of motion of the muscle
- Has a TrP elicited along it
- Can be snapped or rolled under the finger in accessible muscles and a 'twitch response' may be elicited.

A trigger point:

- Is palpable within a taut band
- When palpated is exquisitely tender and pain is referred to a characteristic distant site – a reference zone
- Exhibits a twitch when needled
- May show an autonomic disturbance (or this may be seen at the reference zone), e.g. temperature change, vasoconstriction
- May refer sensory changes other than pain, such as tenderness and dysaesthesia
- Can be 'active' (gives rise to pain on spontaneous movement of the muscle, and restricts range of movement) or 'latent' (painful only when palpated).

Figure 8.1 illustrates the location of TrPs and reference zones.

## Diagnosis

### Clinical presentation

Patients with active myofascial TrPs often complain of a 'muscle strain', with a degree of radiation of pain. Therefore, the pain may be poorly localized and regional. It is often described

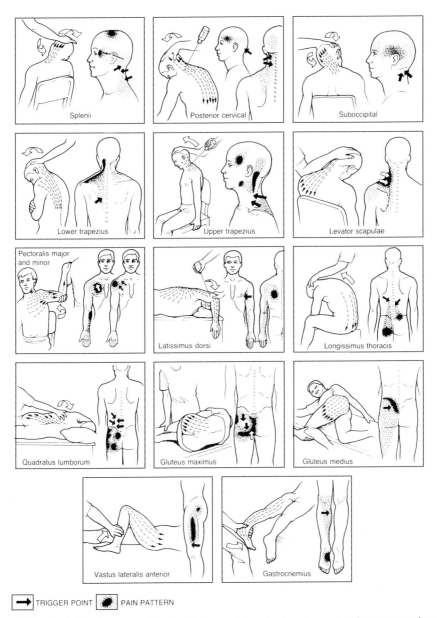

→ TRIGGER POINT ● PAIN PATTERN

**Figure 8.1** Myofacial pain patterns: location of trigger points and pain patterns, stretch positions and spray patterns for muscle groups commonly causing pain patterns seen in pain clinics. The curved white arrows identify the direction of pressure applied to stretch the muscle. The dashed arrows trace the impact of the stream of vapocoolant spray applied to release the muscular tension during stretch.

as a dull, aching pain in the deep tissues, sometimes in both muscles and joints. Sometimes a precipitating factor or activity can be identified. Restriction of joint motion and stiffness, especially in the cervical region, is seen.

Taut bands and TrPs are found. The reference zone for pain following palpation does not follow dermatomal/myotomal boundaries and numbness or paraesthesia may be experienced rather than pain. Latent TrPs may cause some increased muscle tension and limitation of stretch and range of motion. This may contribute to the localized muscle imbalance.

Associated disturbances of autonomic and motor functions can occur. These include abnormal sweating and pilomotor activity and changes in colour and temperature. Other 'neurological' disturbances include proprioceptive dysfunction caused by TrPs, dizziness, tinnitus and distorted weight perception of lifted objects. Weakness, poor coordination and decreased work tolerance of the involved muscle, and spasm of distant muscles may all complicate the clinical picture. Weakness, presumably due to reflex motor inhibition, can be distressing and cause patients to drop objects from their grasp.

Other features include:

- Poor sleep
- Depression and anxiety
- Poor posture
- Common presentation in middle-aged females.

Trigger points are common in the general population and have numerous causes and associations. They may be activated by acute mechanical overload, overuse fatigue, trauma, and by radiculopathy. Visceral disease (ranging from myocardial infarction to gall bladder disease), joint disease and emotional distress may all precipitate the development of a TrP.

## Diagnostic criteria

Clinical criteria for the diagnosis of MPS have been devised. For a clinical diagnosis of MPS, 5 major criteria should be present along with at least 1 of 3 minor criteria.[18]

Major criteria:

- Regional pain complaint
- Pain complaint or altered sensation in the expected distribution of referred pain from a myofascial trigger point
- Taut band palpable in an accessible muscle
- Exquisite spot tenderness at one point along the length of the taut band
- Some degree of restricted range of motion, when measurable.

Minor criteria:

- Reproduction of clinical pain complaint, or altered sensation, by pressure on the tender spot
- Elicitation of a local twitch response by transverse snapping palpation at the tender spot or by needle insertion into the tender spot in the taut band
- Pain alleviated by elongating (stretching) the muscle or by injecting the tender spot (TrP).

## Differential diagnosis

There is a wide differential diagnosis for MPS:

- Head and neck
  - Radiculopathy
  - Cervical spondylosis/degenerative disc disease
  - Thoracic outlet syndrome
  - Destructive/malignant lesion of cervical spine
  - Ménière's Disease

- Torticollis
- Polyneuropathy
- Dental problems
- Earache
- Temporomandibular joint (TMJ) arthropathy
- Migraine and other paroxysmal headaches
- Upper Limb
  - Thoracic outlet syndrome
  - Radiculopathy
  - Brachial neuritis
  - Nerve entrapment syndromes, e.g. carpal tunnel syndrome, ulnar nerve entrapment at elbow or wrist, suprascapular nerve entrapment
  - Complex regional pain syndrome (CRPS)
  - Rotator cuff disease and tendonitis about the shoulder complex
  - Epicondylitis
  - Idiopathic inflammatory myositis/myopathy
  - Referred pain from cardiorespiratory disease
- Lumbar spine and lower limb
  - Radiculopathy
  - Lumbar spondylosis/degenerative disc disease
  - Destructive/malignant lesion of lumbar spine
  - Sacroiliitis
  - Hip and knee arthrosis
  - Greater trochanteric bursitis
  - Iliotibial band syndrome
  - Piriformis syndrome
- Multiple MPS sites
  - A similar differential diagnosis to FMS/CWP.

## Pathophysiology

Many factors have been implicated in the development of MPS and TrPs. Some contributing factors include:

- Chronic mechanical stress
- Posture problems
- Muscle trauma and fatigue
- Chronic infection and inflammation
- Psychological distress
- Chronic sleep problems
- Metabolic disturbances
- Nutritional deficiency.

It has been proposed that MPS and TrPs may occur following some form of muscle injury (in the loosest sense of the term).

- Histological studies have failed to demonstrate significant structural abnormalities in muscle, though sarcolemmal distortions and contraction knots have been proposed as a mechanism to explain muscle contraction at the site of a TrP.
- Electromyography studies, although normal at rest, have revealed bursts of activity (akin to a normal muscle twitch) when a TrP is palpated.

**65**

- Thermographic temperature differences at TrPs, abnormal pressure algometry at TrPs and delayed muscle relaxation and muscle fatigue, mediated via muscle spindle have also been proposed to play a role.
- Botulinum toxin can relieve MPS either via a direct effect on muscle contraction, or via an indirect on the spinal reflex/pain mechanisms.
- The role of the endogenous opioid system is not clear, but the observation that the beneficial effect of TrP injection with local anaesthetic can be blocked by naloxone suggests that peripheral opioid receptors modulate TrP activity.
- Peripheral and central sensitization may be responsible for the development of TrPs and their reference zones. Raised levels of substance P in MPS muscle suggest peripheral activation of the peptidergic nervous system in MPS, implicating the afferent nervous system in the development and perception of myofascial pain.[20]

## Management

Successful management of MPS must include the recognition of underlying postural and biomechanical problems that might increase tension and irritability in a muscle or group of muscles. Thus, myofascial pain can occur in association with many other conditions and injuries of the neuro-musculoskeletal system. Contributing factors, such as exercise patterns, biomechanics and posture, and work practices and ergonomics should be assessed. In addition, as in all chronic painful conditions, psychosocial factors can play an important role. Muscle tension can be increased by anxiety and depression.

A number of approaches are used in MPS, though few have been subjected to robust, well-designed randomized control trials and, for those that have, results are conflicting. Once the underlying factors have been addressed and a muscle-training programme (stretching, flexibility, strengthening and balance) has been planned, local treatments can be employed. These include counter stimulation, 'stretch and spray', local anaesthetic (±corticosteroid) and botulinum toxin injections. Advice from an occupational therapist, physiotherapist and orthotists is often required.

### Counter stimulation
Repetitive action techniques may relieve MPS and include massage, TENS, acupuncture, heat and cold application.

### Stretch and spray[19]
A vapocoolant/local anaesthetic spray is used in conjunction with a passive stretch of the target muscle. This can be repeated several times, allowing time for the painful area to rewarm. This technique may have an immediate effect, but often needs repeating on a daily basis – which frequently cannot be provided due to lack of resources.

- The stretch should be performed with a fluid motion, facilitating muscle relaxation.
- Ethyl chloride or a local anaesthetic spray is used.
- The spray is directed parallel to the muscle fibres in a sweeping motion.
- Applying heat to the painful area after this technique may be helpful.
- The muscle group should be stretched through a full range of motion after the procedure
- Occasionally patients find this technique very uncomfortable and it exacerbates pain and muscle spasm.

### TrP injections
Whether the beneficial effects derive from the needle itself or the local anaesthetic (with or without corticosteroid) is not clear, but this technique can often reduce pain and increase range of motion. Dry needling can be used alone.[21]

- The TrP within the taut band should be identified, palpated and fixed.
- Insert the needle and inject the TrP directly with a small volume (approx. 1 ml) using sterile technique.
- Inserting the needle (and agitating it) may cause a local twitch response (and sometimes referred pain).
- Injection therapy may be repeated two or three times.
- A short-lived response helps to confirm the diagnosis, but suggests perpetuating factors may exist.

## Botulinum toxin type A (Botox, Dysport)

Botulinum toxin type A blocks cholinergic transmission at the neuromuscular junction, denervating the muscle cell. This results in a dose-dependent reduction of hyperactive muscle contraction, which may last for 3 months. In the weeks and months following botulinum toxin injection, a new nerve sprout establishes a new neuromuscular junction, and muscle activity gradually returns. Repeat injections may be required to maintain the clinical effect. There is emerging evidence that this toxin can relieve pain and increases muscle relaxation in MPS.[22,23]

## Analgesia

Medication for myofascial pain syndrome is unlikely to have a major role to play, but may be helpful when administered before stretching or exercise. Muscle relaxants are not effective. Low-dose tricyclic antidepressants may be useful if the patient suffers from sleep disturbance.

# Repetitive strain injury

Repetitive strain syndrome, or repetitive stess injury (RSI), is a chronic pain syndrome that has become a major source of disability at work. Use of the term 'RSI' followed an 'outbreak' of upper limb pains in workers in Australia in the 1980s. Similar historical descriptions of work-related disability have been described in writers, telegraphists and railway workers over the past two centuries.

This regional pain syndrome occurs in the context of repetitive movement, often with a postural constraint, but it is not clear whether there is abnormality or tissue damage in the affected limb. There is a considerable controversy and confusion surrounding the use and meaning of the term itself, the clinical diagnosis, medico-legal issues and the management of these patients with chronic upper limb pain.

The wider context of neck and arm pain in the general population is important to consider:

- These are common symptoms in working people. As Nortin Hadler states: 'Regional arm pain is a ubiquitous, remittent, and intermittent predicament of life'.[24]
- 3.8 million working days were lost in 1995.[25]
- Linking certain activities to a disease is difficult (work or leisure?).
- Relative risks of upper limb problems associated with occupational exposure are low.[26]
- Associations between work, hand and limb usage and pathology are complex and not 'causal'.
- Rigidly defined and prescribed industrial injury – such as work related tendonitis/tenosynovitis, carpal tunnel syndrome and writers cramp – must be considered.

Difficulties encountered when trying to sort through the 'RSI' literature:

- Epidemiological studies have largely been retrospective, cross sectional or purely observational.

- Lack of widely accepted valid and repeatable diagnostic criteria.
- Few diagnostic tests or imaging studies that compliment a diagnostic work-up.
- Physical workloads in the workplace decrease and reporting of upper limb problems and resultant disability continues to rise.
- Furthermore, the Australian epidemic and medico-legal controversy has polarized both lay and medical opinion.

## Diagnosis

### Clinical presentation

In the clinic, patients present with upper limb pain in association with reduced work performance. The complaint may be task specific and may be related to finely controlled repetitive postures. Patients may also experience neck and chest wall pain. The syndrome may follow a discrete soft tissue injury or condition.

- Symptoms that begin in the periphery may often become more proximal.
- Pain is centred in the forearm and wrist, often with poor grip strength.
- Pain symptoms may fluctuate with activity and environmental changes.
- Pain phenomena vary markedly – hyperalgesia, hyperpathia and allodynia.
- Sensory disturbance also occur, such as 'numbness' or 'painful tingling'.
- TPs/TrPs may be present in the cervicobrachial area.
- Vasomotor changes, with skin colour and temperature abnormalities, and swelling may be visible.
- Cramps may be a feature, sometimes developing into dystonia.
- Symptoms of poor sleep, psychological distress and depression may be present.

### Diagnostic criteria

A consensus workshop (convened by the Health and Safety Executive) has agreed diagnostic criteria, for 'non-specific diffuse forearm pain' although this is essentially a diagnosis made by exclusion.[27] A diagnostic examination schedule for upper limb disorders has also been published.[28]

### Differential diagnosis

A careful assessment, with appropriate investigations, is necessary to look for evidence of pathology in the muscle–tendon unit and elsewhere, such as nerve entrapment and referred pains. Unfortunately, in a small but significant minority, a clear diagnosis is not possible and the problem is often labelled RSI or 'non-specific upper limb pain'.

The Differential diagnosis for RSI includes:

- Tendonitis
- Enthesitis
- Arthritis
- Nerve entrapment syndromes
- Referred pain from cervicobrachial region
- Radiculopathy
- Complex regional pain syndrome
- Thoracic outlet syndrome
- Myofascial pain syndrome
- Vascular claudication of the upper limb.

NB: The prescribed industrial diseases (determined by the Industrial Injuries Advisory Council) should be considered and the patient advised accordingly.

# Pathophysiology

Repetitive strain syndrome is a complex condition often related to posture and activity, and shares some features of pain syndromes, CRPS, tendonitis, and muscle–tendon unit dysfunction. However, there is no consistent evidence that comfortable, familiar arm use at home or at work, increases the incidence of upper limb pain. A summary of the proposed mechanisms is given below.

### Arthritis or tendonitis?
- There is little evidence that RSI is due to sub-clinical musculotendinous injury.
- Imaging studies of all modalities (plain X-ray, ultrasound, bone scanning and MRI) do not reveal local musculoskeletal pathology in non-specific upper limb pain.
- There is possible referred pain from neck structures.
- Sex hormones may influence tendon biology and predispose to tendonopathy.
- Neurogenic mechanisms may promote inflammation and influence expression of genes involved in tendon cellular and molecular biology.[29]

### Mechanical/postural?
- Cervical posture has a role.
- Signs of 'adverse neural tension' are common and may reproduce pain.
- Muscle micro-trauma theory.

### Vascular basis?
- Blood flow to the painful limb areas is altered (thermal image changes, abnormal cold stress tests, and abnormal blood flow and pool phases on isotope scan) – though contradictory, with both increases and decreases observed.
- Physiological claudication of forearm muscle – Doppler ultrasound studies suggested that local blood vessel dilatation could be faulty.[30]

### Median nerve damage?
- Mechanical damage to the median nerve at the wrist and possible neuroma formation – MRI scanning has shown reduced median-nerve movement in the carpal tunnel.[31]
- Carpal tunnel syndrome (CTS) now accounts for almost half of the repetitive motion disorders in USA.

### Nervous system dysfunction?
- Peripheral and central neural processing is abnormal.[32]
- There are alterations in the function of both nociceptive and non-nociceptive pathways in RSI limbs (pain threshold, capsaicin flare response and sensory defects).
- Allodynia, hyperalgesia, TPs and TrPs are common.
- Central nervous system pathway abnormalities are well illustrated in both animal and human studies. (Primate RSI model reveals a reduction in cortical sensory feedback information.[33] Human studies – cortical 'event-related' responses are reduced in patients with non-specific upper limb pain.[34])

### Psychosocial phenomena?
- In common with other pain syndromes, psychosocial influences are important in the development and persistence of disability.

- Psychosocial factors such as work organization, job satisfaction, interpersonal relationships, mood and distress are the common factors that dictate reporting and morbidity from upper limb pain, not the task demands.
- Evidence from the 'Australian Epidemic'.[35]

## Management

The principles involved in the management of RSI are no different to those applied when dealing with other musculoskeletal disorders and pain syndromes:

- Recognition of symptoms and acknowledgement of difficulties
- Explanation of possible pain mechanisms and contributing factors
- Simple analgesics and non-steroidal anti-inflammatory drugs (NSAIDs, oral or topical)
- Involvement of the multidisciplinary team
- A regimen of exercise (adequate rest between periods of exercise is essential), education, physical therapy modalities and some pain management strategies
- Physical therapy techniques – heat, cold, TENS, manual release work and mobilization
- Splinting the wrist and hand may be necessary, but not be at the expense of secondary 'disuse' problems such as stiffness and weakness
- Early return to work, with a graded reintroduction to tasks
- Alteration and modification to the workplace to alter physical constraints, which may also alter employee's perception of an 'ergonomically friendly' workstation
- Address contribution from sleep disturbance and mood disturbances
- Novel techniques, such as 'mirror virtual visual feedback' – using a mirror image of the 'normal' limb to promote involvement in exercise programmes and to reduce pain. This has been used in stroke, phantom limb pain, CRPS and regional pain in musicians and is being studied in RSI.

# References

1. Lidbeck J. Central hyperexcitability in chronic musculoskeletal pain: A conceptual breakthrough with multiple clinical implications. *Pain Res Manag* 7: 81–92, 2002
2. Wolfe F, Smythe HA, Yunus MB, et al. The American College of Rheumatology 1990 Criteria for the Classification of Fibromyalgia. Report of the Multicenter Criteria Committee. *Arthritis Rheum* 33: 160–172, 1990
3. MacFarlane GJ, Croft PR, Schollum J, Silman AJ. Widespread pain: is an improved classification possible? *J Rheumatol* 23: 1628–1632, 1996
4. Burckhardt CS, Clark SR, Bennett RM. Fibromyalgia and quality of life: A comparitive analysis. *J Rheum* 20: 475–479, 1993
5. White KP, Speechley M, Harth M, Ostbye T. Fibromyalgia in Rheumatology practice: a survey of Canadian Rheumatologists. *J Rheum* 22: 722–726, 1995
6. Moldofsky H: A chronobiologic theory of fibromyalgia. In: Jacobsen S, Danneskiold-Samsoe B, eds. *Musculoskeletal Pain, Myofascial Pain Syndrome, and Fibromyalgia Syndrome*. 1993, pp. 49–59
7. Moldofsky H, Scarisbrick P, England R, Smythe H. Musculoskeletal symptoms and non-REM sleep disturbance in patients with "fibrositis syndrome" and healthy subjects. *Psychosom Med* 37: 341–351, 1975
8. Wallace DJ, Linker-Israeli M, Hallegua D, et al. Cytokines play an aetiopathogenetic role in fibromyalgia: a hypothesis and pilot study. *Rheumatology (Oxford)* 40: 743–749, 2001
9. Staud R. Evidence of involvement of central neural mechanisms in generating fibromyalgia pain. *Curr Rheumatol Rep* 4: 299–305, 2002
10. Gracely RH, Petzke F, Wolf JM, Clauw DJ. Functional magnetic resonance imaging evidence of augmented pain processing in fibromyalgia. *Arthritis Rheum* 46: 1333–1343, 2002

11. Krag NJ, Norregaard J, Larsen JK, Danneskiold-Samsoe B. A blinded, controlled evaluation of anxiety and depressive symptoms in patients with fibromyalgia, as measured by standardised psychometric interview scales. *Acta Psychiatr Scand* **89**: 370–375, 1994

12. McBeth J, Macfarlane GJ, Benjamin S, Silman AJ. Features of somatization predict the onset of chronic widespread pain: results of a large population-based study. *Arthritis Rheum* **44**: 940–946, 2001

13. Busch A, Schachter CL, Peloso PM, Bombardier C. Exercise for treating fibromyalgia syndrome (Cochrane Review). *Cochrane Database Syst Rev* (3):CD003786, 2002

14. White KP, Nielson WR. Cognitive behavioral treatment of fibromyalgia syndrome: a follow up assessment. *J Rheumatol* **22**: 717–721, 1995

15. Macfarlane GJ, McBeth J, Silman AJ. Widespread body pain and mortality: prospective population based study. *Br Med J* **323**: 662–665, 2001

16. Richards SC, Scott DL. Prescribed exercise in people with fibromyalgia: parallel group randomised controlled trial. *Br Med J* **325**: 185, 2002

17. Goldenberg D, Mayskiy M, Mossey C, Ruthazer R, Schmid C. A randomized, double-blind crossover trial of fluoxetine and amitriptyline in the treatment of fibromyalgia. *Arthritis Rheum* **39**: 1852, 1996

18. Simons DG. Muscle pain syndromes. In: Fricton JR, Awad EA, eds. *Advances in Pain Research and Therapy, vol 17*. New York: Raven Press, 1990, pp.1–41

19. Travell JG, Simons DG: *Myofascial Pain and Dysfunction: The Trigger Point Manual*. Baltimore: Williams & Wilkins, 1983

20. De Stefano R, Selvi E, Villanova M, et al. Image analysis quantification of substance P immunoreactivity in the trapezius muscle of patients with fibromyalgia and myofascial pain syndrome. *J Rheumatol* **27**: 2906–2910, 2000

21. Cummings TM, White AR. Needling therapies in the management of myofascial trigger point pain: a systematic review. *Arch Phys Med Rehabil* **82**: 986–992, 2001

22. Cheshire WP, Abashian SW, Mann JD. Botulinum toxin in the treatment of myofascial pain syndrome. *Pain* **59**: 65–69, 1994

23. Porta M. A comparative trial of botulinum toxin type A and methylprednisolone for the treatment of myofascial pain syndrome and pain from chronic muscle spasm. *Pain* **85**: 101–105, 2000

24. Hadler NM. Coping with arm pain in the workplace. Clin Orthop **351**: 57–62, 1998

25. Jones JR, Hodgson JT, Clegg TA, Elliott RC. *Self reported work-related illness in 1995. Results from a household survey*. London: HMSO, 1998 p. 180.

26. National Institute for Occupational Safety and Health. *Musculoskeletal disorders and workplace factors. A critical review of epidemiologic evidence for work-related musculoskeletal disorders of neck, upper extremity and low back*. Cincinnati, OH: US Department of Health and Human Sciences/NIOSH, 1997

27. Harrington JM, Carter JT, Birrel L, Gompertez D. Surveillance case definitions for work related upper limb pain syndromes. *Occup Environ Med* **55**: 264–271, 1998

28. Palmer K, Walker-Bone K, Linaker C, et al. The Southampton examination schedule for the diagnosis of musculoskeletal disorders of the upper limb. *Ann Rheum Dis* **59**: 5–11, 2000

29. Hart DA, Archambault JM, Kydd A. Gender and neurogenic variables in tendon biology and repetitive motion disorders. *Clin Orthop* **351**: 44–56, 1998

30. Pritchard MH; Pugh N; Wright I; Brownlee M. A vascular basis for repetitive strain injury. *Rheumatology* **38**: 636–639, 1999

31. Greening J, Smart S, Leary R, Hall-Craggs M, O'Higgins P, Lynn B. Reduced movement of median nerve in carpal tunnel during wrist flexion in patients with non-specific arm pain. *Lancet* **354**: 217–218, 1999

32. Harris AJ. Cortical origins of pathological pain. *Lancet* **354**: 1464–1466, 1999

33. Byl NN, Melnick M. The neural consequences of repetition: clinical implications of a learning hypothesis. *J Hand Ther* **10**: 160–174, 1997

34. Gibson SJ, LeVasseur SA, Helme RD. Cerebral event-related responses induced by $CO_2$ laser stimulation in subjects suffering from cervico-brachial pain. *Pain* **47**: 173–182, 1991

35. Hocking-B Epidemiological aspects of 'repetition strain injury' in Telecom Australia. *Med J Aust*. 1987; **147**: 218–222.

# 9 Headache

*Robin S Howard*

Headache is an extremely common symptom and it is estimated that the 1-year prevalence in the general population is 90% with a lifetime prevalence of 99%.[1] The differential diagnosis of headache is extensive, and precise aetiological diagnosis is necessary. Although most primary headaches (migraine, tension-type headache, cluster and other miscellaneous headaches) are benign, they are a cause of considerable morbidity. Secondary headaches are heterogeneous and classification is based on the underlying cause. A variety of epidemiological studies attest to the ubiquitous nature of headaches.[2–6] Classification of headaches and diagnostic criteria have been established by The International Headache Society.[7,8] A number of recent reviews have considered the clinical features and management of headaches.[1,9–13] The major classifications are given in Table 9.1.

## Migraine

Migraine (Table 9.2) is a paroxysmal syndrome characterized by recurrent attacks of headache separated by symptom-free intervals. The headaches are usually associated with nausea and vomiting and preceded by an aura, but the aura may occur without any ensuing headache. The clinical diagnosis of migraine is based on the repetition and characteristics of the attack.[14]

The International Headache Society[7,8] have developed the following diagnostic criteria: the patient must have had five or more attacks of headache lasting 4–72 hours (if untreated) with at least two of four features (unilaterality, pulsating quality, moderate or severe intensity and aggravation with exertion) as well as nausea with or without vomiting, or photophobia and phonophobia. Structural abnormalities or other underlying causes should be excluded. Migraine headaches may be preceded by premonitionary symptoms in 10–15% of patients, which usually develop several hours before the attack but may be present for 1–2 days before the onset of headache. They are often non-specific and may include mood changes, yawning and craving for food.

A variety of factors may trigger migraine attacks. These are summarized in Table 9.3. Investigations, including imaging with CT or MRI, are rarely helpful.[15]

### Migraine with aura

In migraine with aura the headache is immediately preceded by focal symptoms in at least 90%. Most patients experience visual auras – visual hallucinations and scotoma, arising from the occipital cortex, are present in about a third, teichopsia (fortification spectra) in 10% and photopsia (unformed flashes of light) in 25%. Others experience sensory, motor or speech disturbances, which may include temporal lobe phenomena. The headache is unilateral in two thirds and generally intensifies from a dull pain to be throbbing and pulsatile although it may be constant. Migraine aura may occur without the headache (acephalgic migraine) – thus episodes of waxing and waning fortification spectra, scotomas, paraesthesiae and dysphasia may represent migraine phenomena rather than transient ischaemic attacks. The neurological differential

| **Table 9.1** Major categories of headache |
|---|

Migraine
Tension-type
Cluster headaches and chronic paroxysmal hemicrania
Headache associated with head trauma
Miscellaneous headaches not associated with trauma
- Idiopathic stabbing
- Cold stimulus
- Coital
- Benign cough
- Benign exertional

Headache associated with vascular disorders
- Acute ischaemia
- Intracerebral haematoma
- Subarachnoid haemorrhage (SAH)
- Unruptured arteriovenous malformation (AVM)
- Arteritis
- Carotid or vertebral pain
- Venous thrombosis
- Hypertension

Headache associated with non-vascular intracerebral vascular disorders
- High or low CSF pressure
- Intracranial infection
- Inflammatory e.g. sarcoidosis
- Neoplasm
- Intrathecal injection

Associated with substance abuse or substance withdrawal
Associated with systemic causes
- CNS infection
- Metabolic
  - Hypoxia
  - Hypercapnia
  - Hypoglycaemia
  - Dialysis

Local structures
Neuralgia
Trigeminal
Glossopharyngeal
Chronic facial pain

diagnosis for the aura includes other transient neurological events, such as partial epilepsy or transient ischaemic attacks. These can usually be distinguished as migraine-related symptoms tend to have a progressive onset and development.

## Migraine without aura

Migraine without aura is defined by the presence of at least 5 attacks with headaches lasting between 4 and 72 hours. The headache should have at least two of the following features: unilateral location, pulsating quality, moderate to severe intensity and be aggravated by exertion. During the headache there may be photophobia, aurophobia, nausea or vomiting. In some

**Table 9.2** Classification of migraine

Migraine without aura
Migraine with aura
Typical aura
- Prolonged aura
- Familial hemiplegic migraine
- Basilar migraine
- Aura without headache
- Acute onset aura
Ophthalmic migraine
Retinal migraine
Childhood migraine
Complications
- Status migrainosus
- Migrainous infarction

patients the aura may be prolonged and dominate the clinical picture, lasting for longer than 1 hour and occasionally up to 1 week, and in some attacks the headache may fail to develop at all.

### Vertebrobasilar migraine
Vertebrobasilar migraine is characterized by symptoms arising from the brainstem including dysarthria, vertigo, tinnitus, decreased hearing, diplopia, ataxia, impaired coordination, bilateral paraesthesia and episodes of transient loss of consciousness. There may be a transient confusional state, which can last up to several days.

### Retinal migraine
Retinal migraine is due to constriction of the retinal arterioles, which impair vision in one eye, with or without photopsia, usually preceding headache or a dull ache behind the affected eye.

### Familial hemiplegic migraine
In familial hemiplegic migraine transient weakness or paralysis is a rare accompaniment of migraine and usually resolves without infarction. It is a rare condition associated with abnormalities of chromosome 19.

### Migrainous infarction
Migrainous infarction is said to have occurred if the neurological deficit occurs during a migraine attack that is typical of those previously experienced. Ischaemic optic neuropathy and

**Table 9.3** Factors that may trigger migraine attacks

| | |
|---|---|
| Hormonal | Menstruation, ovulation, OC, HRT, pregnancy, menopause |
| Dietary | Alcohol, tyramine (chocolate, cheese. missing meals) |
| Psychological | Stress, periods after stress, anxiety, worry, depression |
| Physical | Glare, flashing lights, altitude, weather |
| Sleep | Lack of, or too much, sleep |
| Drugs | Nitroglycerine, histamine, hydralazine |
| Others | Head trauma, exertion |

retinal artery occlusion are well-defined examples, but the risk of cerebral infarction is less certain. Other causes of infarction must be excluded.

## Management

The management of migraine has been discussed in a number of recent review articles.[16–18] It is essential that patients should receive a full and detailed examination and explanation concerning the nature of migraine. They should be reassured that they do not have an underlying cerebral tumour but should understand that a 'cure' may not be possible. Migraine may be exacerbated by a variety of trigger factors (see Table 9.3), and these factors should be avoided. General lifestyle advice concerning ensuring adequate sleep, regular diet, and limiting tea and coffee may be valuable. Some patients find complementary therapies helpful.[19] The first-line treatment for acute migraine headache is either simple analgesics alone or the combination of analgesic and anti-emetic. During migraine, there is impaired gastric emptying because of stasis and this is helped by a prokinetic antiemetic such as metoclopramide or domperidone, which may be given rectally, further to aid absorption. High-dose dispersible aspirin may be used, but many now prefer a non-steroidal anti-inflammatory drug (NSAID), such as naproxen, given orally or as a suppository, or paracetamol. Fixed drug combinations are less satisfactory. The introduction of triptans has led to a radical change in the management of migraine. They are the most effective agents in interrupting an attack, however, these drugs are expensive, the response is variable and they are often only slightly more effective than appropriate simple analgesia. The triptans are 5-hydroxytryptophan (5-HT) agonists. Sumatriptan may be given subcutaneously and is the most effective, but it is associated with frequent side-effects. Rizatriptan is the most effective given orally but the mouth-dispersible forms have little advantage over tablets, as the drug is not absorbed via the buccal mucosa; naratriptan is the least potent but is well tolerated. All the triptans carry significant side-effects and have incomplete penetrance; there is also a tendency to overuse or misuse.[20–23] There is little role for ergotamine because of its unselective receptor profile, unreliable bioavailability and variable efficacy. Prophylactic medication should be considered if the attacks are frequent, disabling and not responding to acute treatment. In particular, prophylactic treatment should be used for headache that occurs more than twice a month, produces disability lasting more than 3 days or is associated with significant neurological abnormalities carrying the risk of permanent neurological injury.

Drugs effective for preventing migraine attacks include β-blockers devoid of intrinsic sympathomimetic activity, sodium valproate, 5-HT antagonists such as methysergide or pizotifen; and calcium channel blockers, especially verapamil. In some patients tricyclic antidepressants may be useful as adjunct therapy. However, all the prophylactic agents have significant side-effects.

## Tension type headache

Other synonyms for tension type headache (TTH) include stress, tension, muscle contraction, psychogenic and essential headaches. They may be highly variable in their manifestations but are characterized by headache of mild-to-moderate intensity, which is bilateral and either pressing or tight. They may occur at least 10 times and last for between 30 minutes and 7 days. There is no associated photophobia, aurophobia, nausea or vomiting and usually no exertional worsening. Tension headache is usually episodic, but it may develop into chronic daily headache, which is considered to be particularly associated with transformed migraine or analgesic overuse.[24]

The International Headache Classification divides TTH into episodic and chronic varieties, with the episodic form being defined by a frequency of less than 15 headache days each month and the term chronic TTH being used for those patients with 15 or more such headaches each month.[25-29] Chronic daily headache may be considered to be transformed (chronic) migraine, in which classical migraine has increased in frequency.[30,31] The aetiology of TTH is uncertain, but there is evidence for a disorder of pericranial muscles in some patients. Episodic TTH may be difficult to distinguish from migraine, as similar features may be present.

## Management

The first line in managing TTH is sympathetic attention to the history and examination. Providing reassurance that the patient does not have a cerebral tumour or other serious intracranial neurological disorder may be adequate to relieve the headache. It is essential for the patient to realize that the doctor is taking their symptoms seriously. The history and examination is important to exclude excessive scalp and facial contraction, dental malocclusion, refractive errors or cervical spine pain. The management of TTH may involve a psychological, physiological and pharmacological approach.[32-34] Imaging rarely identifies an underlying lesion but, in practice, CT or MRI brain scan may be undertaken either because the physician suspects an underlying lesion or to reassure the patient and their relatives.[35-38]

Acute treatment of TTH may be difficult. Most patients prefer to use NSAIDs such as ibuprofen rather than simple analgesia with aspirin. Others find caffeine, sedatives or tranquillizers to be valuable. The occasional use of anxiolytics is reasonable and relatively safe, but if analgesics are taken daily they may lead to rebound headache as their effect wears off predisposing to chronic daily headache.

### Prophylaxis

Tricyclics are the drug of choice for prophylaxis but their role is difficult to evaluate. Amitriptyline is the most widely used and its effects seem to be independent of its antidepressant activity. The dose should be gradually built up to 100–150 mg per day and any effects may be delayed for several weeks. Clomipramine may be a little more effective, but it is associated with a wider range of side-effects. Dothiepin is also widely used in low dose. If TTH persists, anticonvulsants may be indicated: valuable drugs include valproate (<1500 mg per day), gabapentin and topiramate, but each has significant toxicity and potential teratogenicity. Many patients derive considerable benefit from complementary techniques including relaxation, biofeedback, cognitive behavioural therapy and physical treatments including transcutaneous nerve stimulation (TENS).

# Short-lasting headaches

Short-lasting headaches are summarized in Table 9.4.

## Cluster headaches

Cluster headaches consist of severe unilateral headache associated with prominent autonomic features and a striking circannual and circadian periodicity. Cluster headache attacks consists of a unilateral excruciating pain in the orbital or temporal region, usually lasting between 45 and 90 minutes, although the pain can be present for up to 3 hours. The onset and cessation are abrupt. A range of autonomic features may occur which including lacrimation, nasal congestion, rhinorrhea, facial sweating, miosis, ptosis, eyelid oedema, conjunctival injection and

**Table 9.4** Short-lasting headaches

Prominent autonomic features (trigeminal autonomic cephalgia (TAC))

Cluster headaches
Paroxysmal hemicrania
Short lasting unilateral neuralgiform headache with conjunctival injection and tearing (SUNCT)

No or few autonomic features

Trigeminal neuralgia
Idiopathic stabbing headaches (ice-pick headache)
Benign exertional headache
Coital headache
Hypnic headache

a sense of restlessness. The attacks may be precipitated by alcohol, nitroglycerine, exercise and hyperpyrexia.[39-42] Episodic cluster headaches recur in periods lasting 7 days to 1 year and separated by pain-free periods with remission from 3 months to 3 years. In chronic cluster headaches the pain occurs much more frequently and may be continual.[43]

The first line of treatment includes general measures to remove exposure to precipitants as far as possible and general patient education about the nature of the condition. Management is directed towards suppressing bouts of episodic cluster headache, aborting attacks that still occur and reducing the frequency and severity of painful episodes in those with chronic cluster headaches. Acute attacks may be aborted by the provision of inhaled 100% oxygen by a facemask.[44] Corticosteroids (up to 50 mg per day), often together with an NSAID, are effective in aborting bouts of episodic cluster headache when taken in short courses of 3–4 weeks.[45] Subcutaneous sumatriptan causes rapid headache relief in most patients without the development of tachyphylaxis.[46-49] In some patients clusters occur regularly without remission. Prophylactic treatment may be necessary using methysergide, ergotamine, lithium, or verapamil.

## Paroxysmal hemicranias[50,51]

These headaches occur with a higher frequency and shorter duration of individual attacks than cluster headaches. They respond dramatically well to indomethacin. SUNCT (short-lasting, unilateral, neuralgiform, orbital pain attacks with conjunctival injection, tearing, sweating and rhinorrhea) is a rare syndrome, usually occurring in males. These headaches are of brief duration but can occur frequently, and they are associated with the presence of prominent conjunctival injection and lacrimation. There is often a trigger zone. The headaches are poorly responsive to treatment but lamotrigine and gabapentin have been used.[52-57]

## Pathophysiology of trigeminal autonomic cephalgia

It has been suggested that the pain-producing innervation of the cranium projects through branches of the trigeminal and upper cervical nerves to the trigeminocervical complex, from whence nociceptive pathways pass to higher centres. This implies an integral role for the ipsilateral trigeminal nociceptive pathways in trigeminal autonomic cephalgia (TACs). Goadsby and Lipton[55] have suggested that the pathophysiology of the TACs revolve around the trigeminal–autonomic reflex. In fact, some degree of cranial autonomic symptomatology is a normal physiological response to cranial nociceptive input, and patients with other headache syndromes often report these symptoms. The distinction between the TACs and other headache syndromes is the degree of cranial autonomic activation.

The cranial autonomic symptoms may be prominent in the TACs because of the central disinhibition of the trigeminal–autonomic reflex. Supporting evidence for this comes from positron emission tomography (PET) and functional MRI (fMRI), which show ipsilateral hypothalamic activation. This is specific to cluster headaches and SUNCT; it is not seen in migraine.

# Other conditions associated with headache

## Post-traumatic headache

Acute post-traumatic headache (PTH) may follow significant head trauma associated with loss of consciousness, post-traumatic amnesia or abnormal neurological signs. It appears within 14 days of trauma and settles within 8 weeks of trauma or regaining consciousness. It is often severe and throbbing in quality, associated with nausea, vomiting, photophobia, phonophobia, memory impairment, irritability, drowsiness or vertigo. It is treated as part of the overall management of the head trauma with supportive and symptomatic care, including simple analgesics and anti-inflammatories.[58]

Chronic PTH is a much more common clinical problem. This is present if the headache has continued for more than 8 weeks after regaining consciousness or after trauma. There are several distinct types of post-traumatic headache. A 'vascular' headache may occur, in which there is a pulsating pain made worse by head movements, coughing or straining. Similarly, following local damage to the scalp, pain may appear in the distribution of the vessel supplying the area. Head trauma may occasionally precipitate migraine or cluster headaches, and whiplash has been described as causing basilar migraine but a direct causal association has not been established.

Most patients develop a muscle contraction (tension-type) headache, which persists for many months but may respond to conventional treatments. Anxiety, depression, other psychological factors and the litigation process may exacerbate the headache.

The management of post-traumatic headache is extremely difficult. Patients require close support and often respond well to cognitive behavioural therapy or other forms of psychological input. Symptomatic treatment is best undertaken using the medications used for the management of migraine and cluster headaches.[59]

## Vascular disorders

The causes of headaches due to vascular disorders are summarized in Table 9.5

Acute ischaemic cerebrovascular disease may present with headache. Transient ischaemic attack or stroke are associated with headache in between 15 and 65%, particularly when the vascular event is in the posterior territory. The headache may precede the ischaemic event and is generally ipsilateral to the arterial territory responsible for the stroke, however, the presence of headache does not help to distinguish ischaemic from thromboembolic stroke.

Headache occurs commonly (33–66%)[60] following intracerebral haemorrhage, but this depends on the onset, size and location of the haemorrhage (Figure 9.1). Acute headache is characteristic of the development of an extradural haemorrhage following head trauma, and subdural haematoma may be associated with a fluctuating paroxysmal headache, which occurs before the development of focal neurological signs. Subarachnoid haemorrhage is

**Table 9.5**   Vascular headaches

Migraine and stroke related
- AVM
- MELAS
- CADASIL

Stroke
- Cerebral infarction
- Haemorrhage
  —SAH
  —Subdural
  —Extradural

Carotid and vertebral artery dissection

Cerebral venous thrombosis

Hypertension
- Malignant hypertension
- Phaeochromocytoma
- Pre-eclampsia/eclampsia

AVM, arteriovenous malformation; CADASIL, cerebral autosomal dominant arteriopathy with subcortical infarcts and leukoencephalopathy; MELAS, mitochondrial encephalomyopathy, lactic acidosis, and stroke-like episode; SAH, subarachnoid haemorrhage.

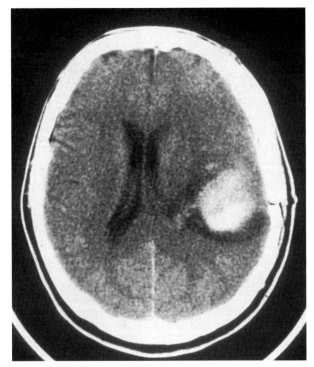

**Figure 9.1**   Intracerebral haemorrhage secondary to middle cerebral artery aneurysm (following decompression).

characterized by the sudden onset of severe and incapacitating headache, which is often occipital and associated with meningism and low back pain. Approximately 25% of patients with an intracranial aneurysm may present with a 'sentinel headache' suggesting intermittent leaking of the aneurysm.[63]

Carotid or vertebral dissection often gives rise to ipsilateral headache or cervical pain, and this may precede the development of neurological symptoms. This is of particular concern for young people as it is often associated with neck trauma, including whiplash injury or chiropractic manipulation of the neck.[64]

Headache is a presenting feature in 75% of patients with cerebral venous thrombosis. The headache is of variable severity and often diffuse, being associated with the development of raised intracranial pressure and papilloedema.[65]

Giant cell arteritis is characterized by the presence of headache, swollen and tender temporal artery, elevated erythrocyte sedimentation rate and the typical pathological features on temporal artery biopsy. The condition occurs in the elderly and responds rapidly to steroids. Headache is the presenting feature in 50%, and it may be unilateral or generalized. Sudden painless loss of vision may be the presenting feature in 15% but visual loss occurs in between 7 and 60% of patients.[66] Urgent treatment with steroids is indicated as soon as possible after the diagnosis.[67]

## Raised intracranial pressure[68–69]

It is unusual for intracranial neoplasms to present with headache; the development of fits, focal neurological deficit or cognitive impairment is more common. Whilst half of patients with cerebral tumours develop headaches, only about 15% will present as headache and this is more common in patients with glioma (Figure 9.2) and cerebral secondaries than with meningioma. The headache is characteristically bilateral although when the headache is unilateral it often occurs on the side of the lesion. It is usually moderate to severe and often worse during the night on waking, possibly due to blockage of venous blood flow in the recumbent position. The headache is classically associated with vomiting and diplopia. Meningeal carcinomatosis occurs in approximately 5% of patients with non-CNS cancers (breast 39%, lung 34%, melanoma 8%, gastrointestinal 5%, genitourinary 4%). Headache is common but usually associated with other neurological features, including progressive cranial nerve palsies and spinal involvement. Benign intracranial hypertension presents with generalized headache associated with visual obscuration and intracranial noises. On examination there is papilloedema and variable visual field defect. It occurs most commonly in the obese and in women aged 20 to 44 years. It may be associated with a variety of medication (vitamin A, tetracyclins, anabolic steroids and steroid withdrawal) as well as venous obstruction either intracranially or in the neck, hypertensive encephalopathy or elevated cerebrospinal fluid (CSF) protein. The condition is treated by managing the underlying cause and reducing CSF pressure, either by repeated lumbar punctures, by optic nerve sheath fenestration and occasionally lumboperitoneal shunting.

## Temporomandibular disorders

Temporomandibular disorders are generally associated with temporomandibular joint (TMJ) dysfunction.[70] The aetiology of these conditions is unknown but they are characterized by tenderness and pain in the TMJ and associated muscles of mastication, trismus, limited or jerky jaw movements and evidence of bruxism. The pain may be felt as temporal headache and is often precipitated by movement and clenching teeth. Signs of internal derangement of the TMJ (subluxation) may include a reduced range of jaw movements, clicking noises and lateral displacement of the meniscus. The aetiology is uncertain; whilst occlusal factors and meniscal

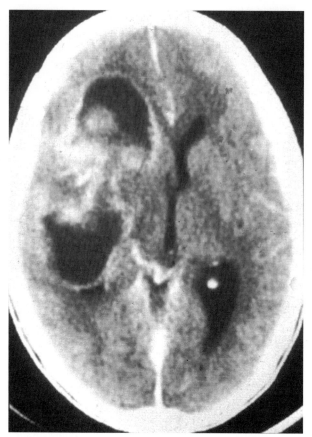

**Figure 9.2** Frontoparietal glioma

displacement have been suggested, in may cases the condition is associated with tension headache, depression, anxiety and stress. The condition should be treated conservatively with antidepressant medication, occlusal appliances and rehabilitation. It usually resolves slowly.[71]

## Trigeminal neuralgia

Trigeminal neuralgia is characterized by recurrent episodes of short-lasting severe, shock-like, stabbing pain, which are unilateral and limited to the distribution of one or more of the divisions of the trigeminal nerve (usually 2nd or 3rd).[9,10] The pain is often triggered by trivial stimuli, such as touch, shaving, teeth-cleaning or chewing. The episodes may occur many times each day and often induce reflex spasms of facial muscles.

The aetiology is unknown, although it is suggested that there may be compression and local demyelination of the trigeminal nerve at the root entry zone due to compression in the posterior fosse, usually by a small tortuous artery or vein. Indeed, surgical decompression of the trigeminal root may be effective in the treatment of chronic trigeminal neuralgia.

The condition may be associated with multiple sclerosis or a benign or malignant tumour in the posterior fossa.

Carbamazepine is effective in improving or resolving trigeminal neuralgia in most patients, but high doses may be necessary with an increased risk of side-effects. Other medication effective in the treatment of trigeminal neuralgia includes baclofen, clonazepam, phenytoin, gabapentin or lamotrigine. For recurrent severe trigeminal neuralgia, thermocoagulation of the Gasserian ganglion or microsurgery has been effective.

## Cervical spine pain

Cervical spine pain occasionally presents as headache. Involvement of the upper three cervical roots causes occipital pain, which may be referred forward to the orbital region. This may occur if there is upper cervical involvement (and in particular instability) following trauma, basilar impression (platybasia) and rheumatoid arthritis. Degenerative changes of the upper cervical spine may also cause occipital headaches, and whiplash injury may also occasionally involve the occipital nerves. Cervicogenic headache is a term used to describe intermittent, recurrent unilateral headaches, lasting from 3 hours to 1 week, associated with degenerative changes in the cervical spine. The headache is usually controlled by treatment of the underlying cervical spondylosis, often with symptomatic treatment, physiotherapy or a collar.[72]

# References

1. Evans RW, Mathew NT. Handbook of headache. Philadelphia: Lippincott Williams and Wilkins, 2000
2. Rasmussen BJ, Jensen R, SchrollM, Olsen J. Epidemology of headache in a general population – a prevalence study. *J Clin Epidemiol* **44**: 1147–1157, 1991
3. Steiner TJ, Stewart WF, Kolodner K, et al. Epidemiology of migraine in England. *Cephalalgia* **19**: 305–306, 1999
4. Lipton RB, Stewart WF, Diamond S, et al. Prevalence and burden of migraine in the United States: data from the American migraine study II. *Headache* **41**: 646–657, 2001
5. Scher A, Stewart WF, Liberman J, et al. Prevalence of frequent headache in a population sample. *Headache* **38**: 497–506, 1998
6. Costillo J, Munoz P, Guitera V, et al. Epidemiology of chronic daily headache in the general population. *Headache* **39**: 190–196, 1999
7. Headache Classification Committee of The International Headache Society. Classification and diagnostic criteria for headache disorders, cranial neuralgias and facial pain. *Cephalalgia* **8**: 1–96, 1988
8. Olesen J. Revision of the International Headache Classification. An interim report. *Cephalalgia* **21**: 261, 2001
9. Goadsby PJ, Lipton RB, Ferrari MD. Migraine – Current understanding and treatment. *N Engl J Med* **346**: 257–270, 2002
10. Lance JW, Goadsby PJ. *Mechanism and Management of Headache, 6th ed.* London: Butterworth-Heinemann, 1998
11. Goadsby PJ. The pathophysiology of headache. In: Silberstein SD, Lipton RB, Solomon S, eds. *Wolff's headache and other head pain, 7th ed.* Oxford: Oxford University Press, 2001, pp. 57–72
12. Olsen J, Tfelt-Hansen P, Welch KMA (eds). *The Headaches. 2nd ed.* Philadelphia: Lippincott-Raven, 2000
13. Steiner TJ, Fontebasso M. Headache. *Br Med J* **325**: 881–885, 2002
14. Ferrari MD. Migraine. *Lancet* **351**: 1043–1051, 1998
15. Goadsby PJ. Migraine, aura, and cortical spreading depression. why are we still imaging in migraine and tension-type headache. *Headache* **35**: 264–268, 1995
16. Silberstein SD. Practice parameter: evidence-based guidelines for migraine headache (an evidence-based review). *Neurology* **55**: 754–762, 2000
17. Steiner TJ, MacGregor EA, Davies PTG. Guidelines for all doctors in the management of migraine and tension-type headache. Available at http://www.bash.org.uk
18. Lipton RB, Stewart WF, Stone AM, et al. Stratified care vs step care strategies for migraine. *JAMA* **284**: 2599–2605, 2000
19. Whitmarsh TE, Coleston-Shields DM, Steiner TJ. Double-blind randomized placebo-controlled study of homoeopathic prophylaxis of migraine. *Cephalalgia* **17**: 600–604, 1997

20. Belsey J. The clinical and financial impact of oral triptans in the management of migraine in the UK. a systematic review. *J Med Econ* **3**: 35–47, 2000
21. Adelman JJ, Lipton RB, Ferrari MD, et al. Comparison of rizatriptan and other triptans on stringent measures of efficacy. *Neurology* **57**: 1377–1383, 2001
22. Ferrari MD, Roon KI, Lipton RB, et al. Oral triptans (serotonin 5-HT,B/ID agonists) in acute migraine treatment a meta-analysis of 53 trials. *Lancet* **358**: 1668–1675, 2001
23. Lipton RB, Stewart WF, Cady R, et al. Sumatriptan for the range of headaches in migraine sufferers. results of the Spectrum study. *Headache* **40**: 783–791, 2000
24. Olesen J. Analgesic headache. A common, treatable condition that deserves more attention. *Br Med J* **310**: 479–480, 1995
25. Silberstein SD, Lipton RB, Sliwinski M. Classification of daily and near-daily headaches: a field study of revised IHS criteria. *Neurology* **47**: 871–875, 1996
26. Goadsby PJ, Boes C. Chronic daily headache. *J Neural Neurosurg Psychiatry* **72**: 2–5, 2002
27. Wang S-J, Fuh J-L, Lu S-R, et al. Chronic daily headache in Chinese elderly. Prevalence, risk factors and biannual follow-up. *Neurology* **54**: 314–319, 2000
28. Li D, Rozen TD. The clinical characteristics of new daily persistent headache. *Neurology* **56**: A452–453, 2001
29. Vanast WJ. New daily persistent headaches – definition of a benign syndrome. *Headache* **26**: 317–320, 1986
30. Mathew NT, Stubits E, Nigam M. Transformation of migraine into daily headache. analysis of factors. *Headache* **22**: 66–68, 1982
31. Ulrich V, Russell MB, Jensen R, et al. A comparison of tension-type headache in migraineurs and in non-migraineurs. a population-based study. *Pain* **67**: 501–506, 1996
32. Fitzpatrick R. Telling patients there is nothing wrong. *Br Med J* **313**: 311–312, 1996
33. Howard L. Telling patients there is nothing wrong. randomised controlled trials are needed. *Br Med J* **313**: 1210, 1996
34. Howard L, Wessely S. Protocol 99PRT/26. Are investigations reassuring or anxiogenic? A randomised controlled trial into the role of neuroimaging in chronic benign headache. URL: http://www.thelancet.com/authorinlol Protocol+review
35. Cala LA, Mastaglia FL. Computerized axial tomography findings in a group of patients with migrainous headaches. *Proc Aust Assoc Neurol* **13**: 35–41, 1980
36. Frishberg BM, Rosenberg JH, Matchar DB, et al. Evidence-based guidelines in the primary care setting: neuroimaging in patients with nonacute headache. URL: http://www.aan.com/public/practiceguidelines
37. Sargent JD, Solbach P. Medical evaluation of migraineurs: review of the value of laboratory and radiologic tests. *Headache* **23**: 62–65, 1983
38. Larson EB, Omenn GS, Lewis H. Diagnostic evaluation of headache. Impact of computerized tomography and cost-effectiveness. *JAMA* **243**: 359–362, 1980
39. Igarashi H, Sakai F. Natural history of cluster headache. *Cephalalgia* **16**: 390–391, 1996
40. Manzoni GC, Micieli G, Granella F, et al. Cluster headache course over ten years in 189 patients. *Cephalalgia* **11**: 169–174, 1991
41. Olesen J, Goadsby PJ. Cluster headache and related conditions. In: Olesen J, ed. *Frontiers in Headache Research, vol 9.* Oxford: Oxford University Press, 1999
42. Kudrow L. Cluster headaches. In: Goadsby PJ, Silberstein SD, eds. *Headache.* New York: Butterworth-Heinemann, 1997, 227–242
43. Silberstein SD, Niknam R, Rozen TD, et al. Cluster headache with aura. *Neurology* **54**: 219–221, 2000
44. Fogan L. Treatment of cluster headache: a double blind comparison of oxygen vs air inhalation. *Arch Neurol* **42**: 362–363, 1985
45. Couch JR, Ziegler DK. Prednisone therapy for cluster headache. *Headache* **18**: 219–221, 1978
46. Ekbom K, The Sumatriptan Cluster Headache Study Group. Treatment of acute cluster headache with sumatriptan. *N Engl J Med* **325**: 322–326, 1991
47. Ekbom K, Waldenlind E, Cole JA, et al. Sumatriptan in chronic cluster headache results of continuous treatment for eleven months. *Cephalalgia* **12**: 254–256, 1992
48. Ekbom K, Krabbe A, Micelli G, et al. Cluster headache attacks treated for up to three months with subcutaneous sumatriptan (6 mg). *Cephalalgia* **15**: 230–236, 1995

49. Gobel H, Lindner A, Heinze A, et al. Acute therapy for cluster headache with sumatriptan. Findings of a one year long-term study. *Neurology* **51**: 908–911, 1998

50. Antonaci F, Sjoastad O. Chronic paroxysmal hemicrania (CPH): a review of the clinical manifestations. *Headache* **29**: 648–656, 1989

51. Russell D. Chronic paroxysmal hemicrania. severity, duration and time of occurrence of attacks. *Cephalalgia* **4**: 53–56, 1984

52. Goadsby PJ, Matharu MS, Boes CJ. SUNCT syndrome or trigeminal neuralgia with lacrimation. *Cephalalgia* **21**: 82–83, 2001

53. Manzoni GC. Gender ratio of cluster headache over the years: a possible role of changes in lifestyle. *Cephalalgia* **18**: 138–142, 1998

54. Pealfield R, Bahra A, Goodsby PJ. Trigeminal-autonomic cephalgias (TACs). *Cephalalgia* **18**: 358–361, 1998

55. Goadsby PJ, Lipton RB. A review of paroxysmal hemicronios, SUNCT syndrome and other short-lasting headaches with autonomic features, including new cases. *Brain* **120**: 193–209, 1997

56. Newman LC, Goodsby PJ. The paroxysmal hemicranias, SUNCT syndrome, and hypnic headache. In: Silberstein SD, Lipton RB, Dalessio Dl, eds. *Wolff's Headache and Other Head Pain.* Oxford: Oxford University Press, 2001 pp. 310–324

57. Pareja JA, Ming JM, Kruszewski P, et al. SUNCT syndrome, duration, frequency and temporal distribution of attacks. *Headache* **36**: 161–165, 1996

58. Young WB, Packard RC. Posttraumatic headache and posttraumatic syndrome. In: Goadsby PJ, Silberstein SD, eds. *Headache.* New York: Butterworth-Heinemann, 1997, pp. 253–278

59. Kelly RE. Post-traumatic headache. In: Vinken PJ, Bruyn GW, Klawans HL, eds. *Handbook of Clinical Neurology. Vol 4.* Amsterdam: Elsevier, 1986, pp. 383–390

60. Edmeads J. Headaches in cerebrovascular disease. In: Vinken PJ, Bruyn GW, Klawans HL, eds. *Handbook of Clinical Neurology. Vol 4.* Amsterdam: Elsevier, 1986, pp. 273–290

61. Vermeulen M, van Gijn J. The diagnosis of subarachnoid haemorrhage. *J Neurol Neurosurg Psychiatry* **53**: 365–372, 1990

62. Edlow JA, Caplan LR. Avoiding pitfalls in the diagnosis of subarachnoid hemorrhage. *N Engl J Med* **342**: 29–36, 2000

63. Wardlaw JM, White PM. The detection and management of unruptured intracranial aneurysms. *Brain* **123**: 205–215, 2000

64. Biosse V, Woimant F, Amarenco P, et al. Pain as the only manifestation of internal carotid artery dissection. *Cephalgia* **12**: 314–317, 1992

65. Bousser MG, Ross Russell R. *Cerebral Venous Thrombosis.* London: W.B.Saunders, 1997

66. Caselli RJ, Hunder GG, Whisnant JP. Neurological disease is biopsy-proven giant cell (temporal) arteritis. *Neurology* **38**: 352–358, 1988

67. Ross Russell RW. Giant cell (cranial arteritis). In Vinken PJ, Bruyn GW, Klawans HL, eds. *Handbook of Clinical Neurology. Vol 4.* Amsterdam: Elsevier, 1986, pp. 309–328

68. Patchell RA. Metastatic brain tumours. *Neurol Clin* **13**: 915–925, 1995

69. Forsyth PA, Posner JB. Headaches in patients with brain tumours: a study of 111 patients. *Neurology* **43**: 1678–1683, 1993

70. Zakrzewska JM. Facial palsy: Neurological and non-neurological. *J Neurol Neurosurg Psychiatry* **72**: 27–32, 2002

71. Forsell H, Kalso E, Koskela P, et al. Occlusal treatments in temporomandibular disorders: a qualitative systematic review of randomised controlled trials. *Pain* **83**: 549–560, 1999

72. Edmeads J. The cervical spine headache. *Neurology* **38**: 1874–1878, 1988

# 10 Facial Pain

## Joanna M Zakrzewska

Orofacial pain is common and the commonest causes are dental whereas all the other causes are rare. Some non-dental pain will present in a similar way, and patients will often consult a dentist thinking they have a dental cause for their pain. Pain in the orofacial region can be divided into three main groups (Table 10.1), which determine referral pathways.[1] Patients with musculoligamentous and soft tissue pain need to be referred to the secondary dental sector; patients with dentoalveolar pain can generally be managed in the primary dental care sector; and neurological and vascular pains need to be referred to neurologists or pain specialists. All patients, especially those with non-dental pain, need a very careful assessment that includes a detailed history and measurement of the disability and coping strategies on scales such as the 'brief pain inventory' and 'McGill pain questionnaire' as detailed in Chapter 5.

## Overall clinical features

As with all patients with pain, a careful history is essential. Important distinguishing features of the pain are:

- localized or diffuse
- intra- or extraoral
- bilateral or unilateral
- preauricular or over the maxillary sinus
- stimulated by hot, cold, sweet or biting (or unstimulated)

| **Table 10.1** Classification of facial pain (adapted from Hapak[1]) | | |
|---|---|---|
| Musculoligamentous/ soft tissue | Dentoalveolar | Neurological/vascular |
| Temporomandibular (TMJ) disorders | Dentinal | Trigeminal neuralgia |
| Myofascial | Periodontal | Glossopharyngeal neuralgia |
| Salivary gland disease | Pulpal | Nerve compression |
| Burning mouth | Dental abscess | Cluster headache |
| Atypical facial pain | Cracked tooth syndrome | Post herpetic neuralgia |
| Atypical odontalgia | Thermal sensitivities | Temporal arteritis |
| Oral ulcerations | Osteomyelitis | Pre-trigeminal neuralgia |
| Blistering conditions | Maxillary sinusitis | Referred pain – cardiac |
| Erosive lichen planus | | |
| Infections – actinomycosis | | |
| Cancer | | |

- intermittent or continuous
- mild or severe.

Nasal and eye symptoms need to be elicited. It is important to take a short dental history to determine whether the patient is a regular attender, how important dental health is to them, what their oral hygiene habits are and whether there is any history of trauma to the face.

Examination includes an extraoral examination, cranial nerve examination in some instances, presence or absence of lymphadenopathy and any other swellings. Intraoral examination requires a good light and a means of retraction with either a wooden spatula or dental mirrors to improve visibility. The soft tissues need to be examined separately from the hard tissues (teeth and jaws) and the areas to examine are shown in Table 10.2.

**Table 10.2** Examination of the oral cavity and associated structures

Intraoral soft tissue examination includes the following areas looking for red, white patches or ulcers

- Lips upper and lower outer and inner to the buccal sulcus.
- Right and left buccal mucosa, stretched and at rest
- Tongue, dorsum, ventral surface, lateral borders
- Floor of mouth and lingual sulci which may need retraction of the tongue
- Palate hard and soft
- Oropharynx, fauces, tonsils, uvula, posterior wall of nasopharynx
- Salivary function – colour, quality and viscosity of saliva, flow, swelling of glands, patency of ducts
- Presence of odour

Examination of hard tissues and musculature

- Measurement of maximum opening from incisive tips of incisors either in mm or fingers lower limit 35 mm for women, 40 mm for men, lateral excursion is normally 8 mm in either direction
- Assess range of movements – right, left, forward and any deviations
- Palpation of joint for crepitations and tenderness
- Palpatation and testing of function of muscles at their origin and insertion on each side temporalis, masseter, medial and lateral pyterygoid
- Looking for evidence of bruxism intra orally and trigger points

Overall state of dentition

- Number of teeth in each arch
- Lack of teeth in each arch, unerupted, partially erupted, submerged
- State of the teeth – caries (broken down), broken teeth, roots, wearing down of tooth substance, mobility, tilted teeth, partially erupted, response of teeth to percussion
- Presence of bridges, fixed appliances, removable appliances
- Examine the appliance in and out of the mouth – type design, age, fit, retention, occlusion, relationship to soft tissue,
- Gingival tissues – colour, swelling, abcessed, pocketing, recession of gingiva from teeth
- Alveolar ridges – overlying mucosa colour, texture, tenderness, degree of resorption, mobility of mucosa, retained roots
- Overall oral hygiene – presence of plaque, calculus

# Overall investigations

## Radiological investigations

- Orthopantomogram (OPG), which is a full-mouth radiogram showing the dentition, mandible and part of the temporomandibular joint (TMJ) and floor of maxillary antrum. If this radiography is not available then right and left lateral obliques are needed.
- Occipitomental radiograms at a variety of angles will show the maxilla and paranasal sinuses.
- Intraoral radiograms are useful for individual teeth to look for periodontal diseases, caries, cysts and abscesses; salivary stones can be seen on occlusal radiograms.
- Sialography is used to show salivary stones and disease, and this can be followed by ultrasound.
- Computed tomography (CT) and magnetic resonance imaging (MRI) may occasionally be needed.

## Dental tests

- Vitality tests are used as an indirect way to test whether the pulp has a blood supply and hence is vital. Thermal and electrical testing is done and the results must be interpreted in the light of other features.
- Percussion of the tooth with a blunt instrument to test whether it is painful or not shows the presence of inflamed periapical tissues. Sometimes a local anaesthetic is useful to identify the tooth causing the problem.
- Fiber-optic transillumination and laser fluorescence are some other sophisticated tests that can be used. The former is useful in maxillary sinusitis.

## Laboratory tests

- In some instances, infective organisms are present and these then need to be cultured.
- Biopsy of oral lesions may be necessary to establish a diagnosis.
- Some autoimmune diseases such as Sjögren's Syndrome, scleroderma need to be confirmed by assessing the autoimmune profile.
- Other haematological and biochemical tests may be indicated based on the history as many systemic diseases present intraorally.

# Dentoalveolar pain

The main causes and guidelines on management of dental pain are shown in Table 10.3.

- Pulpitis occurs when dental pulp or dentine is exposed, due to either caries (decay) or trauma, and results in an inflammatory process in the pulp. The pain is provoked by cold, hot and sweet stimuli. In the initial phases the pain is difficult to localize and disappears on removal of stimuli. At this stage the tooth can probably still be salvaged but as the pain becomes more localized and continuous so the pulp will need to be removed or the tooth extracted. If pulpitis is left untreated an infection will develop at the apex leading to periodontitis. As the periodontal fibres have both pain and pressure sensitive nerve endings the pain becomes localized and the tooth is extremely sensitive to touch. This can in turn lead to an acute abscess, which can result in an extraoral swelling, fever and malaise.

**Table 10.3** Dental causes of pain: principal features and management

| Aetiology | Pain features | Provoking factors | Relieving factors | Associated features | Management |
|---|---|---|---|---|---|
| Tooth hypersensitivity | Sharp, localized, mild to moderate, stimulation evoked | Thermal, tactile, chemical, osmotic | Removal of stimulus | Attrition, erosion | Coverage of exposed dentine with fluoride, potassium salts or toothpaste |
| Reversible pulpitis | Sharp, poor localization, mild to moderate, stimulation evoked | Hot, cold, sweet | Removal of stimulus | Caries, restorations | Remove caries, temporary filling till pain free |
| Irreversible pulpitis | Sharp, throbbing, poor localization, severe, intermittent/ continuous | Hot, chewing, lying flat | Initially cold | Deep caries | Remove pulp or extract tooth |
| Periapical periodontitis | Deep, boring, localized, moderate to severe, continuous | Biting, touch | Removal of stimulus | Swelling, mobility | Drain through pulp cavity or extract tooth |
| Acute apical abscess | Continuous, boring, moderate to severe | Touch, biting | None | Mobile tooth, swelling extra- or intraoral, fever | Drain, remove pulp or extract tooth, may need antibiotics |
| Lateral periodontal | Deep aching, localized, continuous, moderate to severe | Biting | None | Deep pockets, mobile teeth, redness, pus | Curettage and drainage |
| Chronic pulpitis | Dull, poor localization, intermittent, mild | None | None | Sinus next to tooth, caries | Clean canal or extract tooth |
| Cracked tooth syndrome | Sharp, localized, moderate to severe, intermittent | Biting, 'rebound pain' | None | Natural opposing tooth | Remove restoration, adjust occlusion, new restoration |
| Pericoronitis | Throbbing, localized, moderate to severe, continuous | Biting | None | Fever, malaise, operculum over partially erupted tooth, opposing tooth | Irrigation with saline, extraction of upper tooth, antibiotics |
| Dry socket | Throbbing, gnawing, localized, moderate to severe, continuous | None | None | 4–5 days post-extraction, loss of clot, exposed bone | Irrigation, eugenol-based dressing |

All patients need to see a dentist, as treatment with antibiotics alone will produce a sterile abscess. Dental pain is often difficult to control, and drainage of the abscess or root canal is the most effective way of achieving pain relief.

- A cracked tooth can be very difficult to diagnose; it is often mistaken as atypical odontalgia or chronic idiopathic facial pain and needs to be looked for carefully.
- Thermal sensitivities of teeth are fairly common and need to be recognized. Patients can have the exposed part of the dentine painted with varnish or can apply toothpaste overnight to the area.
- Pericoronitis is an infection of a flap of gingival round a partially erupted or impacted tooth, most commonly the lower wisdom tooth (last molar). It can be associated with systematic signs and ultimately the tooth will need extracting. (For indications for extraction of wisdom teeth, see Worrall[2]).
- Dry sockets occur most frequently in the mandible, and patients will recognize the pain as being of dental origin as it occurs within 2 or 3 days of an extraction.

### Maxillary sinusitis
Sinusitis, especially maxillary sinusitis, is extremely common, and it is not gender or age specific. The infection in most cases is due to bacterial causes and the common organisms are *Haemophilus influenzae* and *Streptococcus pneumoniae*.

## Clinical features

History of previous upper respiratory tract infection, dental extraction of maxillary molar or long term use of vasoconstrictor nasal sprays.

- Report of coloured nasal discharge
- No improvement on use of decongestants
- Site and radiation – cheek, zygomatic bone
- Character – dull, boring, pressing, throbbing, deep pain
- Severity – mild to severe
- Duration and periodicity – days or weeks, continuous
- Provoking factors – bending, head movements
- Relieving factors – none
- Associated factors – presence of coloured discharge, abnormal transillumination.

## Investigations

Radiograms are probably only needed in complicated cases and those failing to respond to treatment as underlying systemic disease or carcinoma may be present. Plain radiograms such as occipitomental (Waters view) should be used first and then CT if the infection fails to heal.

## Management

The latest evidence-based treatment recommendations can be found in the Cochrane Library or a regularly updated article in Clinical Evidence (e.g. Del Mar and Glasziou[3]).

- Nasal decongestants are of limited use.
- Antibiotics in those patients with bacterial maxillary sinusitis: penicillin V, amoxycillin are most commonly used for 7–10 days.
- One small randomized controlled trial has shown that intranasal steroid use improved symptoms of acute sinusitis over 21 days in patients taking antibiotics.

### Infective causes

*Actinomycosis* is extremely rare and will often present with other oral lesions such as facial sinus.

## Osteomyelitis

### Aetiology and predisposing factors

Osteomyelitis is rare in the developed world and most often occurs in mandible due to poor blood supply. It is seen in patients who have or had:

• Extensive dental infections
• Severe facial trauma
• Paget's disease
• Previous radiotherapy to the jaws
• Immunological deficiency.

### Clinical features

• Pyrexia and malaise
• Severe, continuous throbbing pain, which is felt deep in the bone
• Pus discharging either intraorally or out of the face
• Often loose, infected teeth that are painful to bite on
• Maybe numbness and trismus
• Cervical lymphadenopathy.

### Investigations

• Radiograms – typically show 'moth-eaten' appearance, the normal bony trabecular pattern is lost and areas of radio-opaqueness represent sequestra
• Swabs for microscopy and culture.

### Management

• Intravenous antibiotics
• Debridement and removal of sequestra once infection has settled.

### Soft tissue lesions

Many of the soft tissue lesions listed in Table 10.1 cause pain, but there are always intraoral lesions present, which will result in the patient being referred either to oral physicians or oral and maxillofacial surgeons. The pain is often localized, of a sharp or burning quality and is made worse by sharp or sour foods. Oral cancer rarely presents with severe pain, mainly presenting as ulcers, white or red patches or large lumps.

## Salivary gland disease

The common conditions are mumps, parotiditis and salivary calculi. Calculi typically cause pain in the gland in relation to meal times and swellings may also be present. The pain is well localized, lasts for hours or days and is of a drawing, pulling character. Chronic obstruction can lead to damage to the gland itself and this can be ascertain by sialography. Calculi can be removed surgically or by lithotripsy and, as a final resort, by removal of the gland.

# Temporomandibular joint pains or myofascial pain

### Definitions
There are a vast number of terms used to describe pain arising in the joints or masticatory muscles. The International Association for the Study of Pain definition is 'aching in the muscles of mastication, sometimes with an occasional brief severe pain on chewing, often associated with restricted jaw movement and clicking or popping sounds'. However, many patients do not have any abnormal clinical findings and, in these, the simple definition of chronic or intermittent pain of the TMJ and/or of its associated musculature is most appropriate.[4] The pain may be caused by internal derangement of the disc or by muscles.

## Aetiology

This remains unknown but several theories have been suggested:

- Psychogenic – can be related to other bodily pains, depression and anxiety or personality disorders, females appear to be at increased risk[5]
- Occlusal abnormalities – parafunctional activities could contribute
- Traumatic – meniscal displacement within the joint is relatively rare.

## Clinical features

- Site – TMJ and associated musculature
- Radiation – associated muscles, temple, neck
- Character – dull, aching, occasionally sharp
- Severity – mild to moderate
- Duration – weeks to years
- Periodicity – continuous, but can be intermittent or worse on wakening or at the end of the day
- Provoking factors – jaw movement, eating, stress
- Relieving factors – jaw rest, tricyclic drugs
- Associated factors – limited mouth opening, deviation on opening, TMJ parafunction, occasional clicking, anxiety.

## Examination

Some or all of these features may be present:

- Pain upon palpation of the TMJ
- Pain upon palpation of the muscles of mastication
- Decreased mouth opening
- Altered lateral jaw movements
- Clicking of the TMJ
- Crepitus of the TMJ.

## Investigations

Radiograms, MRI and CT scans are now commonly used in TMJ assessment. The use of radiograms is limited by its 2-dimensional image (unless tomographic techniques are employed).

## Management

The prevailing recommendation of the American Dental Association is that only conservative, reversible forms of treatment should be undertaken as, in general, the condition is self-limiting (although it may last for 2–3 years).

- Reassurance with a careful explanation is essential as patient education is crucial.
- Exercises and avoiding opening the mouth wide are often useful, but there are no randomized controlled trials in this field.
- Physical therapy such as heat and ultrasound have been tried, but there are no controlled trials.
- Bite guards can be made to fit the upper or lower jaw, but there are no randomized controlled trials that provide enough evidence for their use.[6]
- Psychological therapy (e.g. cognitive behaviour therapy, stress management) have been shown to be effective as they enable patients to gain more control over their pain and to see their pain in a broader context.
- Antidepressants have been shown in three randomized controlled trials to be effective
- Analgesics such as NSAIDs have not been shown to be effective.

## Burning mouth syndrome

### Definition

Burning mouth is said to be a symptom of other disease when local or systemic factors are found to be implicated and their treatment results in resolution of burning mouth. Burning mouth syndrome (BMS) is an intraoral burning sensation for which no medical or odontological causes can be found and in which the oral mucosa is of grossly normal appearance. Many will also have subjective dryness, paraesthesia and altered taste.

## Clinical features

- Duration – mean time to development 3 years, builds up gradually
- Periodicity – some patients have continuous symptoms, in others the sensation builds up over the day being worse in the evening
- Character – may be described as a pain or discomfort, burning, smarting, tender and annoying
- Site – often more than one site: tongue (most common), cheeks, gingiva, palate
- Radiation – remains in the mouth
- Severity – ranges from mild to moderate
- Provoking factors – tension, fatigue
- Relieving factors – sleep, cold foods, distraction
- Associated factors – taste changes, mood changes, tongue thrusting, dryness
- Examination – no gross changes found, although may be some dryness.

## Differential diagnosis

- Denture stomatitis – redness under denture sometimes, may be symptom of uncontrolled diabetes

- Atrophic candidiasis – generalized redness in the palate, could be related to inhaler use, antibiotics, post-radiotherapy, immunocompromised patients, allergy
- Geographic tongue – presents as changing red patches surrounded by white elevated margins on the dorsum of the tongue, may be associated with candidiasis and so cause burning
- Fissured tongue – is considered a variation of normal, seen often in patients with dry mouths but may indicate Sjögren's syndrome
- Dry mouth, lack of pooling in the floor – consider drugs, anxiety, Sjögren's syndrome.

## Investigations

- Full blood count and differential
- Iron status – serum ferritin
- Vitamin B12 and red cell folate levels
- Random blood glucose or glycosylated Hb
- Salivary flow
- Oral swabs
- Oral biopsy
- Allergy testing
- Denture functioning
- Immunological – rheumatoid factor, complement, antinuclear factor.

## Management

This is initially based on reassurance and correction of all contributing factors. Assessing patients' drug therapy is important as many drugs cause xerostomia, which can then lead to candidiasis and burning. Patients who complain of dry mouth may be offered a variety of saliva substitutes, which have not been evaluated in randomized controlled trials.

If treatment of all local causes does not result in resolution and there are no signs of oral mucosal disease then you can assume the patient has BMS. To date there have been no high quality randomized controlled trials reported in this field so making management difficult.[7] The only treatment that has shown some benefit is cognitive behaviour therapy. Others have attempted to give female patients hormone replacements or massaged oestrogen locally but none are conclusive. Vitamin replacements have been tried but the trials are inconclusive. Antidepressants are used but often patients with BMS have not been analysed separately from other facial pain patients so their individual outcomes are not known. Treatments for BMS have been the subject of a Cochrane review, and there is also an article in Clinical Evidence, which is regularly updated.[7]

There is little work on prognosis but it would appear that the condition lasts for several years. Patients need empathy, coping skills and support.

# Atypical facial pain/chronic idiopathic facial pain

Atypical facial pain (AFP) is a controversial diagnosis and not formally recognized by the International Association for the Study of Pain.[4]

### Definition
The definition given by the International Headache Association is persistent 'facial pain that does not have the characteristics of any cranial neuralgias and is not associated with physical signs or a demonstrable organic cause'. The International Headache Association provide some diagnostic criteria.[8]

## Clinical features

- Duration – often 2–21 years
- Periodicity – varies from constant daily pain to months that are pain free
- Character – deep poorly localized pain, many pain words are used to describe the pain including vicious, throbbing, stabbing, nagging, burning
- Site – any part of the face, does not follow an anatomical distribution
- Radiation – to many parts of the face, head and neck
- Severity – varies from mild to severe
- Provoking factors – stress, cold weather, chewing, head movements, life events[8]
- Relieving factors – warmth and pressure, medication
- Associated factors – may follow trauma/dental treatment to area, altered sensation, often pains in other parts of the body including back pain, irritable bowel syndrome, pruritus, tinnitus, and may be associated with anxiety, depression, personality disorders
- Examination – usually no abnormal findings are detected, except for pain upon palpation of the area.

## Differential diagnosis

When bilateral and extensive the diagnosis is fairly easy, but unilateral cases do present a problem as many of the conditions listed in Table 10.1 under neurological and vascular would need to be considered.

## Investigations

Some radiograms may be necessary to rule out dental pain.

## Management

A biopsychosocial model of care is essential using a holistic approach. Patients with shorter histories and who have seen fewer specialists tend to do better.

- Acknowledge reality of pain and show empathy.
- Encourage control and reduce catastrophizing.
- Assess and reduce the effect of life events and stressors on the pain.
- Provide cognitive behaviour therapy, which may include relaxation, distraction, and positive thinking. There is evidence for the effectiveness of this treatment.[9]
- Antidepressants have been shown to be effective in randomized controlled trials, and treatment may need to be continued for 1–2 years.[10,11]
- Provide patient information and education.

# Atypical odontalgia

### Definition
Atypical odontalgia is a variant of AFP, localized to the teeth or tooth; some consider it to be a variant of phantom tooth pain.

## Clinical features

- Duration – months to years
- Periodicity – usually continuous, but may last from a few minutes to hours

- Character – severe throbbing, aching
- Site – teeth and gingivae
- Radiation – to other teeth
- Severity – varies from mild to severe
- Provoking factors – hot and cold, dental treatment, pressure on tooth
- Relieving factors – none
- Associated factors – hypersensitivity to heat and cold, emotional problems.

## Examination

Teeth may be sound, restored, endodontically treated or extracted. Teeth that are clinically sound are vital and tender to thermal stimuli.

## Differential diagnosis

Any of dental causes listed in Table 10.3.

## Investigations

Dental radiograms and dental tests may need to be done if not done already.

## Management

Counselling and avoidance of unnecessary pulp extirpations and extractions
Rest of management as for AFP.

# References

1. Hapak L, Gordon A, Locker D, Shandling M, Mock D, Tenenbaum HC. Differentiation between musculoligamentous, dentoalveolar, and neurologically based craniofacial pain with a diagnostic questionnaire. *J Orofac Pain* **8**: 357–368, 1994
2. Worrall S. Impacted wisdom teeth. *Clinical evidence* 7: 1244–1247, 2002
3. Del Mar C, Glasziou P. Upper respiratory tract infections. *Clinical evidence* 7: 1391–1399, 2002
4. Merskey H, Bogduk N. *Classification of Chronic Pain. Descriptors of Chronic Pain Syndromes and Definitions of Pain Terms. 2nd ed.* Seattle: IASP Press, 1994
5. Drangsholt M, LeResche L. Temporomandibular disorder pain. In: Crombie IK, Croft PR, Linton SJ, LeResche L, eds. *Epidemiology of Pain*. Seattle: IASP, 1999, pp. 203–233
6. Forssell H, Kalso E, Koskela P, Vehmanen R, Puukka P, Alanen P. Occlusal treatments in temporomandibular disorders: a qualitative systematic review of randomized controlled trials. *Pain* **83**: 549–560, 1999
7. Buchanan AG, Zakrzewska JM. Burning Mouth Syndrome. *Clinical evidence* 7: 1239–1243, 2002
8. Anonymous. Classification and diagnostic criteria for headache disorders, cranial neuralgias and facial pain. Headache Classification Committee of the International Headache Society. *Cephalalgia* **8(Suppl 7)**: 1–96, 1988
9. Madland G, Newton-John T, Feinmann C. Chronic idiopathic orofacial pain: I: What is the evidence base? *Br Dent J* **191**: 22–24, 2001
10. Newton-John T, Madland G, Feinmann C. Chronic idiopathic orofacial pain: II. What can the general dental practitioner do? *Br Dent J* **191**: 72–73, 2001
11. McQuay HJ, Tramer M, Nye BA, Carroll D, Wiffen PJ, Moore RA. A systematic review of antidepressants in neuropathic pain. *Pain* **68**: 217–227, 1996

# Further Reading

Birnbaum W, Dunne SM. *Wright Oral Diagnosis. The clinician's guide.* Oxford: Wright 2000

Chestnutt IG, Gibson J. (ed) *Churchill's Pocketbook of Clinical Dentistry. 2nd edition.* London: Churchill Livingstone, 2002

Sharav Y. Orofacial pain. In: Wall P, Melzack R, eds. *Textbook of Pain.* London: Churchill Livingstone, 1999, pp. 711–737

Zakrzewska JM, Hamlyn PJ. Facial pain. In: Crombie IKCPR, Linton SJ, LeResche L, Von Korff M, eds. *Epidemiology of Pain.* Seattle: IASP, 1999, 171–202

Zakrzewska JM (ed) *Assessment and management of orofacial pain.* Amsterdam: Elsevier, 2002

# 11 Neck Pain

## Nicholas L Padfield

Thirty five percent of us have suffered at one time or another from neck pain. The prevalence quoted in one paper was 10% of the adult population.[1] Happily, the majority of times it is transient, acute and resolves. However, there are a number of patients for whom this is not the case. The neck contains the most mobile part of the vertebral column with some 40 bony articulations with supporting ligaments, muscles and synovial membranes. Because of its mobility the neck is particularly susceptible to trauma and degeneration of the bones with their discs and articular surfaces, and the soft tissues comprising muscles, ligaments, blood vessels and nerves. Although it is very common, over the age of 30 years, to see radiological changes indicative of cervical spondylosis, severe disability and loss of function is far less common than with the lumbar spine. Indeed, it has been known for a long time that asymptomatic abnormalities of the cervical spine may be found in up to 80% of patients. This underlines the fact that it is very difficult to ascribe radiological changes to clinical syndromes per se – they often only act to confirm the clinical picture.

## Clinical assessment

When assessing a patient complaining of neck pain, always have in mind:

- The structures that may be involved, i.e. bones, muscles, nerves, blood vessels, ligaments, joint capsules, discs
- The pathological process, i.e. traumatic, degenerative, infective, inflammatory, neoplastic and metabolic
- The genesis of the pain, i.e. if due to a road traffic accident, ascertain the speed and direction of impact; if occupational, what are the actual physical demands on the body; if metabolic, does the condition (e.g. osteoporosis or osteomalacia) require treatment in its own right
- The psychological impact, especially if litigation is in progress.

## History

As with any pain, the speed of onset and duration, especially after any precipitating event, along with the character and periodicity should indicate the likely pathologic process. The site and radiation along with provoking and relieving factors (e.g. the effects of specific movements and positions) should indicate the likely structures involved. The medical history (e.g. post-menopause, renal disease, endocrine disease) should indicate likely relevance of coexisting significant medical disease. The patient's body language and use of descriptors will indicate the psychological impact, and the involvement in litigation may alert the clinician to hidden agendas.

# Examination

Stand your patient upright undressed to underwear. Look specifically at:

- Posture – abnormal curvature of spine, thoracic kyphosis, loss of cervical lordosis, loss of lumbar lordosis, scoliosis, position of shoulders, position head is held
- Skin and hair – altered pigmentation and distribution, sweating, abnormal hair growth and altered blood flow anywhere from head to fingers
- Muscles – wasting, spasticity, trigger points, excessive lengthening or shortening and any change in the full range of movement achievable
- Fingernails – trophic changes, splinter haemorrhages, nicotine staining, dirt, abnormal nail biting
- Joints – cervical facet joints where compression reproduces pain on the affected side, check movement of shoulders and arms in all directions
- Nerves – check for adverse upper limb tension, get the patient to perform a Valsalva manoeuvre, which by raising intrathecal pressure may also suggest significant cervical disc protrusion, adhesions around nerve roots, lateral canal stenosis; a positive Adson's sign may indicate thoracic outlet syndrome.

# Investigation

Thus far you should have an idea whether there is the need for further investigation. Remember to confine your investigations to only those upon whose results you are likely to act. Therefore, pain lateral and anterior posterior cervical spine views should indicate osteophyte formation and extraosseous calcification and may confirm facet joint sclerosis, spondylolisthesis, loss of cervical disc height, abnormal vertebral curvature such as loss of lordosis and the rare diffuse idiopathic skeletal hyperostosis. Plain views through the open mouth demonstrate the atlantoaxial joint. Barium studies outline the soft tissues in front of the vertebral column and confirm dysphagia resulting from significant osteophyte formation. Further investigation such as magnetic resonance imaging (MRI) may be indicated to define cervical disc protrusion, lateral canal stenosis, the significance of a spondylolisthesis and, rarely, extensive scarring or adhesions around nerve roots.

Metabolic studies such as bone densitometry may be indicated to monitor the progress of treatment of osteoporosis.

Nerve conduction studies and electromyography may be indicated in the case of radiculopathy, such as thoracic outlet syndrome or neuropathic myopathies.

Autoantibodies should be screened when an inflammatory arthritis is suspected, as a rheumatological cause may need treating in its own right.

Table 11.1 shows the common sources of neck pain; it is far from exhaustive but sorts conditions into logical groups, all of which may require different and sometimes specific treatments.

# Specific syndromes

There are some particularly common conditions that are easy to diagnose and have particular features in presentation and in their subsequent management. They make good examples of the pain clinician's assessment and treatment strategies. Evidence for the efficacy of treatments will be given where available.

| Table 11.1 Sources of neck pain | |
|---|---|
| Bones and ligaments | Cervical spondylosis |
| | Rheumatoid arthritis |
| | Ankylosing spondylitis |
| | DISH (Diffuse idiopathic skeletal hyperostosis) |
| | Ossification of the posterior longitudinal ligament |
| | Metastatic disease |
| | Repetitive strain injury |
| Nerves | Radiculopathy – entrapment, disc prolapse |
| | Myelopathy |
| | Brachial plexus – thoracic outlet syndrome, brachial plexus neuropathy |
| | Cervical neuralgia |
| Muscular | Whiplash |
| | Myofascial pain |
| | Cervical dystonia |
| | Fibromyalgia |
| | Myalgic encephalitis |
| | Polymyalgia rheumatica |
| Referred pain | Head, (teeth, ear, temperomandibular joint) |
| | Thoracic viscera: heart, lung, aorta |
| | Abdominal viscera: gall bladder, oesophagus (hiatus hernia) |
| | Cervical lymphadenopathy |
| | Intracranial causes (space occupying lesions, tumour, aneurysm infection/inflammation – meningism) |
| | Shoulder – acromioclavicular joint, subacromial compression, suprascapular, subscapular and biceps tendonitis |

## Traumatic

### 'Whiplash'

Cervical strain is associated with rapid flexion and extension injury. Although cord damage can occur, it is the soft tissue that bears the brunt of the injury. There has been change in opinion about the genesis of the chronic pain that can so frequently arise as a result of a much greater understanding of the biomechanics of the cervical vertebral column.[3] Also, traditionally the cervical disc has been considered in much the same way as the lumbar disc, but anatomical studies show that it is morphologically quite different in that it does not have a circular annulus fibrosis but rather a crescentic one that tapers out from thick bands anteriorly to thin paramedian fibres orientated vertically.[4]

Following injury and starting at the head there can be ocular trauma with lens dislocation and detachment of the retina, temporomandibular joint damage particular to the meniscus. In the neck, the discs can be damaged by abnormal anterior separation while the zygapophyseal joints can be impacted, resulting in an S-shaped deformity affecting the upper and lower vertebral levels with relative sparing of the middle ones.[5] In addition to the discs, the supporting muscles, tendons and ligaments of the neck are most commonly traumatized, which may be associated with damage to the nerve roots directly or through increased pressure by subsequent muscle spasms.[6]

Common causes are road traffic accidents, falls, high-velocity sports injuries and electrocution. As patients age they become more susceptible to injury.

Initially, patients may present with pain and stiffness in the shoulder girdle, hoarseness or dysphagia, headache and various complex regional pain type syndromes. Absence of neurological signs may be taken as a good indicator of minimal or no cord or spinal damage. However, even with apparently minimal symptoms and signs patients should be followed up for several days following the incident.[7]

Muscles and ligaments heal within 4–6 weeks depending on age and nutritional status, whereas the intervertebral discs, being avascular, heal much more slowly. If there is any suspicion of a cervical spinal injury then lateral plain X-rays must be taken of the entire cervical spine.

**Treatment**  Provided there is no spinal injury, physiotherapy can be used, including mild cervical traction and 'stretch and spray' (see Chapter 8).

Dry needling of trigger points, particularly in the sternocleidomastoid muscle, is the best initial treatment with concomitant administration of non-steroidal anti-inflammatory drugs (NSAIDs).

Soft cervical collars are of no proven benefit and may 'label' a patient as a victim leading to cognitive issues.

Since injury may involve the scalene, levator scapulae, sternocleidomastoid and posterior cervical muscles along with muscles in the lower back and the glutei exhaustive examination for tender trigger points should be made. These must be treated early as, if neglected or overlooked, they will cause exacerbations of the problems in the neck and shoulders converting the problem to a chronic one.

If it does not settle within 4–6 weeks and the zygapophyseal joints continue to be significant pain generators, posterior branch blocks of the affected levels should be done. A counsel of perfection is to perform these on separate occasions using local anaesthetics with different durations of action, comparing them with a placebo response to normal saline.[8] If the pain is significantly improved then these joints should be 'denervated' by radiofrequency lesions – (described in the appendix) intra-articular injection of steroid was shown not to be any more effective than local anaesthetic in a randomized trial.[9]

There is class 2 evidence from a randomized placebo controlled trial, which demonstrated resolution of psychological distress of whiplash patients following treatment by radiofrequency neurotomy.[10]

Some clinicians would also advocate provocative discography to test for pain generators at different vertebral levels. The results, however, can be equivocal, probably because of the morphology of the cervical disc; the procedure is very painful and to proceed to intradiscal radiofrequency thermocoagulation, in the absence of good evidence of benefit, is not recommended at the moment by the author. This has been shown to be unhelpful in one randomized trial for back pain,[11] but there is a need for more trials in the neck because of the different disc morphology.

**Outcome**  Usually, 85% of those injured are back at work within 3 months, and 75% of cases do not result in litigation. However, when symptoms persist longer than 6 months it is likely to run a chronic course and is frequently associated with post-traumatic syndromes comprising stress and anxiety, balance problems, narrowing of the visual fields, insomnia, confusion and memory loss. These are particularly common in those patients who have residual injuries, socioeconomic stresses, depression, anger and adjustment problems and the complicating problem of litigation, especially when it is particularly protracted.

They unfortunately often present late to the pain clinician, by which time they have developed many cognitive issues, behavioural disorders and even overt depression, all of which can prove difficult to manage. Cognitive behavioural therapy is the mainstay of treatment and anger management is often appropriate. Occasionally, the psychological picture can change dramatically if cervical facet denervation significantly reduces the pain, as these patients appear to be psychologically distinct from non-traumatic headache patients, for example.[12]

## Degenerative

### Cervical spondylosis

Changes are more common in the lower cervical spine and begin with the development of osteophytes in the vertebral bodies. The facet joints are progressively involved. Intervertebral disc degeneration may lead to loss of disc height. Progression of the disease may lead to radiculopathy. Rarely, there may be involvement of sympathetic nerves leading to dysphagia, vertigo and visual disturbances. This may also occur due to vertebrobasilar insufficiency.

Symptoms include:

- Pain initially diffuse, more localized if nerve roots are involved, which may be referred to the face or to the anterior chest
- Restriction of neck movement with discomfort on attempting the full range
- Stiffness
- Multiple root constriction may lead to sensory loss in the hands and forearms in a pattern not conforming to a peripheral nerve, can affect the face, tongue and shoulder
- Spinal cord compression, myelopathy
- Sympathetic involvement – dysphagia, vertigo and visual disturbances
- Vascular – vertebrobasilar insufficiency due to compression or coincident atheroma
- Headache – occipital is common in upper cervical disease.

On examination, there can be lower cervical tenderness and associated spasm. Deep trigger points may be found if there is facet joint involvement, or superficial ones in myofascial disease. There is limitation of both active and passive movement.

Investigations will be determined by the clinical symptoms. Radiographs of the lateral cervical spine as well as open mouth views will help confirm the problem and act as a baseline. Diagnostic changes include subchondral bone density, osteophyte and pseudocyst formation and narrowing of the joint spaces. The onset of radiculopathy or myelopathy indicate that MRI should be undertaken as there may need to be corrective surgery in the case of instability or significant root impingement from canal stenosis, or intervertebral disc prolapse.

**Treatment**   Treatment will depend on the manner in which an individual patient is affected. As this is an episodic and gradually progressive disease one has to think of long-term management. Initially, physiotherapy may be indicated to strengthen weak neck muscles and improve mobility. The majority of meta-analyses of manipulative therapy only indicate a short-term improvement of a few weeks in most cases following physical therapy,[13,14] thus emphasizing the importance of lifestyle changes in order to live with this pain. One meta-analysis undertaken in 1996 reviewing conservative measure for mechanical neck pain concludes that, in general, conservative interventions have not been studied in enough detail to assess efficacy or effectiveness adequately.[15]

- NSAIDs should be used to treat the initial inflammation – they should not be used continuously long term as the patients are usually elderly and would run serious risks from nephropathy and catastrophic gastric haemorrhage.
- Cervical epidural injections of 40 mg triamcinolone with 20 mg lignocaine diluted in normal saline to a total volume of 6 ml are frequently beneficial.
- Injection of involved zygapophyseal joints and trigger points with Depot methyl prednisolone preparations and local anaesthetic give significant symptom relief but more

importantly facilitate physiotherapy, which may take the form of heat treatment, massage, cervical traction and exercises.

- Although osteoarthritis comprises a heterogeneous group of diseases, glucosamine at a dose of 500 mg three times a day (TDS) has been shown to be as effective as ibuprofen without the gastrointestinal morbidity for knee pain.[16] It is tempting to suggest trying it in cervical spondylosis.

## Inflammatory

### Rheumatoid arthritis

Rheumatoid arthritis occurs in 5% of British women. In the neck, the upper cervical spine is the most commonly involved area, seen in up to 80% of patient's X-rays. Of particular vulnerability is the atlantoaxial joint, where subluxation of the odontoid peg may occur spontaneously or during manipulation of the neck and was found in 25% of patients in one hospital-based study.[17] Less commonly, lateral, posterior[18] and vertical subluxation of the joint may also occur, and subluxation of the second or third cervical vertebrae.

Pain may be localized to the neck or referred to the occiput or retro-orbital areas from the upper cervical nerve roots, and it is exacerbated by movement. Myelopathy may occur at any level. Other features of rheumatoid arthritis should be sought in making the diagnosis, particularly peripheral joint involvement, rheumatoid nodules and evidence of vasculitis with subungual splinter haemorrhages. Serial X-rays show soft tissue swelling, periarticular osteoporosis, and loss of joint space, erosions and deformity. The diagnosis may be suspected from the finding of a high erythrocyte sedimentation rate (ESR) and, in 80% of cases, a positive rheumatoid factor.

**Treatment**   Treatment is of the underlying disease process, with NSAIDs in high doses during acute exacerbations and opioids only if absolutely necessary. Physiotherapy may be useful after acute episodes. If there is subluxation of a joint, a collar or surgical stabilization may be indicated.

**Outcome**   The prognosis is reasonable in the majority of patients and even 50 years ago in a study of rheumatoid arthritis patients over a 10 year period only 11% became completely disabled.[19]

### Ankylosing spondylitis

Ankylosing spondylitis is a disease that predominantly affects men. It has an incidence of 2 per 100 000 in Caucasians, and 95% have the human leukocyte antigen HLA-B27. Ankylosing spondylitis affects mainly the axial skeleton, particularly the sacroiliac joints, and also the neck. Onset is usually in early adult life. It is primarily an inflammatory process occurring at the margins of bone where tendons, ligaments and joint capsules adhere. Bony erosion occurs initially, but healing leads to bone formation at the site and loss of flexibility.

Clinical features are gradual onset of pain and morning stiffness improved by exercise, with diminished movements of the neck. This may initially be episodic; but rigidity eventually becomes marked. Limitation of range of movements affects the whole spine, with loss of normal lumbar lordosis, and there is pain on springing of the sacroiliac joints. In established ankylosing spondylitis, complications arise such as iritis, aortic incompetence, amyloidosis and a restrictive pulmonary abnormality due to the involvement of the thoracic cage. Neurological damage may occur due to an increased vulnerability to spinal trauma.

Radiographic changes show loss of definition of joint margins, erosions and then sclerosis of the whole joint. Sacroiliac involvement is necessary to make the diagnosis. The ESR may be raised acutely, as may plasma viscosity. Although HLA-B27 is almost universal in ankylosing spondylitis patients, it should be remembered that only 1% of HLA-B27 carriers develop the condition, possibly due to an infective trigger.

**Treatment**   Treatment is conservative, with NSAIDs and physiotherapy aimed at maintaining an upright functional posture. Local trigger points may occur and should be treated with local anaesthetic or steroid mixtures as above.

**Outcome**   In addition to mechanisms, it is also important to consider specific tissues when unravelling the complexities of neck pain.

## Nerve entrapment and compression

Nerve entrapments cause pain and motor or sensory loss, and they may occur from the spinal cord through nerve roots out to peripheral nerves, giving different clinical pictures.

### Myelopathy

Cervical myelopathy occurs due to cord compression, most commonly in the lower cervical spine because the spinal cord is slightly larger in this region. The clinical features are of a lower motor neuron lesion at the level of compression, with upper motor neuron signs below this. Sensory disturbances are common but differ from those seen in a radiculopathy by being non-dermatomal in pattern.

There are two main presentations:

- Acute cervical myelopathy – with a sudden onset, often in young patients due to cervical disc prolapse or to trauma
- The less acute form – onset over weeks rather than hours, may present with clumsiness, or gait disturbances. This is often due to cervical spondylosis, but can be caused by other degenerative diseases of the bones, tumour, haematoma and infection. Some elderly patients with narrowed cervical canals develop cord compression on flexion of the head.

The differential diagnosis of a compressive myelopathy is one of secondary radiation, or primary disease of the spinal cord, classically syringomyelia. More marked positional symptoms may be due to an inflammatory myelopathy, such as multiple sclerosis.

If the onset of a myelopathy is suspected in a patient being treated for neck pain, urgent investigation, including MRI, is indicated. Anteroposterior X-ray views showing narrowing of the cervical canal diameter increase the likelihood of a diagnosis of cord compression, but if negative do not exclude large space-occupying lesions.

### Radiculopathy

Compression of the nerve roots within the neck may occur secondary to many conditions affecting this area, but some particular patterns of involvement predominate:

- Acute radiculopathy is most commonly due to trauma or disc prolapse in young patients and may occur at any cervical level.
- Radiculopathy due to cervical spondylosis usually affects the middle or lower cervical nerve roots and occurs in an older population. The development of an acute radiculopathy in this group may be precipitated by minor trauma if the intervertebral foramen is already narrowed with osteophytes.

- Chronic radiculopathy may arise insidiously or persist after an acute episode. It is usually due to degenerative diseases of the cervical skeleton. However, caution should be exercised when there is a suspicion of malignancy, as differentiation of involvement with tumour from coexisting degenerative disease can be difficult.

The clinical features are of a dermatomal distribution of pain and sensory disturbance in the neck, shoulder and arm. The pain is typically neuropathic in character, with a persistent burning and/or intermittent lancinating component. Tenderness may be noted at the site of pathology. Symptoms can be increased by stretching the root with any manoeuvre that depresses the shoulder on the affected side, such as carrying a heavy weight. They will also be increased by increasing intrathecal pressure, e.g. coughing, sneezing, the Valsalva manoeuvre and sometimes by lateral flexion to the affected side, rotation away from the involved side or compression of the spine from above, which all cause narrowing of the intervertebral foramen. Conversely, symptoms may be relieved by shoulder abduction, reducing tension on the nerve root. The diagnosis may be made by electromyography (EMG) or evoked potentials. MRI may demonstrate impingement and differentiate between tumour recurrence and degenerative change.

**Treatment**   Treatment is of the underlying cause where appropriate, or by conservative measures such as NSAIDs and physiotherapy, including cervical traction and soft collar support of the neck. Neuralgic components can be treated with anticonvulsants. As in many conditions of the neck, severe pain may lead to secondary muscle spasm, and then trigger point injections may be appropriate.

### Thoracic outlet syndrome

The subclavian vessels and the lower trunk of the brachial plexus may be compressed as they leave the neck. The most common cause is a cervical rib, either a complete anatomical rib or a fibromuscular band. About 1 in 200 of the population have bilateral cervical ribs, but only 10% give rise to symptoms of thoracic outlet syndrome. This may be due in part to poor posture. Thoracic outlet syndrome may also be due to a fracture of the clavicle or first rib, or mechanical factors, including the habitual lifting of heavy weights on one shoulder, and bodybuilding leading to compression by hypertrophied muscle.

Symptoms include pain in the neck, shoulder or upper arm, which tends to be intermittent and is often associated with movement, particularly when lifting objects overhead. Patients tend to be young and more commonly female. Sensory disturbances occur in the lower dermatomes of the brachial plexus, typically C8 and T1. Weakness of the small muscles of the hand may occur, and in 10% of cases there is vascular occlusion of the upper limb, which may present as Raynaud's phenomenon, venous thrombosis or swelling of the arm after exercises. The confirmatory clinical test is to have the patient hold their arms out at 90° externally rotated angled posteriorly for 3 minutes; if the radial pulses remain normal but the usual pain or paraesthesiae are produced, the test is considered to be positively indicative of thoracic outlet syndrome.

Investigations to confirm the diagnosis include X-rays of the cervical spine, EMG, somatosensory evoked potentials and MRI. Treatment is initially conservative with exercises to improve shoulder girdle posture. Surgery to divide the band or resect the cervical rib may be indicated if vascular symptoms predominate, but vasomotor symptoms may persist postoperatively, and then chemical or surgical sympathectomy is indicated.

## Neuropathies

Cervical neuralgia is rarer than facial neuralgia. It may arise from the glossopharyngeal nerve or the dorsal rami of the upper cervical nerve roots (C2–4); the sensory distribution of each nerve root (and potential areas of referred pain) are shown in Table 11.2.

| Table 11.2 Sensory distribution of nerve roots | |
|---|---|
| Nerve root | Cutaneous supply |
| C1 | Suboccipital muscles, no cutaneous supply (absent in 50–70% of the population) |
| C2 | Supplies the majority of the greater occipital nerve, skin over occiput |
| C3 | Supplies the majority of the lesser occipital nerve, some of the greater occipital nerve, the greater auricular nerve and some of the skin near the midline below the occipital protuberance |

Glossopharyngeal neuralgia is a rare condition similar to trigeminal neuralgia but affecting the ninth cranial nerve. The pain is a severe paroxysmal lancinating pain occurring in the throat, ear and upper neck. It occurs in elderly patients, and may be provoked by swallowing and speech.

The ventral roots of C5 to T1 form the brachial plexus. These may be involved in a brachial plexus neuropathy occurring in middle-aged patients, and may have a familial, viral or toxic aetiology. Pain in the shoulder girdle progresses over a few weeks, then resolves spontaneously, but is followed by rapidly progressive patchy sensory and motor loss in the upper limb, which may be bilateral. Recovery takes several months, with 90% complete recovery by 3 years, although the condition may recur. Treatment for this when intractable is problematic. Twenty consecutive patients with intractable pina in the cervical region were treated with a radiofrequency lesion of the dorsal root ganglion on level C4, C5 or C6. Electromyography and sensory evoked potentials were recorded before and 3 weeks after the lesions. Side-effects were studied at 3 weeks, 6 weeks and 3 months afterwards. The most common side-effect was burning pain in the dermatome of the affected nerve root, but except in one patient all these side-effects had disappeared in 6 weeks. They concluded that there were no long term signs of deafferentation but that the pain did tend to recur after 6–9 months.[20] There are now exciting developments in the use of pulsed radiofrequency with the object of treatment without neurological damage.[21]

## Muscles

Muscles can be damaged by occupations where eccentric contractions generate a higher force per active fibre[22] but at a lower metabolic cost than other types of muscle activity.[23] Recent evidence increasingly indicates connective tissue damage,[24] which may cause pain along with the inflammatory process.

### Viral polymyositis
Myalgia is a feature of severe acute viral infection notably by Influenza A and B and Coxsackie A and B. A syndrome of muscle cramps, aching and fatigability has been described and designated 'benign post-infection polymyositis'.[25] The symptoms may persist for 2 years.

### Polymyalgia rheumatica
This affects principally women over the age of 55 years, and it is characterized by pain and stiffness of the proximal muscles of the shoulder girdle. The response to steroids is usually immediate and dramatic.[26]

### Myalgic encephalitis
Myalgic encephalitis is characterized by a diffuse muscle pain, exacerbated by exercise and associated with loss of concentration and sleep disturbance. A proportion of patients relate it

to a viral illness. It occurs most commonly in young to middle aged women.[27] Some patients will recover in a few months whilst others progress to become chronic invalids.[28]

On objective testing there is no evidence of muscle wasting, weakness or abnormal fatigability, due to either central or peripheral mechanisms,[29] neither is there consistent histochemical or metabolic change.

**Treatment**   Treatment consists of graded exercises, although the patients complain that exercise makes it worse,[30] and some benefit has been reported by dietary supplementation with fatty acids.[31]

### Cervical dystonia
Cervical dystonia or spasmodic torticollis is a condition characterized by an intermittent abnormal posturing of the head due to painful involuntary contraction of the neck muscles. It may rarely be secondary to cerebral injury, neurodegenerative disease such as Wilson's disease, or trauma. Onset is most common in middle-aged adults. Rotation of the head commonly occurs due to contraction of sternocleidomastoid, trapezius or splenius, but lateral flexion and extension may also occur.[32] The muscle posture relaxes during sleep. Tremor is also common, occurring in 70% of one series. The disease remits and recurs. Eventually contractures develop, and there is the risk of a secondary radiculopathy or myelopathy.

**Treatment**   Treatment with anticholinergics reduces muscle tone, and surgery can be used to release contractures. However, specific treatment with botulinum toxin (which prevents acetylcholine release) has been shown to cause a marked improvement in 76% of patients in one study.[33] The effects last on average 9 weeks, but have been successfully repeated many times.[34]

## Repetitive strain injury (overuse syndrome)

This is a 'basket' term for pain developing as the consequence of some repetitive occupation. Although changes in muscle biopsy specimens have been reported,[35] there has been no firm confirmation of any neurological or rheumatological abnormalities.[36] Indeed, in large studies, a group of patients always appears who complain of pain in which no abnormalities are found despite exhaustive testing.[37]

It should be suspected in patients who:

• Perform a repetitive task
• Maintain a fixed position for long periods of time
• Lift above or below a mechanically strenuous height
• Perform a tedious monotonous task
• Perform a similar task to one that has caused disability in others.

**Treatment**   Treatment is centred on occupational changes where a full ergonometric assessment of the work station[38] may be indicated. Cognitive behavioural therapy may also be indicated where there are obvious psychological issues.

## Referred pain

### Myofascial pain
The neck and shoulders often contain numerous latent points that result in pain when challenged by physical and emotional stresses. A vicious cycle is set up when pain leads to spasm

in local muscles, leading to ischaemia resulting in changes in the extracellular environment and release of algesic agents, which in turn lead to an increase in motor and sympathetic activity and then other 'trigger points' flare up contributing to the cycle.[39] This often persists even after the initial problem has resolved.

The situation is compounded when tissues damaged by an earlier injury become prone to react to new insults. Thus a patient, who is often older, with an established pool of repeated injuries will be susceptible to experiencing pain out of proportion to any new insult.[40] It is important to note that neck trigger points often are associated with gluteal trigger points even though the patient may be unaware of overt pain in these muscles.

**Treatment**   Treatment consists of injection of local anaesthetics and normal saline with the addition of steroids, the use of vasocoolants and the insertion of a solid needle (dry needling) in order to break the pain cycle.

There is new work being researched in the field of laser therapy and the use of electromagnetic fields.

## Fibromyalgia

Although fibromyalgia is a part of a more widespread pain syndrome, the neck is often involved with trigger points along the sternocleidomastoid and in the nuchal insertions of the splenius muscles into the occiput. The guidelines for diagnosing the condition have been defined at a consensus meeting hosted by the American Society of Rheumatologists, the details of which are dealt with elsewhere in this book.

Briefly, fibromyalgia is associated with disorders of sleep where many patients exhibit an alpha-delta electroencephalogram pattern, which diminishes the restorative stages 3 and 4 of non-REM sleep.[41] There is a correlation between cognitive dysfunction, psychological distress and disturbed sleep in these patients. Psychological disorders per se do not seem to be intrinsically related to the fibromyalgia syndrome, but they may adversely affect coping mechanisms.

**Treatment**   The mainstays of treatment are cognitive behavioural therapy, education and support. Patients need to ensure sleep hygiene (i.e. regularly planned periods of rest during the night rather than during the day) and regular low-grade exercise. Indeed, this is a group of patients who cannot afford NOT to exercise.

Tricyclic antidepressant drugs in low doses can be helpful with disordered sleep, and if there is associated 'restless legs' then L-DOPA can be beneficial. Trigger point injections with local anaesthesia and steroids combined with stretches and physiotherapy, including massage. Lastly, in suitable patients opiates should be considered with appropriate supervision.

**Outcome**   Remission can be variable and depends on an effective multidisciplinary approach to management. Granges *et al.* report a 24% remission rate after 2 years.[42]

## Summary

Pain can be referred to the neck from almost any of the structures in the upper body, in particular from the heart, temporomandibular joints and teeth, or due to malignancy. Differential diagnosis must be made on clinical grounds with referral to the appropriate specialist. However, proven referred pain may still present difficult management problems and result in re-referral to the pain specialist.

Neck pain often arises from structural components or nerves within the neck, and is very common, in part due to the unique relationship between structure and function. Degenerative conditions and trauma are the most frequent causes. Treatment is aimed at symptom relief and improvement of functional ability, with NSAIDs and physiotherapy being mainstays of management, although patient participation in any treatment programme is essential.

# References

1. Wilson PR. Chronic neck pain and cervicogenic headache. *Clin J Pain* 7: 5–11, 1991
2. Conlon PW, Isdale IC, Rose BS. Rheumatoid arthritis of the cervical spine. *Ann Rheum Dis* 25: 120–126, 1966
3. Bogduk N, Mercer S. Biomechanics of the cervical spine.1: Normal kinematics. *Clinical Biomechanics* 15: 633–648, 2000
4. Mercer S, Bogduk N. The ligaments and annulus fibrosus of human adult cervical intervertebral discs. *Spine* 24: 619–626, 2000
5. Bogduk N, Yogonandran N. Biomechanics of the cervical spine Part 3: minor injuries. *Clin Biomechanics* 16: 267–227, 2001
6. Johnson G. Hyperextension soft tissue injuries of the cervical spine – a review. *J Accident Emergency Med* 13: 3–8, 1996
7. Borchgrevik GE, Kaasa A, McDonagh D, Stiles TC, Haraldseth O, Lereim I. Acute treatment of whiplash neck sprain injuries. A randomised trial of treatment during the first 14 days after a car accident. *Spine* 23: 25–31, 1998
8. Lord SM, Barnsley l, Wallis BJ, Bogduk N. Chronic cervical zypoapophyseal joint pain after whiplash. A placebo-controlled prevalence study. *Spine* 21: 1737–1744, 1996
9. Barnsley L, Lord SM, Wallis BJ, Bogduk N. Lack of effect of intraarticular corticosteroids for chronic pain in the cervical zygoapophyseal joints. *N Engl J Med* 330: 1047–1050, 1994;
10. Wallis B, Lord SM, Bogduk N. Resolution of psychological distress of whiplash patients following treatment by radiofrequency neurotomy: a randomised, double-blind, placebo controlled trial. *Pain* 73: 15–22,1997
11. Barendse GA, Van Den Berg SG, Kessles AH, Weber WE, Van Kleef M. Randomised controlled trial of percutaneous intradiscal radiofrequency thermocoagulation for chronic discogenic back pain: lack of effect from a 90-second 70°C lesion. *Spine* 26: 287–292, 2001
12. Wallis BJ, Lord SM, Barnsley L, Bogduk N. The psychological profiles of patients with whiplash-associated headache. *Cephalgia* 18: 101–105, 1998
13. Hurwitz El, Aker PD, Adams AH, Meeker WC, Shekelle PG. Manipulation and mobilisation of the cervical spine. A systematic review of the literature. *Spine* 21: 1746–1759, 1996
14. Koes BW, Assendelft WJ, Van der Heijden GL, Bouter LM, Knipschild PG. Spinal manipulation and mobilisation for back and neck pain: a blinded review. *Br Med J* 303: 1298–1303, 1991
15. Aker PD, Gross AR, Goldsmith CH, Peloso P. Conservative management of mechanical neck pain: systematic overview and meta-analysis. *Br Med J* 313: 1291–1296, 1996
16. Muller-Fassbender H, Bach GL Haase W, et al. Glucosamine sulfate compared to ibuprofen in osteoarthritis of the knee. *Osteoarthritis Cartilage* 2: 61–69, 1994
17. Mathews JA. Atlanto-axial subluxation in rheumatoid arthritis – a 5 year follow up. *Ann Rheum Dis* 33: 526–531, 1974
18. Brunton RW, Grennan DM, Palmer DG, de Silva RTA. Lateral subluxation of the atlas in rheumatoid arthritis. Br J Radiol 51: 963–967, 1978
19. Duthie JR, Thompson M, Wier MM, Fletcher WB. Medical and social aspects of the treatment of rheumatoid arthritis with special reference to factors affecting prognosis. *Ann Rheum Dis* 14: 133–149, 1955
20. Van Kleef M, Spaans F, Dingemans W, Barendse GA, Floor E, Sliujter ME. Effects and side effects of a percutaneous thermal lesion of the dorsal root ganglion in patients with cervical pain syndrome. *Pain* 52: 49–53, 1993
21. Higuchi Y, Nashold BS Jr, Sliujter ME, Cosman E, Pearlstein RD. Exposure of the dorsal root ganglion in rats to pulsed radiofrequency currents activates dorsal horn lamina 1 and 11 neurons. *Neurosurgery* 50: 850–855. 2002

22. Abbott BC, Bigland B, Ritchie JM. The physiological cost of negative work. *J Physiol* **117**: 380–390, 1952
23. Menard MR, Penn AM, Lee JE, Dusik LA, Hall LD. Relative metabolic efficiency of concentric and eccentric exercise determined by 31P magnetic resonance spectroscopy. Arch Phys Med Rehab **72**: 976–983, 1991
24. Brown SJ, Child RB, Day SH, Donnelly A. Indices of skeletal muscle damage and connective tissue breakdown following eccentric muscle contractions. *Eur J Appl Physiol* **75**: 369–374, 1997
25. Schwartz MS, Swash M, Gross M. Benign post-infection polymyositis. *Br Med J* **2**: 1256–1257, 1978
26. Bird HA, Esselinck W, Dixon A StJ, Mowat AG, Wood PHN. An evaluation of the criteria for polymyalgia rheumatica. *Ann Rheum Dis* **38**: 424–439, 1979
27. Behan PO, Bakheit AMO. Clinical spectrum of post-viral fatigue syndrome. In: Behan PO, Goldberg DP, Mowbray JF, eds. Post viral fatigue syndrome. *Br Med Bull* **47**: 793–809, 1991
28. Wessely S, Newham DJ. Virus syndromes and chronic fatigue. In: Vaeroy H, Merskey H, eds. *Pain Research and Clinical Management, Vol 6. Progress in fibromyalgia and myofascial pain.* Elsevier, Amsterdam, pp. 349–360
29. Rutherford OM, White J. Human quadriceps strength and fatigability in patients with post-viral syndrome. *J Neurol Neurosurg Psychiatry* **54**: 961–964, 1991
30. Edwards RHT. Muscle fatigue and pain. *Acta Medica Scand (suppl)* **711**: 179–188, 1986
31. Behan PO, Behan WM, Horrobin D. Effects of high doses of essential fatty acids on the post viral fatigue syndrome. *Acta Neurol Scand* **82**: 209–216, 1990
32. Jankovic J, Leder S, Warner D, Schwartz K. Cervical Dystonia: clinical findings and associated movement disorders. *Neurology* **41**: 1088–1091, 1991
33. Anderson TJ, Rivest J, Stell R, et al. Botulinum toxin treatment of spasmodic torticollis. *J Royal Soc Med* **85**: 524–529, 1992
34. Poewe W, Schelosky L, Kleedorfer B, Heinen F, Wagner M, Deuschl G. Treatment of spasmodic torticollis with local injections of botulinum toxin. One year follow-up in 37 patients. *J Neurol* **239**: 21–25, 1992
35. Fry HJH. Overuse syndrome of the upper limb in musicians. *Med J Austral* **144**: 182–185, 1986
36. Barton NJ, Hooper G, Noble J, Steel WM. Occupational causes of disorders in the upper limb. *Br Med J* **304**: 309–311, 1992
37. Simons DG, Manse S. Understanding muscle tone as related to clinical muscle pain. *Pain* **75**: 1–17, 1998
38. Khalil T, Abdel-Moty E, Steele-Rosomoff R, Rosomoff H. The role of ergonomics in the prevention and treatment of myofascial pain. In: Rachlin ES, ed. *Myofascial pain and fibromyalgia.* St Louis, Mosby, 1994
39. Zimmerman M. Peripheral and central nervous mechanisms of nociception, pain and pain therapy: facts and hypothesis. P.3 In: Bonica JJ, Liebeskind JC, Albe-Fressard DG, eds. *Advances in Pain Research and Therapy. Vol 3.* Philadelphia, Lippincott Raven, 1980, p.3
40. Sola AE. Treatment of myofascial pain syndromes. In: Benedetti, Chapman R and Moricca G et al, eds. *Advances in Pain Research and Therapy.* New York, Raven Press. p. 13, 1984
41. Drewes AM, Gade K, Nielsem KD, et al. Clustering of sleep electroencephalographic patterns in patients with the fibromyalgia syndrome. *Br J Rheumatol* **34**: 1151–1156, 1995
42. Granges G, Zilko P, Littlejohn GO. Fibromyalgia syndrome: assessment of the severity of the condition 2 years after diagnosis. *J Rheumatol* **21**: 523–529, 1994

# 12 Thoracic Pain

## Jane Hazelgrove and Peter Rogers

Thoracic pain is a neglected area; it could be classified in many ways. One difficulty in considering a classification is that thoracic pain is an extremely heterogenous group of conditions, including many syndromes involving pain referred from beyond the thoracic region.

Pain can arise from the chest wall, viscera within the chest, the vertebral column and related structures, or be referred from above or below the thorax.

An immediate area of concern is to ensure the patient's pain is not potentially life-threatening, such as an expanding aortic aneurysm or angina pectoris, which require urgent specialist referral. Symptoms that should alert the clinician are predictable, but necessitate a thorough clinical history and examination:

- Fever, chills, sweats
- Lymphadenopathy
- Weight loss
- Bruits, significant murmurs or pericardial rub
- Angina on exertion or at rest
- Pain localized to a single site and worsening
- Limitation of chest movement
- Pain radiating to the mid-thoracic spine
- Pain radiating to the axilla, left or both arms, neck
- Haemoptysis
- Unexpected laboratory findings.

The International Association for the Study of Pain (IASP) has developed a classification system.[1] This system is useful as an internationally accepted classification of disease entity, so all pain physicians refer to the same disease process. The authors feel that a classification corresponding to the fifth axis of the IASP code, i.e. aetiology, is more practically helpful when discussing thoracic pain in particular.

It is impossible to be comprehensive, but an attempt will be made to cover the more commonly encountered conditions.

## Musculoskeletal syndromes

### Thoracic facet pain

Pain arising from the thoracic facet joints is often poorly localized and dull in nature. It tends to be paravertebral, extending laterally as far as the posterior axillary line and inferiorly for up to two and a half segments lower than the pathological level. It is exacerbated by rotation and extension of the back. Pain from the thoracocervical junction and upper thoracic joints tends to be more dispersed, with much overlap radiating around upper limb girdle and down to inferior edge of the scapula. Pain from thoracolumbar joints radiates out to the iliac crest. The condition is often secondary to disc degeneration, vertebral collapse and scoliosis. The radiological existence of Schmorl's nodes or Scheuermann's disease is thought to predispose to early degenerative changes. Pain referral patterns from provocative intra-articular injections have been described in detail.[2,3]

If conservative therapy fails then the sequence of diagnostic blockade of the joints followed by radiofrequency (RF) lesioning of the medial branches of the posterior primary rami (MBPPR) at segments above and below the joint would lead to improvement in symptoms. It was thought that the MBPPR ran at the junction of the superior articular facets and the transverse process. This assumption was proved to be wrong by an anatomical study[4].

The MBPPR arise 5 mm from the lateral margin of the intervertebral foramina. They pass dorsally, inferiorly but mainly laterally leaving the intertransverse space and crossing the superolateral corner of the transverse process before ramifying onto the multifidus muscle. The upper thoracic MBPPRs have a small cutaneous distribution. At T11 and T12 the relations are more like the lumbar region (i.e. at the junction of the superior articular facet and transverse process). There are no randomized double-blind controlled studies concerning blockade or denervation of the thoracic facets. Studies to date have used erroneous anatomy, whereby the needle placements have been up to 11 mm away from the nerves. However, reasonable results have been obtained.[5] Present feeling is that with such soft anatomical landmarks the nerves need to be located by electrostimulation. The most recent description is still quite vague in that a 22g, 10.5 cm Sluijter-Mehta cannula with a 5 mm active tip is placed 'some millimetres' lateral to the junction of the superior articular process and the transverse process. Localization by passing a current at 50 Hz should give paravertebral tingling at less than 1 V. Paravertebral muscle twitching should be observed by stimulating at 2 Hz at less than 1 V. Lesions are made at 80°C for 60 seconds.

## Costovertebral and costotransverse joint pain

Little is known about the pathology of these joints. There are no clinical studies. Pain from these joints is likely to be similar to facet joint pain; it can be sharp and stabbing. Innervation of the costovertebral joints is from the sympathetic chain and continuation of the nerve plexi of the anterior longitudinal ligament. The costotransverse joints have supply from the lateral branches of the posterior primary rami.

There is no evidence base for diagnosis or treatment. Standard conservative measures, reassurance and local joint injections have all been tried with varying results.

## Intervertebral disc and segmental thoracic pain

The incidence of intervertebral disc protrusion increases towards the lower end of the thoracic spine, with the last mobile segment above the thoracolumbar junction most common.[6] Thoracic prolapsed intervertebral disc disease is relatively rare, and it is typically associated with radicular symptoms but also with myelopathy. Patients usually recover spontaneously. The injection of steroids into the thoracic epidural space is thought to be therapeutic, but it has not been evaluated formally. Surgical management is only required in 2% of cases.

## Benign thoracic pain

This condition affects young women. They complain of pain and tenderness in the midthoracic spine, which radiates around the chest wall. Typically pain is in the interscapular region, and there may be associated skin hyperaesthesia. The pain is worse on movement.

A magnetic resonance imaging (MRI) study in 1989 found 90% of the patients had evidence of intervertebral disc dehydration with no evidence of prolapse.[7] They suggested that impaired shock absorption could be a cause of the pain. Treatment is conservative with reassurance.

## Fybromyalgia and trigger points

The American College of Rheumatology criteria for diagnosis stipulated pain on palpation in 11 of 18 tender point sites. Six of these sites are related to the chest wall, i.e. second rib at the costochondral junction. Pain is widespread and is associated with fatigue, morning stiffness, sleep disorders, paraesthesia, headaches, depression and anxiety. There are no specific laboratory abnormalities; it is generally encountered in middle age with a preponderance of females. There may be a genetic predisposition; a neuroendocrine deficiency is suspected with decreased cortisol, 5-hydroxytryptamine (5-HT; serotonin) and growth hormone production.[8] Autonomic dysfunction exists with decreased cholinergic tone and impaired catecholamine production.

Treatments include graduated physiotherapy or hydrotherapy, aerobic exercises, improving sleeping habits, pain management programmes, tender point injections, tricyclic antidepressants, non-steroidal anti-inflammatory drugs (NSAIDs), sex hormones and decreased carbohydrate intake. Patients often find reference to the Internet useful.

## Myofascial pain syndromes

There are a variety of specific myofascial pain syndromes that cause subacute or chronic chest wall pain. They present with tenderness, trigger points, stiffness, muscle spasm, limitation of movement and, occasionally, autonomic dysfunction. They develop gradually and often cause anxiety as they are perceived by the patient to be of a serious nature. They are often the result of poor posture, continuous or repetitive movements. Examples include:[9]

- Pectoralis major muscle syndrome
- Serratus anterior muscle syndrome
- Sternalis syndrome
- Precordial catch syndrome – sharp catch/stitch in precordial area/apex that is worse on deep breathing. The aetiology is unknown and exercise may improve symptoms.

### Treatment
- Reassurance
- Local anaesthetic (LA) and steroid injections
- Hot packs
- Progressive stretching exercises
- Trigger point injections
- Elimination of overuse of the muscle.

## Slipping rib syndrome/twelfth rib syndrome

Slipping rib syndrome presents as a dull ache, or an intermittent stabbing pain. It is associated with hypermobility of the anterior end of a costal cartilage of the 8th, 9th or 10th ribs.[1] There may be a history of minor trauma or repetitive constrained movements. The costal cartilage slips superiorly, impinging on the intercostal nerve. Classically, hooking the cartilage forwards may reproduce pain with a click. In the authors experience, tenderness on manipulation of the ribs is more common. Movement such as rotation or flexion of the thorax aggravates the pain. It is important to exclude gastrointestinal disease and psychiatric disorders.

Twelfth rib syndrome is a similar condition to slipping rib syndrome. There is loin pain with sharp attacks often radiating to the groins. As above, movement aggravates it. Manipulation of the 11th or 12th ribs can reproduce the pain.

Practically, these two syndromes cause similar symptoms, which tend to pursue an indefinite course.

## Treatment

- Reassurance and simple analgesia
- Avoid provocative postural movements
- Local anaesthetic ± steroid injected into the costochondral junction or intercostal nerves (these may be diagnostic or therapeutic)
- Neurolytic or differential neural blockade with 5% lignocaine, pulsed radio frequency lesioning, cryolysis or phenol applied to the intercostals, paravertebral nerves or dorsal root ganglion (DRG)
- Rib excision preserving the intercostal nerve.

There is no evidence base for any treatment.

## Costosternal syndrome

Costosternal syndrome is a relatively common cause of chest pain especially in women, and needs to be distinguished from cardiac pain. It is of unknown origin but could be related to overuse. Pain or tenderness is found on palpation of one or more of the costosternal joints (typically 2nd to 5th). It can present similarly to Tietze's syndrome (see below), but without the swelling.

## Xiphodynia

Xiphodynia is a spontaneous anterior chest wall pain with tenderness of the xiphisternum. It is of unknown aetiology, and usually disappears spontaneously without any specific treatment over weeks or months. Treatments include local anaesthetic injections and analgesics. Very rarely, surgical excision is required.

## Forestier's disease or DISH syndrome

In Forestier's disease, or DISH syndrome (diffuse idiopathic skeletal hyperostosis), there is ligamentous calcification especially of the anterior longitudinal ligament, although the posterior longitudinal ligament can be involved.

Distinctive radiographical changes occur, such as osteophytes entering the ligaments and joining up with osteophytes from above. The facet joints and intervertebral discs are spared. Spinal cord compression and fractures can occur, possibly necessitating interventional therapy.

## Referred musculoskeletal pain

Cervical disc disease and degenerative changes at the cervicothoracic junction can refer pain to the chest or mimic angina.

# Inflammatory syndromes

## Ankylosing spondylitis

Ankylosing spondylitis (AS) progresses to involve the thoracic spine. The thoracolumbar junction is frequently involved. The disease process involves both synovial and cartilaginous joints, as well as sites of tendon and ligamentous attachment. The involvement of costal joints often causes painful inspiration with limited thoracic expansion. Treatments include analgesics and physiotherapy.

## Tietze's syndrome

Tietze's syndrome is an uncommon though well known condition of unknown aetiology. It can be acute or chronic, presenting as a firm to hard painful swelling of the 2nd or 3rd costochondral junction (usually a single lesion). The pain is worse on inspiration and lying prone. The swelling distinguishes it from other chest wall syndromes. Laboratory investigations are usually negative. Treatments include analgesics (e.g. NSAIDs), local anaesthetic with steroid injections, and physiotherapy. The condition is usually self-limiting dissipating after a few years; rib biopsy can be required for reassurance.

## Rheumatoid arthritis

Rheumatoid arthritis is mentioned here only for completeness. It is far more common in the cervical and lumbar spine.

# Metabolic syndromes

## Osteoporosis

The risk of developing a fracture after 50 years of age is 40% in women and 15% in men, (the lifetime fracture risk). These fractures result in pain that tends to subside after a few months. Any secondary degenerative changes can of course prolong the duration of symptoms. A diagnosis of osteoporosis (OP) is not always obvious, and measurement of bone mineral density is required. Radiographically, the presence of deformed vertebrae is more reliable for the diagnosis than the appearance of apparent low density bones.

### Treatment
Treatment is two-fold: firstly, the prevention of further fractures and, secondly, symptomatic pain relief. It includes:

- Hormone replacement therapy (HRT)
- Biphosphonates (etidronate, alendronate, risedronate)
- Raloxifene
- Testosterone therapy – men
- Calcium/vitamin D (calcitriol)
- Calcitonin
- Epidural steroids
- Vertebroplasty.

Bone formation can be stimulated with parathyroid hormone (daily injections).

## Paget's disease

Paget's disease is a disorder resulting in bone remodelling, and it rarely occurs in the thoracic vertebrae. There is increased osteoclastic activity, but there is an overall weakening of the spine, and vertebral collapse may occur. Increases in bone bulk can cause radicular pain and spinal stenosis. Treatment is with bisphosphonates, which inhibit mature osteoclast activity, thus reducing the rate of bone resorption.

# Malignancy

In the UK, over 35 000 people die each year from bronchial carcinoma – the third most common cause of death and increasing in women. Pain is a presenting feature in approximately 37%. It is often described as fullness within the chest, however, it can be pleuritic with invasion of the ribs/pleura. Severity can increase such that opioids become ineffective. Two-thirds of patients with metastatic disease have pain, skeletal metastases being the most common. The specialist pain management decisions are based on the nature and origin of the pain (e.g. neuropathic or bone pain).

Malignant chest pain usually presents in three ways. There may be local invasion of ribs and/or pleura and/or intercostal nerves, (formally referred to as costopleural syndrome). There may be local infiltration of other bones or vertebral secondary deposits. Finally, there can be a brachial plexus infiltration such as in Pancoast's syndrome.

Wide ranges of cancerous conditions causing thoracic pain are referred to pain management specialists (Table 12.1).

## Mesothelioma

Mesothelioma accounts for 1300 deaths per year in the UK. The incidence is likely to increase until 2025. The median survival from presentation is 12–18 months. Patients usually present with pain and breathlessness. The pain is often difficult to manage. Radiotherapy can decrease pain intensity, but it does not prolong survival. Early recourse to interventional treatment is recommended. Although intrathecal or intercostal phenol has been used, the most consistently successful treatment is percutaneous cordotomy.

## Other sources of invasion of the chest wall

Other lung tumours can invade the pleural cavity and chest wall, as can breast and rib tumours. Adenocarcinoma is the most common lung tumour that invades the chest wall.

| Table 12.1 Tumours resulting in thoracic pain | |
| --- | --- |
| Primary tumours | Secondary tumours |
| Mesothelioma | Lung metastases |
| Lung carcinoma, especially bronchial (including Pancoast's tumour) | |
| Vertebral lymphoma | Vertebral metastases |
| Vertebral haemangioma | |
| Breast cancer | |
| Oesophageal/abdominal tumours | |
| Multiple myeloma | Other bone metastases (e.g. ribs) |

Very severe chest and back pain will often require escalating doses of opioids. This pain is notoriously difficult to manage, and many pharmacological and interventional techniques have been applied to such patients. Tumour invasion of intercostal nerves can result in neuropathic pain.

## Treatment

Pharmacological:

- NSAIDs ± codeine
- Tricyclics
- Anticonvulsants
- Strong opioids/slow release preparations.

Interventions include:

- Radiotherapy
- Intercostal nerve blockade (including neurolytic)
- Paravertebral nerve block*
- Interpleural catheters*
- Intrathecal opiates/implantable delivery pumps
- Intrathecal phenol*
- Stellate ganglion blockade
- Cordotomy.*

*These interventions are discussed in detail below.

## Pancoast's syndrome

Pancoast's syndrome is most commonly due to squamous cell or adenocarcinoma arising from the superior pulmonary sulcus. Any apical tumour can result in the symptoms described below. Invasion of the inferior parts of brachial plexus occurs as it passes from the neck to the arm. In particular, the lower nerve roots are involved, i.e. C7, C8, T1 and T2. In addition to severe pain, the patient reports weakness and pain in the shoulder and arm (especially in the ulnar nerve territory). The forearm and medial border of the hand are especially affected. There may be features of hyperpathia and dysaesthesia. It may be associated with a Horner's syndrome. There can be phrenic nerve and recurrent laryngeal nerve involvement, the latter causing a hoarse voice. Spinal cord compression can occur. The locality of the tumour implies it is inoperable. The pain is notoriously difficult to treat – 80–100% of patients report pain, which occurs early (deep, aching) and may become severely neuralgic and incapacitating.

Breast carcinoma primaries and radiotherapy can also cause brachial plexopathy.

## Treatment

Pharmacological:

- NSAIDs ± codeine
- Tricyclics
- Anticonvulsants
- Strong opioids/slow release morphine.

Interventions:

- Neurolytic blocks (phenol/alcohol) including brachial plexus

- Cervicothoracic sympathetic blocks
- Cordotomy*
- Dorsal root entry zone (DREZ) lesioning
- Intrathecal opioids
- Intrathecal phenol/alcohol.*

*These interventions are discussed in detail below.

## Vertebral tumours and metastases causing pain/collapse/pathological fractures[10–12]

The most common primary tumours associated with boney metastases are those of breast, lung, prostate, thyroid and kidney, and myeloma. Primary tumours of the vertebrae are rare, haemangiomas being the most common. Metastases usually present as localized pain with or without radicular symptoms. Vertebral collapse may result in nerve entrapment or spinal cord compression. Hypercalcaemia is often an additional problem. Diagnosis can prove difficult as vertebral bodies can appear radiographically normal with as much as 50% bone loss. Bone scans and MRI are more useful.

### Treatment
Pharmacological:

- Conventional analgesics
- Oral biphosphonates – delay the progression of osteolytic bone lesions, decrease pain, reduce hypercalcaemia and hypercalciuria
- Disodium clodrinate.

Interventions:

- Epidural steroid/phenol
- Paravertebral nerve blocks*
- Percutaneous vertebroplasty*
- Palliative radiotherapy.

*These interventions are discussed in detail below.

Radiotherapy is effective for treating painful boney metastases that do not respond to analgesics – it is said that up to 80% of patients achieve substantial pain relief.[12] Radiotherapy may prevent pathological fracture by treating osteolytic lesions, and is the treatment of choice in spinal cord compression.[13]

## Radiotherapy pain

Side-effects of radiotherapy are usually restricted to localized site. Late complications of radiotherapy include damage to the peripheral and central nervous system, resulting in plexopathy, neuropathy and spinal cord damage. Treatment is with antidepressants and anticonvulsants.

## Breast cancer pain

Breast cancer pain is a rare presenting symptom of breast cancer – only 7% of breast cancer patients have mastalgia as their only symptom.

# Iatrogenic causes of pain

## Post-surgical pain

In a recent UK epidemiological study from Northern Britain, surgery was found to contribute to pain in 22% of patients attending chronic pain clinics.[14]

## Post breast surgery pain

Wide variations in incidence of post breast surgery pain are quoted, 1 year after surgery[15] (Table 12.2).

Pain occurs along the breast scar, anterior chest wall, in the axilla and ipsilateral arm. It is intermittent and described as tender, aching, stabbing, sharp or shooting. It is also often movement related, which accounts for an increased incidence of frozen shoulder observed following breast surgery.

The mechanisms of pain production are not fully understood. Possibly the most common cause in post-mastectomy syndrome is injury to the intercostobrachial nerve. This is a branch of the second intercostal nerve that supplies the axilla and medial upper arm. Complex regional pain syndrome (CRPS) type II has been reported. Radiation-induced plexopathy or neuritis are encountered. Long thoracic, thoracodorsal and lateral and medial pectoral nerves may also be injured at surgery or be compressed by implants. Dysaesthetic scar pain due to deafferentation, mechanosensitivity, neuromas and axonal sprouting also occur. Tissue and nerve ischaemia, lymphoedema, capsule formation and scarring are additional mechanisms. Many post-mastectomy patients become depressed, which exacerbates symptoms.

### Treatment
- Clear instructions to move shoulder (make circles with elbow)
- Amitriptyline
- Capsaicin
- Simple analgesics
- Anticonvulsants (gabapentin)
- Transcutaneous electrical nerve stimulation (TENS)
- Intercostal cryolysis, DRG lesions

## Post-thoracotomy pain (PTP)

Post-thoracotomy pain (PTP) is common some time following surgery (e.g. 1 month). Usually this pain subsides over the first year, although mild residual pain is often present. Richardson *et al.* found particular risk factors included lower thoracic incisions for benign oesophageal disease, and chest drain insertion, whilst rib removal for accessing the thorax

| Table 12.2 Incidence of post breast surgery pain 1 year after surgery | |
|---|---|
| Procedure | Incidence |
| Mastectomy | 31% |
| Mastectomy and reconstruction | 49% (mainly with implants: submuscular > subglandular) |
| Breast reduction | 22% |
| Breast augmentation | 38% |

reduced the risk of pain.[16] Katz *et al.* found aggressive successful management or early post-operative pain reduced the risk of long-term PTP.[17] It is likely that intercostal nerve damage may contribute to the syndrome as sensory changes correlate with the emergence of PTP, indicating a neuropathic element.[18] Some patients report changes in sudomotor and skin blood flow changes implicating involvement of the sympathetic nervous system.[19]

## Treatment
- Analgesics and conservative therapy
- TENS
- Sympathectomy[20]
- Interpleural catheter insertion*
- Stereotactic RF dorsal root gangliolysis.

* Intervention discussed below.

## Pain following sternotomy and internal mammary artery dissection

Sternotomy scar pain is not common. It is often associated with hyperalgesia of the skin. Occasionally, there is localised discomfort from wires. The latter condition is extremely rare. Nerve injury occurring during arterial dissection is the likely cause.

# Infective

## Post-herpetic neuralgia

Post-herpetic neuralgia is dealt with in more detail in Chapter 22. It is a condition affecting the older population. Treatments commonly are instigated in the Primary Care setting. Refractory cases are referred for advanced pain management techniques.

## Treatment
Pharmacological:

- First line
  - Antiviral medication
  - Amitriptyline
- Second line
  - Anticonvulsants (carbamazepine, gabapentin)
  - Capsaicin cream
  - Lignocaine 5% patches
- Others
  - Interpleural catheter*
  - Paravertebral block*
  - RF of the DRG
  - Intercostal nerve block (including neurolytic agents).*

*These interventions are discussed below.

## Bornholm's disease (epidemic pleurodynia, epidemic myalgia)

Bornholm's disease can affect patients of any age, although children and young adults are more commonly affected by this acute infection caused by the Coxsackie B virus. They report severe epigastric or lower thoracic pain. It is easily diagnosed during an epidemic – sporadic cases are more of a challenge. Treatment is symptomatic, symptoms quickly resolve.

# Visceral

Patients with chest pain are often extremely anxious and much reassurance is required. Cardiac and oesophageal disease can mimic each other, and can often coexist. The close proximity of the heart and oesophagus adds to the occasional difficulty in differentiation. Exercise-induced chest pain, radiating to the arms, jaw etc, or the presence of significant risk factors, should lead to a cardiac series of investigations first (common sense dictates).

## Angina

Angina is included here for completeness and to emphasize its importance. The reader is referred to Chapter 25.

## Oesophageal pain

Oesophageal pain tends to be central, radiating through to the back. Reflux symptoms tend to respond to advice, such as stopping NSAIDs, losing weight, or taking antacids/proton pump inhibitors etc.

Nutcracker oesophagus and diffuse oesophageal dysmotility can result in severe pain. Diagnosis can be very difficult and is usually one of exclusion. Oesophageal tonometry can help, and specialist centres offer 24-hour recording. Treatment is usually with glyceryl trinitrate, calcium channel blockade or stelazine. It can be associated with other chronic pain conditions such as irritable bowel syndrome or fibromyalgia.

### Other treatment
- Tricyclic antidepressants
- Psychology
- Balloon dilation.

Anticholinergics are not useful.

## Referred pain

Thoracic pain may be referred from the abdomen (e.g. gall bladder, pancreas, peptic ulcer etc.). The shoulder girdle muscles derive innervation from the cervical region. Pain originating from the cervical or shoulder region, can be perceived in the pectoral or periscapular region.

# Psychological disorders

A significant proportion of referrals to chest clinics do not have significant ischaemic heart disease.[21] Non-cardiac organic causes, such as those discussed in this chapter, must be excluded. There remain those patients who suffer emotional disorders, which may be associated with functional symptoms. Such conditions include depression, extreme anxiety or panic attacks, which may have been triggered by very stressful life events. Signs of depression include hopelessness, poor sleep, lack of interest or concentration, irritability etc. It is worth exploring what the patient believes to be the cause of their pain, and try to establish what they think about when the pain occurs. This can expose abnormal health beliefs. These patients with non-cardiac chest pain must be treated promptly as they often rapidly develop substantial disability. In addition, the treatment must be appropriate. The belief that they have ischaemic heart disease is supported by the medical profession prescribing anti-anginal medication and referring them to specialist units. This reinforces the concept of this being a life-threatening condition. Consequently, reassurance and counselling is important from the outset of contact, as is a full explanation of actions taken. Once cardiac causes have been excluded, some patients will improve. Others, especially those with more severe symptoms, may need following up. They may require referral for psychological opinion if they are depressed, especially anxious, suffer panic attacks or have abnormal health beliefs. Treatment approaches include cognitive behavioural therapy and medication (5-HT reuptake inhibitors, tricyclic antidepressants).

# Specific treatments referred to in text above

## Cordotomy (cervical percutaneous cordotomy)

Cordotomy is the ablation by radiofrequency lesions, of the pain fibres in the spinothalamic tract in the anterolateral column of the white matter of the spinal cord. The procedure leads to loss of pain and temperature sensibility on the side contralateral to the lesion. This is because incoming sensory fibres decussate within a few segments of entering the spinal cord. The tract is located by advancing a needle under X-ray control at the anterior portion of the C1/2 space. Cerebrospinal fluid (CSF) is obtained on penetration of the dura. The dentate ligament is outlined using a water-soluble dye. An electrode is placed through the needle anterior to the dentate ligament. The impedance in CSF is approximately 350 $\Omega$. As the electrode is advanced into the spinothalamic tract, the impedance is seen to rise to above 1000 $\Omega$.

Correct needle placement must be confirmed as follows. Electrical stimulation at 100 Hz should produce contralateral sensations, and at 2 Hz should produce no ipsilateral motor stimulation. The lesion(s) are then made. Almost 90% of patients have effective relief of unilateral pain.

Complications, although uncommon, include ipsilateral weakness, bladder dysfunction, spinal headache, occipital neuralgia and respiratory difficulties.

Death in the first week after cordotomy is 1–4%. This usually occurs when patients are treated too late in the course of their malignancy. If the patient is likely to live for more than 18 months, there is a likelihood of serious dysaesthesia (anaesthesia dobrosa).

## Percutaneous vertebroplasty

Percutaneous vertebroplasty was first described in the mid-1980s in France. It is an effective treatment for lesions of the vertebral body, and it is usually offered following a multidisciplinary discussion.

### Indications:
- Osteolytic metastasis
- Multiple myeloma
- Painful or aggressive vertebral haemangiomas
- Fibrous dysplasia of vertebral body
- Osteoporotic vertebral collapse
- Vertebral lymphoma.

Dion describes the lifetime risk of a vertebral fracture for white women in the USA to be 16%, and 5% for men.[22] Most vertebral fractures are said to occur between T8 and L2. The technique is still evolving but, essentially, an 11-gauge bone trocar is advanced, with fluoroscopy or computed tomography (CT) guidance, along the pedicle, into the anterior third of the vertebral body. Venography is often performed to give an indication of the likely spread of the bone cement. Methyl methacrylate cement is prepared and mixed with barium powder. This is injected using 1 ml syringes until the vertebra is filled. Lately, custom-made devices are available for this purpose. It may require up to 5 ml cement. Timing is critical as the operator has approximately 5–7 minutes before the cement sets. Lateral views of the spine are recommended to ensure that the cement is not leaking into the epidural space or intervertebral foramina.

Dramatic improvements in debilitating pain can be seen in more than 80% of patients over 2 or 3 days. There is strengthening of the vertebral body itself. In addition, kyphoscoliosis development is prevented, there is an improvement in quality of life and a reduction in analgesics used. The mechanism of analgesia is not yet clear, and a direct heating effect on nerves is a possibility. The procedure is not without it's risks, including:

- Leakage of the methyl methacrylate
- Compression of the spinal cord requiring emergency decompression – risk in osteoporotic patients < cancer patients (1% and 5–10% respectively).
- Disc space leakage, anterior epidural leakage, foraminal leaks, paravertebral leaks
- Infection, osteomyelitis
- Pulmonary embolus
- Rib fractures.

When vertebroplasty is used for pathological fractures/vertebral collapse that is secondary to malignancy, concurrent radiation therapy is given as tumour growth continues despite cement injection.

## Interpleural catheters

Interpleural blockade is used acutely for postoperative pain and fractured ribs. The longer-term use as intermittent injections or infusions in hospital or in a home setting has proven useful for post-herpetic neuralgia and upper limb CRPS.

Advanced cancer patients with less than 3 months to live have also benefited when conventional techniques have failed. Success has been reported in brachial plexopathies, and invasive wall tumours when the pain is unilateral, and also in patients with oesophageal cancer pain.

Using fluoroscopy an 18-gauge Tuohy needle is used to contact the 7th or 8th rib at, or just lateral to, its posterior angle. The needle is directed off the superior edge of the rib and a loss-of-resistance technique is employed to locate the interpleural space. A reinforced catheter is advanced 10 cm into the space. Tunnelling is optional. Analgesia is obtained by infusion of intermittent injections of local anaesthetic. Phenol has also been used to good effect. Injections are made in the lateral position with the patient bad side up. For plexopathies, a higher level of injection is chosen and these are performed as before, but with the patient in a head-down position. Complications include pneumothorax (<5%), Horner's syndrome, infection, phrenic nerve blockade and local anaesthetic toxicity.

Pleural phenol therapy has been reported for the treatment of terminal chronic oesophageal cancer pain.

## Subarachnoid phenol

Dogliotti first described subarachnoid chemical neurolysis over 70 years ago.[23] Pain relief is achieved with segmental neurolysis using either hypobaric alcohol or hyperbaric phenol. In the peripheries, careful positioning is required in an attempt to block the sensory branch and not the motor branch of the somatic nerves involved. This is not so critical in the thoracic region as the loss of a few intercostal nerves is not as serious as losing lumbar or sacral nerve roots.

Suitable patients are those who have an established diagnosis of cancer pain. The life expectancy should be less than 1 year, and the pain should be unresponsive to radiotherapy, chemotherapy and the World Health Organization analgesic policy. The pain should be unilateral, and localized to two to three dermatomes, or possibly sclerotomes. Informed consent should be obtained.

Increased accuracy and better results have been obtained in the thoracic region by Naguro *et al.* using fluoroscopy.[24] The patient is placed in the lateral position with the painful side dependent. A lateral approach is made with a spinal needle with the point angled downwards towards the segments to be blocked. Hyperbaric water-soluble radio-opaque dye is injected so that the spread of the dye can be adjusted by the tilt of the operating table. The object is for the dye to remain at the targeted level. Phenol in 10% glycerine (0.2 ml) is injected at one or more levels. The patient remains in this position for at least 30 minutes. The success rate was 85%. It is difficult to establish success rate for intrathecal neurolysis as different investigators have used different tools to gauge success. However, overall, 75% of patients should have beneficial effects.[25] Complications are unusual at the thoracic level, but would include all those discussed in Chapter 29.

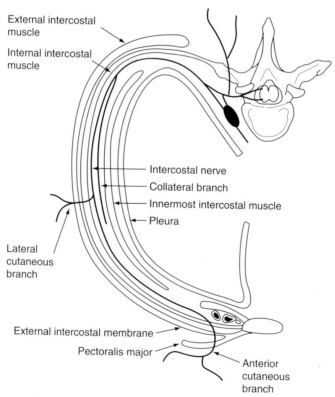

Figure 12.1 Intercostal nerve

## Intercostal and paravertebral nerve blockades

Used diagnostically, intercostal and paravertebral nerve blockades can help distinguish abdominal wall pain from visceral pain. Using fluoroscopy, these blocks can define the exact segments of the painful pathology (Figure 12.1). Rarely do they give long-term benefit, and some form of neurolytic block is anticipated. Indications include rib metastases, tumour infiltration of the chest wall, 12th rib and slipping rib syndromes, and some painful postsurgical scar pains. There is an incidence of neuritis following neurolysis, so it is the authors' practice to start by using lignocaine 5% and progressing via cryolysis to phenol blocks.

Lignocaine 5% has been shown to have neurolytic properties, and case reports have shown that refractory cases of post-herpetic neuralgia have obtained up to 9 months of pain relief.

Cryolysis of the intercostal nerves is unreliable and cumbersome. The anatomy of the intercostal nerves is quite variable with much more branching than is generally appreciated. The classical subcostal position of the nerve is relatively uncommon.[26] The authors find more consistent anatomy paravertebrally, where the nerve can be frozen in the superior part of the intervertebral foreman. Neuritis is not a frequent problem following cryolysis. Phenol tends to be used intercostally for malignant pain. For safety and accuracy, needles are placed subcostally under X-ray control at the posterior angle of the rib. Radio-opaque dye can help precision and location. A 6% aqueous solution of phenol is usually used, care is taken to flush the agent from the needle so that a subcutaneous track of phenol is not produced.

# References

1. Merskey H, Bogduk N. *Classification of Chronic Pain: Descriptions of Chronic Pain Syndromes and Definitions of Pain Terms. 2nd edn.* Seattle: IASP Press, 1994.
2. Dreyfuss P, Tibiletti C, Dreyer S. Thoracic zygapophyseal joint pain patterns. A study in normal volunteers. *Spine* 19: 807–811, 1994
3. Fukui S, Ohseto K, Shiotani M. Patterns of pain induced by distending the thoracic zygapophyseal joints. *Reg Anesth* 22: 332–336, 1997
4. Chua W and Bogduk N. The surgical anatomy of thoracic denervation. *Acta Neurochir* 136: 140–144, 1995
5. Stolker R, Vervest A, Groen G. Electrode positioning in thoracic percutaneous partial rhizotomy; an anatomical study. *Pain* 57: 241–251, 1994
6. Singer KP. *Pathomechanics of the Ageing Thoracic Spine.* Lawrence D, ed. Advances in Chiropractic. St Louis: Mosby, pp. 129–153, 1997
7. Bruckner FE, Leung AWL. "Benign thoracic pain" syndrome: role of magnetic resonance imaging in the detection and localisation of thoracic disc disease. *J Roy Soc Med* 82: 81–83, 1989
8. Dessein PH, Shipton EA, Cloete A. Fibromyalgia as a syndrome of neuroendocrine deficiency: a hypothetical model with therapeutic implications. *Pain Rev* 4: 79–89, 1997
9. Bonica J. *The Management of Pain. Vol 2. 2nd edn.* Philadelphia: Lea and Febiger, pp. 1114–1145, 1990
10. Lahtinen R, Laakso M, Palva I. Randomised placebo controlled multicentre trial on clodrinate in multiple myeloma. *Lancet* 340: 1049–1052, 1992
11. Luzzani M, Vidili MG, Risotto R, et al. Disodium clodronate in the treatment of pain due to bone metastasis. *Intl J Clin Pharm Res* 4: 243–246, 1990
12. Bates TD. The management of bone metastases; radiotherapy. *Palliative Med* 1: 117–120, 1987
13. Saarto T, Tenhunen M, Kouri M. Palliative radiotherapy in the treatment of skeletal metastases. *Eur J Pain* 6: 323–330, 2002
14. Crombie IK, Davies HTO, Macrae WA. Cut and thrust: antecedent surgery and trauma among patients attending a chronic pain clinic. *Pain* 76: 167–171, 1998
15. Wallace MS, Wallace AM, Lee J, et al. Pain after breast surgery: a survey of 282 women. *Pain* 66: 195–120, 1996
16. Richardson J, Sabanathan S, Mearns AJ, et al. *Pain Clinic* 7: 87–97, 1994

17. Katz J, Jackson M, Kavanagh BP, et al. *Clin J Pain* **12**: 50–55, 1996
18. Benedetti F, Vighetti S, Ricco C, et al. Neurophysiologic assessment of nerve impairment in postero-lateral and muscle sparing thoracotomy. *J Thor Cardiovasc Surg* **115**: 841–847, 1998
19. Gotoda Y, Kambara N, Sakai T, et al. The morbidity, time course and predictive factors for persistent post-thoracotomy pain. *Eur J Pain* **5**: 89–96; 2001
20. d'Amours RH, Reigler FX, Little AG. Pathogenesis and management of persistent post-thoracocotomy pain. *Chest Surg Clin N Am* **8**: 703–722, 1998
21. Bass C, Mayou R. ABC of psychological medicine. *Chest Pain Br Med J* **325**: 588–591, 2002
22. Dion JE. Percutaneous vertebroplasty. *Medica Mundi* **45**: 20–28, 2001
23. Dogliotti AM. Traitment des syndromes douloreux de la peripherie par l'alcoholisation subarachnoi-dienne des racines posterieures à leur émergence de la moelle epineri. *Presse Med* **39**: 1249–1252, 1931
24. Nagaro T, Yamauchi Y, Ochi G, et al. Subarachnoid phenol block under fluoroscopy in the management of thoracic cancer pain. *Pain Clinic* **4**: 205–208 1991
25. Patt RB, Cousins MJ. Techniques for neurolytic blockade. In: Cousins MJ, Bridenbaugh PO, eds. *Neural Blockade*. Philadelphia, Lippincott. pp. 1007–1061, 1998
26. Hardy PAJ. Anatomical variation in the position of the proximal intercostal nerve. *Br J Anaesthesia* **61**: 338, 1988

# 13 Abdominal Pain

*Nicholas L Padfield*

Abdominal pain is one of the most common causes of patients seeking medical help. It affects all ages yet, in the majority of cases, no obvious cause is found. In one study, less than 5% of young patients required admission to hospital.[1] Patients can arrive in the pain clinic after extensive investigation, and the clinician must be ready for considerable psychological issues. In order to effectively assess a patient and subsequently plan appropriate and effective pain management, it is essential to consider the anatomy of the abdominal contents and their nerve supply, and to have a comprehensive knowledge of relevant medical and surgical diseases. There has been a huge expansion in the basic science of visceral nociception, which has benefited our understanding of pain mechanisms. But somatic disorders like myofascial pain can mimic visceral problems.

## Anatomy

### Innervation of the abdominal viscera

Unlike the somatic tissue, the viscera are innervated by two sets of primary afferent fibres that project to distinct regions in the neuraxis. Vagal afferent fibres originating from the nodose ganglia provide innervation from the oesophagus to the transverse colon and project centrally to the nucleus of the tractus solitarius. The remainder of the large bowel receives fibres from the afferent fibres originating from the sacral dorsal root ganglia, which project centrally to the sacral spinal cord. The entire gastrointestinal (GI) tract is also innervated by the afferent fibres in the splanchnic nerves projecting to the T5–L2 segments of the spinal cord. These coalesce to form the greater, lesser and least splanchnic nerves, which synapse in the ganglia of the coeliac plexus along with the vagal afferents. Each thoracic sympathetic ganglion is connected to the corresponding spinal nerve by preganglionic (white) and postganglionic (grey) rami communicantes. In addition to carrying afferent sympathetic fibres to the celiac plexus, the splanchnic nerves also carry efferent fibres, which pass via the grey rami communicantes from the sympathetic ganglia to the corresponding somatic nerves.

Principle organs and their segmental innervation:

- Pancreas          T5–11
- Stomach           T6–9
- Duodenum          T6–8
- Jejunum           T9–11
- Gallbladder       T6–9 mostly (some from T10 to T12)
- Liver             T6–11
- Kidney and ureter T10–12 and L1–2

The peripheral terminals of these afferent fibres innervate all layers of a viscus (vagal/pelvic to mucosa; thoracolumbar, pelvic to muscle and serosa). However, they have no end organs or morphological specialization, unlike their somatic counterparts.

Viscerosensory axons are almost exclusively thinly myelinated Aδ-fibres and unmyelinated C fibres. There appear to be two distinct types of receptor: the high-threshold receptors that respond to mechanical stimuli within the noxious range, and the low-threshold receptors that encode the stimulus intensity in the magnitude of their discharges across the range from innocuous to noxious.[2]

The distribution of these fibres varies among organs. High-threshold exclusively innervate organs from which pain is the only sensation (e.g. ureter, kidney, lungs, heart) but there are relatively few of them in organs that provide innocuous and noxious sensations (e.g. colon, stomach, bladder). There are also data suggesting that the abdominal viscera also have 'silent' nociceptive afferents that can be sensitized by inflammation.[3]

Studies suggest that the two nerves that innervate a particular organ serve different functions.

- Vagal afferents do not convey painful stimuli directly but can have a neuromodulatory role.[4]
- Pelvic afferents from the lower bowel though are the predominant pathway mediating sensations from the rectum.

The role of pelvic splanchnic nerves projecting to the lumbar spinal cord remains poorly understood. It has recently been suggested that inflammation alters the central processing of afferent thoracolumbar input. Similar observations have recently been made in model of visceral hyperalgesia.[5]

# Pathophysiology

## Peripheral sensitization

In the presence of inflammation, tissue injury and local ischaemia injury, visceral afferents become sensitized and respond to previously innocuous stimuli. Both low- and high-threshold receptors usually signal acute visceral pain. However, these and previously silent receptors can be sensitized to produce pain. Inflammatory mediators produced locally can augment and perpetuate the transmission of noxious stimuli.[6] This is partially mediated by Tetrodotoxin (TTX)-resistant sodium channels, which are expressed in virtually all colonic and bladder afferents, and the current density recorded from these channels increases following tissue inflammation or the application of inflammatory mediators.[7]

Sensory motor disturbances remain after peripheral inflammation subsides.[8]

Colonic afferents when compared with somatic show a greater percentage containing neuropeptides, especially substance P, calcitonin gene-related peptide (CGRP), somatostatin and vasoactive intestinal peptide (VIP). To date, no differences have been reported in colonic afferents that project into the pelvic and splanchnic nerves.

Colonic afferents in the pelvic nerves contain many receptors, including amino acid receptors[9] and opioids receptors.[10] Colonic afferents are inhibited by κ- and not μ- or δ- opioid agonists and peripheral administration of κ-agonists is anti-nociceptive.

## Central mechanisms

Visceral afferents comprise 10% of all afferent inflow to the spinal cord, and they terminate in laminae I, II, V and X. Viscerosomatic and viscerovisceral convergence have been demonstrated anatomically and electrophysiologically in both the dorsal horn and the supraspinal centres.

The low density of visceral nociceptors, along with the functional divergence of visceral input, may explain the poorly localized nature of visceral pain. The central projections of the pelvic sacral and thoracolumbar splanchnic include not only the spinothalamic, the spinohypothalamic, the spinosolitary, the spinoreticular, the spinoparabrachial and other tracts but also, interestingly, the dorsal columns.

One difference between the dorsal column fibres and those of the spinothalamic tracts is that they travel on the ipsilateral side before converging on the nucleus gracilis and the nucleus cuneatus thence internal arcuate fibres transmit nociceptive fibre input to the contralateral side of the ventroposterolateral thalamic nuclei. There is increasing evidence from animal work that the dorsal column fibres are more important in visceral nociception than the spinothalamic tract or the reticulospinal tract. This fact has opened up new means of treating visceral pain. Dorsal column stimulation has recently been shown to significantly reduce neuronal responses to colonic distension.[11] A midline myelotomy has been used to treat visceral cancer pain successfully with neurological sequelae.[12]

## Central sensitization

Unlike in somatic tissue where N-methyl-D-aspartate (NMDA) receptors contribute to the central sensitization following tissue inflammation or injury, they can signal acute noxious stimuli in the absence of inflammation (such as distension of the ureter) and also contribute the process of central sensitization following innocuous colorectal distension. The contribution of NMDA receptors to the signalling of innocuous colonic stimuli leads to speculation that excessive activity at these receptors, in the absence of inflammation, could produce central sensitization leading to visceral hyperalgesia associated with irritable bowel syndrome.

## History and examination

In order to make a diagnosis, a thorough description of the pain and associated symptoms must be elicited from the patient. This must include:

- The site and radiation
- Character – colicky, constant, burning, aching, sharp or dull, good or poor localization
- Duration and frequency of painful episodes
- Periodicity – especially any relation to diurnal rhythm, food, alcohol, stress or emotion and the effect of sleep
- Any consistent aggravating or relieving factors and, of course, bowel habit
- Previous surgery or illnesses – including diabetes, vasculitis, other chronic disease like systemic lupus erythematosus (SLE), rheumatoid arthritis, peripheral and visceral vascular disease and other illnesses that refer pain to the abdomen, such as inferior myocardial infarction, pleurisy, vertebral column disease, acute porphyria
- Family and social history – alcohol and substance abuse (which may indicate a functional cause); previous psychiatric treatment
- Current medication and any history of allergy, which may indicate a reversible iatrogenic cause.

Inspection of the abdomen will reveal any previous surgical scars, cachexia, visible peristalsis, distension, visible pulsation from an enlarged aortic aneurysm and vascular abnormalities like caput medusae. Gentle palpation may reproduce the pain in the case of nerve entrapment or elicit tenderness or guarding if there is underlying visceral disease. Organ enlargement or masses such as an aortic aneurysm may also be discovered.

Carnett's test is useful in differentiating pain of abdominal wall origin from intra-abdominal causes (Figure 13.1). The point of maximum tenderness is elicited with the patient lying supine. The arms are placed across the chest and the abdominal muscles tensed; if palpation

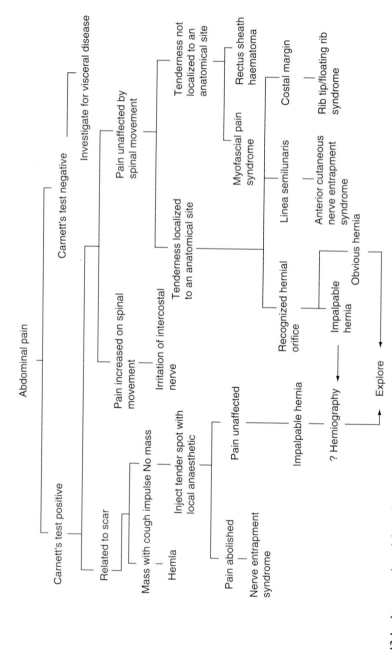

**Figure 13.1** An approach to abdominal wall pain

of the tender spot is now more painful, the test is positive and the likely cause arises from the abdominal wall, if negative then a visceral cause should be sought.

# Differential diagnosis

## Extra-abdominal sources

The most common extra-abdominal causes are listed in Table 13.1. It should be possible to differentiate these from intra-abdominal causes. Treatment will be centred on managing the systemic disease or condition.

- Angina/myocardial infarction – apart from the classic distribution down the left arm and into the jaw this can be experienced as pain in the epigastrium especially in association with inferior infarcts and irritation of the diaphragm. Unexplained indigestion in a patient with coronary artery disease risk factors, such as diabetes, hyperlipidaemia, hypertension, obesity and a history of cigarette smoking, should be investigated cardiologically.
- Vertebral column disease – intrinsic disease such as myeloma and other space-occupying pathologies (i.e tumour, pus or blood in the lower thoracic and upper lumbar spine) may refer pain to the abdomen. They would also be accompanied by constitutional upset, such as loss of weight, sweating, anaemia, malaise and tiredness.
- Fractured ribs – in the absence of a history of trauma, these will occasionally pose a diagnostic challenge. They may well be the result of pathological fractures in osteoporotic ribs or through tumour secondary deposits. It is, therefore, important not to accept a plain thoracic radiograph, which does not show the lower ribs clearly, as such fractures will commonly be in the lowest ribs.
- Spinal tumours – intramedullary tumours can frequently cause diagnostic challenges. The value of magnetic resonance imaging (MRI) at the appropriate vertebral level can thus not be overemphasized. But the pain clinician must, of course, think of it!
- Pleuritic pain – this can occasionally be referred to the hypochondrium on the affected side. There may well be other constitutional signs to aid diagnosis.
- Haemolytic crisis – sickle cell disease can often cause a multitude of signs and symptoms, depending on the blood vessels involved. Sickle cell patients, though, will always have had a long history of crises hospital admissions and, as a result, this will be an easy diagnosis.
- Acute porphyria – a rare condition, often associated with a family history to aid diagnosis.
- Lead poisoning – common in children eating old lead paint. There may be the characteristic 'lead lines' in the gums if this has been happening for some time.
- Pyogenic sacroiliitis – there will be other constitutional signs of fever, sweating and general malaise, and pelvic springing will be exquisitely painful.

| **Table 13.1**    Extra-abdominal causes of abdominal pain |
| --- |
| Angina/ myocardial infarction |
| Vertebral column disease |
| Fractured ribs |
| Spinal tumours |
| Pleuritic pain |
| Haemolytic crisis |
| Acute porphyria |
| Lead poisoning |
| Pyogenic sacroiliitis |

## Intra-abdominal causes

### Hollow organ dysfunction

The following groups of diseases will for the most part be dealt with by other disciplines, but occasionally there will be a patient who presents in an untypical way and the pain clinician must be aware of potentially treatable diseases that require dealing with rather than the physical sensation of pain. These diseases are summarized in Table 13.2.

A lot of the pain is by distension of a viscus, and consideration of the mechanisms of visceral pain elucidated at the beginning of this chapter should provide a rational basis for management. The length of time the condition has been present may indicate neuropathic processes rather than nociceptive pain from physical causes.

- Oesophageal disease – especially lower oesophagus, reflux, adenocarcinoma (unfortunately often a late sign)
- Gastric ulceration/cancer – pain is often food-intake related
- Biliary disease – may be accompanied by jaundice, history of fat intolerance
- Bowel obstruction – often accompanied by abdominal distension. The acute abdomen requires a surgical opinion, but chronic adhesions are often referred to the pain clinician and can be a management challenge
- Diverticular disease – usually requires management of an isolated segment by surgery, or medical management. Only intractable cases find their way to a pain clinician and, again, careful consideration of pain mechanisms and genesis should lead to a rational management approach.
- Renal pelvic or ureteric calculus or blood – usually such patients will only be referred by a urologist after stones have been dealt with and underlying biochemical disorders, such as hyperuricaemia, treated. A considerable proportion of patients following nephrectomy complain of loin pain, which can be particularly refractory to treatment.
- Ileitis – causes a deep abdominal aching and distension, which can be nociceptive inflammatory and neuropathic.
- Crohn's disease
- Irritable bowel – toxins/pharmacological, environmental.

### Solid organ dysfunction

A summary of solid organ dysfunction that can cause abdominal pain is given in Table 13.3.

- Hepatic tumour, inflammation, distension – the pain associated with this is usually due to the distension of the capsule. Abdominal palpation will often reveal an enlarged liver. If

---

**Table 13.2**  Intra-abdominal causes of abdominal pain: hollow organ dysfunction

Oesophageal disease
Gastric ulceration/cancer
Biliary disease
Bowel obstruction
Diverticular disease
Renal pelvic or ureteric calculus or blood
Ileitis
Crohn's disease
Irritable bowel
    Toxins/pharmacological
    Environmental

| **Table 13.3** | Intra-abdominal causes of abdominal pain: solid organ dysfunction |
|---|---|

Hepatic tumour, inflammation, distension
Pancreatic (acute/chronic)
Pancreatic tumour
Renal tumour/inflammation
Perisplenitis
Hypersplenism

an anterior approach coeliac plexus block is contemplated, it is imperative to ascertain if there is distension and increased pressure in the biliary system since this would increase the likelihood of causing biliary peritonitis by the passage of the needle during the procedure. Such patients should have been worked up before a clear diagnosis is made. Puncturing an undiagnosed hydatid cyst would have disastrous consequences, for example.

- Pancreatic (acute/chronic) – the diagnosis is classically confirmed by significantly raised serum amylase associated with severe epigastric pain radiating to the back. It is commonly associated with gall stones and binge consumption of alcohol. Patients can often be poorly nourished and have borderline personalities, all of which issues need addressing every bit as much as the pain itself. The pain tends to be relapsing if the pancreatitis proceeds to a chronic course. It can be extraordinarily difficult to manage. It tends to be unresponsive to opiates, but some help can be gained with treatment with NMDA antagonists; dorsal column stimulation may be helpful – but only in very carefully selected cases where psychological issues, lifestyle and diet have all been optimized. In the chronic form, the use of CREON pancreatic enzymes, along with dietary advice on content and frequency of meals, can offer worthwhile help in the day-to-day management of this pain. The much advocated employment of coeliac plexus block and splanchnic nerve blocks are to be deprecated in the authors opinion. Since this is likely to be a case of visceral neuropathy, further nerve damage is illogical as a treatment and certainly causes a significant morbidity in its own right. There have been enough cases of transverse myelopathy following posterior approach coeliac plexus block to warrant careful scrutiny of the evidence that such treatment is not only effective but lasting in the case of chronic pancreatitis.
- Pancreatic tumour – by the time this is diagnosed, pain treatment is usually palliative as the patient's life expectancy is usually measured in months. This being the case, a neuro-destructive lesion of the coeliac plexus is indicated, which can be very effective in treating this pain especially if there has been tumour invasion of the coeliac plexus.
- Renal tumour/inflammation – the pain associated here is the result of stretching the renal capsule or the collecting system. It is almost certainly a neuropathic pain by the time it produces the intractable relentless pain that we see in the pain clinics. There was a fashion for instilling a capsaicin preparation into the collecting systems, on the rationale that reducing the substance P levels would reduce the pain experienced. Unfortunately, it rarely worked and patients undergoing this treatment had to have epidural local anaesthetic infusions as the pain produced was completely unresponsive to opiates. It still remains a very difficult pain to treat. Paravertebral steroid and local anaesthetic injections at the appropriate levels can offer a measure of relief, but it tends to be incomplete and short lasting. Pulsed radiofrequency treatment of the appropriate dorsal root ganglia is showing some promise, but it is still very early days in the full evaluation of this novel form of treatment. At least, though, it is not destructive but neuromodulatory. Spinal cord stimulation has not proven to be helpful as it is extremely difficult to produce appropriate well-matched paraesthesia coverage of the painful area.

**135**

- Perisplenitis – the pain is produced by distension of the splenic capsule. If no relief is obtained with medication, NSAIDs and Tricyclic antidepressants (TADs), then paravertebral injection of local anaesthetic and depot steroid preparations at the appropriate level can be helpful. A trial of dorsal column stimulation may be worthwhile in intractable cases, but success or failure will depend on the ability to produce paraesthesiae coverage of the pain.
- Hypersplenism – again the pain is the result of distension of the capsule. However, hypersplenism as part of a generalized reticulosis may require treatment of the underlying condition and, once that is controlled, may cease to be so painful.

## Abdominal wall

The following causes of abdominal pain are summarized in Table 13.4.

- Scar pain/nerve entrapment – it is important to differentiate between neuroma formation and cicatrisation and, therefore, constriction around previously healthy nerves. Both may require surgical exploration and release if appropriate. When surgery is not indicated then local infiltration with local anaesthetic and steroid may be helpful. Stretching exercises of the appropriate quadrant may also help. In intractable cases that are not helped by medication such as NSAIDs, TADs or gabapentin, local anaesthetic and steroid infiltration of the appropriate dorsal root ganglion should be tried and then if helpful, followed by/pulsed radiofrequency treatment to the appropriate dorsal root ganglion.
- Post-herpetic neuralgia – this can be very refractory to treatment and is dealt with in Chapter 22.
- Hernias – these should be obvious from abdominal examination and require surgical correction. The problems occur when they are small, and so easily missed, especially the rare Spigelian hernia.
- Myofascial syndrome – this is discussed in Chapter 10. However, it can lead to a lot of diagnostic difficulty when not part of a generalised and well-recognized pattern. Patients will frequently have numerous accompanying psychological issues, not least because their attendant physicians have tended to overlook the pain, or to treat it as psychogenic.

## Vascular

Vascular causes of abdominal pain are summarized in Table 13.5.

- Occlusion – vascular events are usually sudden and often catastrophic. There will usually be other diagnostic indicators in the history, such as diabetes, heavy smoking, obesity, hyperlidaemias. They will present as an acute abdomen and need urgent investigation and management by the on-call surgical team. Rarely, a chronic form can present as abdominal angina where pain is precipitated by large meals. Diagnosis is confirmed by mesenteric arteriography; this is sometimes called the superior mesenteric artery syndrome.
- Sickle cell anaemia – this more commonly affects hips, shoulders and spine, but will occasionally cause splenic infarct leading to sudden-onset left hypochondrial pain. Treatment

**Table 13.4** Abdominal wall causes of abdominal pain

Scar pain/nerve entrapment
Post-herpetic neuralgia
Hernias
Myofascial syndrome

| Table 13.5 Vascular causes of abdominal pain |
| --- |
| Occlusion |
| Superior mesenteric artery syndrome |
| Sickle cell anaemia |
| Splenic infarct |
| Collagen vascular disorders, acute rheumatoid, polyarteritis nodosa |

is geared towards treating the sickle cell crisis, i.e. fluids, warmth, analgesia and maybe oxygen.

- Collagen vascular disorders, acute rheumatoid, polyarteritis nodosa – this may cause pain within the abdominal wall itself or vascular ischaemia leading to abdominal angina. Treatment will be initally geared to controlling the acute phase of the polyarteritis with steroids, and even immunosuppressants, with general measures for controlling the pain such as patient-controlled opiates, since these patients will necessarily be hospitalized.

## Miscellaneous

The following disorders are summarized in Table 13.6.

- Diabetic autonomic neuropathy – the diagnosis will be suggested when there is a history of long-standing, frequently poorly controlled, diabetes mellitus, postural hypotension, other peripheral neuropathies etc. Treatment is for visceral neuropathic pain and can be very difficult.
- Tabes dorsalis – easily overlooked as it is not considered because the perception of tertiary syphilis is a rare entity. Abdominal pain is also a manifestation of other genitourinary diseases such as HIV (see Chapter 31).
- Vitamin deficiencies – these will often be accompanied by malnutrition, alcohol abuse and sleeping rough. Thiamine deficiency may be accompanied by peripheral neuropathies and is treated with thiamine 100 mg daily, but patient compliance in this particular population can be a major issue. Pellagra is characterized by the three Ds – Dermatitis, Diarrhoea and Dementia – and is occasioned by B6 deficiency, which is likely to be dietary. B12 deficiency is an issue in vegans as there are few natural vegetarian sources of this vitamin. Apart from neuropathy there will be haematological manifestations like macrocytosis; treatment comprises hydroxocobalamin 1000 μg monthly.
- Porphyria – the diagnosis is confirmed by the presence of urinary porphyrins. It is likely that there will be other signs and symptoms of porphyria to aid diagnosis.

| Table 13.6 Miscellaneous causes of abdominal pain |
| --- |
| Diabetic autonomic neuropathy |
| Tabes dorsalis |
| Vitamin deficiencies |
| Porphyria |
| Mesenteric lymphadenitis |
| Peritonitis |
| Maldigestion syndromes, carbohydrate maldigestion, enzyme deficiencies |

- Mesenteric lymphadenitis – this is more commonly a problem in children and is accompanied by a suggestive history of a viral illness and other evidence of constitutional upset.
- Peritonitis – this is often a late presentation of a complication of bowel/hollow viscus perforation. It requires urgent surgical exploration.
- Maldigestion syndromes, carbohydrate maldigestion, enzyme deficiencies – there is often a family history to aid diagnosis. In addition to pain there will be constitutional upset, and the particular problem will be elucidated by intestinal biopsy.

## Investigations

The patient should have some baseline screening tests performed, if only to exclude serious organic and systemic disease. These would include:

- Full blood count
- Erythrocyte sedimentation rate
- Urea and electrolytes
- Blood glucose
- Liver function test
- Serum calcium
- Serum amylase
- Urine analysis.

Further investigation depends on the findings of these tests, which may indicate further investigation with referral to another specialist, though it is usual for these to have already been performed prior to referral to the pain clinic. They are summarized in Table 13.7.

## Psychological causes

Occasionally abdominal pain will have no organic cause found after exhaustive investigation. True psychogenic pain is rare, but it will be more likely to be picked up when routine psychometric testing is employed as part of a routine pain patient work-up. Patients with psychogenic pain are often depressed or give a history of a traumatic event leading to inappropriate fears and beliefs. Often, specific stressors can be found that are related to family or work. Clearly the treatment lies in cognitive behavioural therapy, which is dealt with in Chapter 32.

| Table 13.7  Further investigation in undiagnosed abdominal pain | |
|---|---|
| Suspected source of origin | Investigation |
| Upper gastrointestinal tract | Oesophagoduodenoscopy |
| | Barium swallow/meal/follow through |
| Renal Tract | Plain abdominal X-ray, intravenous urography |
| | Cystoscopy/ureteroscopy |
| Liver and biliary tree | Ultrasound |
| | Cholangiography/cholecystogram |
| | Endoscopic retrograde choledochopancreatogram |
| Pancreas | Computed tomography |
| | ERCP |
| Abdominal viscera | Angiography |

# Summary

When dealing with abdominal pain, a pathophysiological process should always be sought. Often, the pain clinician will make a likely hypothesis as to the mechanism/genesis of the pain and will treat the mechanisms accordingly. Technical details of splanchnic nerve block, coeliac nerve block, paravertebral nerve block, pulsed radiofrequency treatment can be found in the appendices and are not listed here.

# References

1. Stevenson RJ. Abdominal pain unrelated to trauma. *Surg Clin N Am* **65**: 1181–1121, 1985
2. Sengupta JN, Gebhart GF. Characterization of mechanosensitive pelvic nerve afferent fibres innervating the colon of the rat. *J Neurophysiol* **71**: 2046–2060, 1994
3. McMahon SB, Koltzenberg M. Silent afferents and visceral pain. Pharmacological approaches to the treatment of chronic pain: new concepts and critical issues. In: *Progress in Pain Research and Management Vol 1*. Fields H and Liebeskind J eds. Seattle: IASP Press, pp. 11–30, 1994
4. Ness TJ, Fillingim RB, Randich A, Backensto EM, Faught E. Low intensity vagal nerve stimulation lowers human thermal pain thresholds. *Pain* **86**: 81–85, 2000
5. Lin C, Al-Chaer ED. Primary afferent sensitization in an animal model of chronic visceral pain. *The Journal of Pain* **3(2) suppl 1**: 27, 2002
6. Cervero F, Laird JM. Visceral pain. *Lancet* **353**: 2145–2148, 1999
7. Traub RJ, Gold MS. Differences in the excitability of two populations of DRG neurones innervating the colon. *Soc Neurosci Abstr* 2000
8. Yoshimura N, Seki S, Novakovic SD, et al. The involvement of the tetrodotoxin-resistant sodium channel nav1.8(pn3/sns) in a rat model of visceral pain. *J Neurosci* **21**: 8690–8696, 2001
9. Lin C, al-Chaer ED 2002
10. McRoberts JA, Coutinhon SV, Marvison JC, et al. Role of peripheral N-methyl-D-aspartate (NMDA) receptors in visceral nociception in rats. *Gastroenterology* **120**: 1737–1748, 2001
11. Su X, Sengupta JN, Gebhart GF. Effects of kappa opioids receptor-selective agonists on responses of pelvic nerve afferents to noxious colorectal distension. *J Neurophysiol* **78**: 1003–1012, 1997
12. Broussard RF, Kawasaki M, Al-Chaer ED. The dorsal column of the spinal cord facilitates spinal neuronal sensitisation associated with colorectal hypersensitivity in an animal model of the irritable bowel syndrome. *Gastroenterolgy* **118**: 53–55, 2000
13. Kim YS, Kwon SJ. High Thoracic midline dorsal column myelotomy for severe visceral pain due to advanced stomach cancer. *Neurosurgery* **46**: 85–90, 2000

# 14 Male Urogenital Pain

*Nicholas L Padfield*

The pelvic viscera have a complex innervation not only from both the sympathetic and parasympathetic autonomic nervous system but also from the somatic sensory system.

Whilst chronic genital pain is well referenced in the medical literature, it is still poorly understood, frequently misdiagnosed and always debilitating for the patient. Female urogenital pain is addressed in Chapter 15 so I shall attend to male urogenital pain in this chapter.

It is an embarrassing pain for a man, and very isolating, as it is often difficult or impossible to discuss it with family members or friends. Such patients have often suffered for some time before plucking up the courage to discuss it with a health care provider. The pain clinician referred such a patient will often find that they have been extensively investigated and no obvious organic lesion has been found. The situation is further compounded by the fact that the pain felt in these regions may not arise from the organs themselves but may be referred from elsewhere, and that local pathology may be minimal or absent. Consequently, such patients are not only embarrassed but frustrated and often depressed. An understanding of the mechanisms of the likely genesis of the pain and an explanation in terms that mean something to the sufferer will go a long way to mitigating their distress.

To arrive at such a working diagnosis requires a detailed knowledge of the anatomy and physiology of the pelvic organs.

## Anatomy

### Autonomic sympathetic and parasympathetic

The pelvic viscera do not signal pain from direct trauma but only by distension or traction. Various hyperalgesic states can exist that change the functions of neurones and the recruitment of receptors. There are almost no Aδ fibres in the pelvic viscera. The autonomic pathways derive from the dual projections from the thoracolumbar and sacral segments of the spinal cord that converge primarily into discrete plexuses, which then provide fibres that extend throughout the retroperitoneum and pelvis.

#### Thoracolumbar outflow

Preganglionic projections to the celiac plexus and the superior hypogastric plexus comprise the presacral nerve. The celiac plexus, which lies on the anterior aorta at the level of the L2 vertebral body, provides innervation to the adrenal, renal pelvis and ureter, as well as some sympathetic outflow to the testes along the course of the internal spermatic vessels. The superior hypogastric plexus, the presacral nerve, at the bifurcation of the aorta provides the majority of the sympathetic input to the pelvic urinary organs and genital tract. In addition to this route the thoracolumbar preganglionic fibres synapse on the postganglionic nerves in sympathetic chain ganglia that commingle with autonomic sacral nerve projections, as well as with pelvic somatic neuronal pathways.

### Sacral outflow

Preganglionic **efferents** arise mostly from the intermediolateral cell column – the sacral parasympathetic nucleus at sacral levels.

The **afferent** fibres cell bodies are contained in the corresponding dorsal root ganglia.

The parasympathetic outflow from the sacral nerves S2–4 consists of preganglionic fibres. Within the pelvis the inferior hypogastric plexus is the major autonomic relay station to the visceral structures of the pelvis, receiving sympathetic fibres from the superior hypogastric plexus and parasympathetic fibres from the presacral nerves form the sacral plexus.

## Somatic sensory

The somatic sensory supply to the pelvis comes from efferent fibres originating from Onuf's nucleus in the ventral horn, and afferents having cell bodies in the dorsal root ganglia. Sacral nerve roots emerge from the spinal cord to form the sacral plexus from which arises the pudendal nerve, the primary afferent and efferent somatic supply to the various pelvic viscera and the pelvic floor musculature.

- Kidney – (T11–L2) thoracolumbar outflow along renal artery and vagus
- Ureter:
  - upper $1/3$ – renal and aortic plexuses from thoracolumbar outflow
  - middle $1/3$ – superior hypogastric (presacral plexus)
  - lower $1/3$ – inferior hypogastric (pelvic plexuses)
- Bladder and proximal urethra – hypogastric plexus (autonomic) and pudendal (somatic)
- Prostate, seminal vesicles and prostatic end of the vas deferens – the terminal portion of the hypogastric ganglion and plexus and the anterior part of the inferior hypogastric plexus
- Testis, and epididymal end of vas deferens – superior (from the spermatic vessels, T10–L1) and inferior spermatic plexuses from the inferior hypogastric plexus
- Epididymis (caudal) – superior spermatic plexus
- Epididymis (corpus) – inferior spermatic plexus
- Cremaster and parietal and visceral tunica vaginalis – (L1–L2) genital branch of the genitofemoral nerve
- Penis – dorsal nerve, branch of the pudendal nerve (S2–S4) provides the sensory supply, and branches from the inferior hypogastric plexus provide the autonomic supply. The glans has an abundant supply of free nerve endings and thinly myelinated A$\delta$- and unmyelinated C fibres. Vibrotactile finger thresholds are significantly lower than penile thresholds in patients with primary premature ejaculation,[1] and these thresholds have been shown to be reduced in men suffering from premature ejaculation.[2]

However, there is certainly likely to be a more complex nerve supply for any individual organ from somatic and autonomic sources and the nerves supplying each organ are likely to be carrying all types of fibres. Hence, the innervation of the pelvic viscera is highly complicated, and it can be very difficult to pinpoint the pain generator with prognostic local anaesthetic blocks to individual nerves such as the pudendal or genitofemoral.

## Treatment

General measures will be applicable in most cases when there is no specific pathology that predicates treatment.

## Nerve blocks

When a particular pain falls into a definite dermatomal distribution, it may be worthwhile performing a diagnostic dorsal root ganglion block at that level. If this produces pain relief then it may be either worth repeating or treating with pulsed radiofrequency treatment. It may respond to a pudendal nerve block if the quality of the pain appears to be somatic and in the appropriate distribution.

It may appear to be a visceral pain subserved by a particular plexus or nerve that may be amenable to a prognostic block. Again, should this be successful in reducing the pain, it may be worth repeating. Neurolytic blocks are only indicated, in the author's opinion, when the patient's life expectancy is likely to be shorter than the time to develop neuropathic pain.

## Medication

Simple analgesics (e.g. paracetamol) taken regularly can be helpful. If there appears to be an inflammatory component to the pain then a course of non-steroidal anti-inflammatory drugs (NSAIDs) may prove beneficial. If it appears that there is visceral hyperalgesia then drugs like amitriptyline, carbamazepine, lamotrigine and gabapentin may prove beneficial. The newer 5-HT5 receptor antagonists, such as alosetron, may be helpful in conditions such as interstitial cystitis or ureteric pain. Individual conditions are discussed in greater detail in the following section. It is important, though, to consider the whole patient's physical condition as the presence of coexisting medical disease may preclude the use of certain drug groups (Viz asthma, renal disease, upper gastrointestinal disease and NSAIDs.)

## Psychological therapy

Patients suffering from urogenital pain frequently have psychological issues that need to be addressed. They can be depressed, impotent, have low self efficacy, be socially isolated, divorced or unemployed. They may have inappropriate fears and beliefs pertaining to their condition, which can be very difficult to change. The neurobiophysiology of the generation of orgasm lies outside the scope of this chapter but is excellently reviewed elsewhere.[3] However, male patients may well cite pain as the reason for sexual impotence, and genuine functional disturbance of the sexual apparatus per se needs investigating by a urologist. However, in the absence of physical causes, a review of the patient's medication may reveal treatment with drugs known to affect arousal and orgasm. The antidepressants in particular inhibit orgasmic sensation and ejaculation.[4] Carbamazepine can block testosterone production resulting not only in testicular atrophy but also gynaecomastia and galactorrhoea. Carbamazepine has been reported as causing ejaculatory failure.[5] Often, behavioural therapy teaching coping strategies and altering sexual behaviour and practice can go a long way to reduce the distress of their pain. Education, in terms that have meaning to the patient, about their condition or more importantly allaying their particular fears about, for instance, cancer or other serious issues may go a long way to reducing their distress. Relaxation techniques and anger management may lead to significant gains in re-establishing personal relationships and, therefore, improving their quality of life.

# Commonly seen chronic pain syndromes of the urogenital tract

## Kidney and ureter pain

There are few chronic non-malignant pain syndromes of the upper urinary tract. Most pain is acute, colicky and associated with distension of the urinary tract by an obstructing lesion or infection. The referred pain is from the costovertebral angle down into the groin and testicle. In one report, after lithotripsy for calculosis pain thresholds remained lower for up to 8 months.[6] This suggests a visceral pain mechanism that has caused changes higher up in the CNS.

## Loin pain/haematuria syndrome

Loin pain/haematuria syndrome describes those patients who experience recurrent attacks of unilateral or bilateral loin pain accompanied by microscopic haematuria and in whom no cause can be found. It appears to be more frequent in women than men and the diagnosis is one of exclusion.[7] Various treatments have been tried from transcutaneous electrical nerve stimulation (TENS) and analgesics, often in large doses, to more drastic surgery such as renal denervation, nephrectomy or autotransplantation. One study reported 65% pain relief lasting several months with irrigation of the renal pelvis and ureter with capsaicin solution. It appeared to work by causing degeneration of the afferent fibres of the ureter and renal pelvis.[8] The treatment requires general anaesthesia, and it is often associated with extreme aggravation of the pain so, as a result, it is not generally employed.

A new treatment, pulsed radiofrequency treatment applied to the dorsal root ganglia of T11 and T12 looks very promising as it is minimally invasive and neuromodulatory. It is in the process of evaluation.

## Bladder pain

Bladder pain may occur as part of several different disease processes, such as chronic bacterial infection, chemical cystitis, irradiation cystitis and neoplastic disease. They require treatment in their own right and lie outside the scope of this text. However interstitial cystitis is a chronic, painful and often very debilitating disease, which gets referred to the pain clinician as a last resort. Its pathophysiology is largely unknown. It is characterized by pelvic and suprapubic pain and urinary symptoms such as frequency and urgency and in females dyspareunia, which may be relieved by voiding. It is nine times more common in females. Various aetiologies have been considered, including immunodeficiency, infection, lymphatic/vascular insufficiency, glycosaminoglycan layer deficiency, presence of toxic urogenous substance, neural factors and mast cell disorders.[9,10]

In men with prostate pain, 60% may have an association with interstitial cystitis.[11,12] It is likely to be a urinary epithelial dysfunction with a single pathophysiological process. The common etiology and pathology have been further confirmed by the potassium sensitivity test.[13]

When it comes to treatment, many things have been tried but there is no consensus and, as yet, no evidence base for guidance.

Surgery to remove or modify the bladder, laser therapy, hydrodistension, urethral dilatation, infusions of dimethyl sulphoxide, silver nitrate, heparin, chlorpactin and hyaluronic acid have been tried. Oral medication, such as tricyclic antidepressants, calcium channel blockers and antihistamines, have been tried along with pentosanpolysulphate sodium (a mild anticoagulant with properties of a sulphated glycosaminoglycan and an affinity for mucosal membranes). Acupuncture, TENS, behavioural interventions and acid-lowering diets have been advocated. Recently, sacral nerve electrical stimulation by placing two spinal cord stimulating electrodes caudally into the sacral epidural space to achieve effectively peripheral nerve stimulation of the sacral nerves has been reported as successful in a few cases. This may be another case for evaluation of pulsed radiofrequency treatment to the relevant dorsal root ganglia. Clearly there is no consistent treatment modality, yet, that is reliable, consistent, reproducible and can be validated. The pain clinician can only be sympathetic and honest about the problem and gauge, as well as possible, the best likely path to tread – i.e. interventional, medication and or behavioural.

## Prostate pain

Prostate pain may arise from acute or chronic bacterial infection, a non-bacterial infection/inflammation (viral, autoimmune or allergic) or, in the absence of abnormal physical signs, prostatodynia.[14] It is characterized by urgency, burning pain on micturition, an aching pain in the back, groin and suprapubic regions and tenderness on palpation of the prostate. There may also be poor stream and voiding difficulties. The bacterial infection can be difficult to eradicate and, therefore, what starts off as an acute infection can frequently progress to a chronic one characterized by relapses and remissions caused by the persistence of the pathogen in the prostate despite numerous courses of antibiotics. Sixty four percent of patients with presumed prostatic pain have chronic abacterial prostatitis.[15] They have excessive inflammatory cells in the prostatic secretions despite negative cultures of the urinary tract and prostatic secretions. It does respond quite well to NSAIDs.

About a third of patients with presumed prostate pain have prostatodynia – no associated urinary tract infection, no pathogens in prostatic fluid cultures and no excessive inflammatory cells in the prostatic secretions. Such patients are young to middle aged and experience variable symptoms of painful and difficult micturition and pain in the pelvic area – the perineum, groin, testicles, low back and suprapubic areas. Interestingly the prostate is rarely tender on palpation. Urodynamic studies have shown some patients with prostatodynia to have a spastic dysfunction of the bladder neck and prostatic urethra. The high intraprostatic pressure generated by smooth muscle spasms can in turn cause intraprostatic reflux and a chemical prostatitis. Alpha adrenergic blockers such as prazocin can be helpful.[16] Transurethral microwave hyperthermia has been suggested for non-bacterial prostatitis and prostatodynia.[17]

## Testicular pain

Although there are well-documented causes for chronic testicular pain from direct trauma, infection and torsion, there can also be chronic constant or intermittent pain for which no organic cause can be easily found. Pain can be referred from T10 to S4 in the spine, the retroperitoneal space, the intra-abdominal cavity, the pelvic cavity and the external genitalia themselves. Disc prolapse, tendinitis of the insertion of the inguinal ligament or the adductor tendons into the pubis may masquerade as testicular or spermatic cord pain. Consequently magnetic resonance imaging (MRI) of the spine and abdominal and pelvic cavities may be indicated to eliminate a physical cause arising from these structures, if not immediately apparent.

Previous surgery, trauma or intermittent torsion (even during sexual intercourse) may be relevant. Pain may occur at or after ejaculation in association with prostatitis or epididymitis, and it can last for several days making sexual intercourse difficult. There is evidence that the sympathetic nervous system may be involved when this is the case. Continuous testicular pain may be the result of a spermatocoele, hydrocoele or varicocoele and other scrotal swellings should be investigated by ultrasound, which will confirm a solid tumour. This would then be explored surgically. A case has been made for spermatic cord denervation for orchialgia refractory to nonsurgical means.[18] Both acute and chronic infection should be ruled out with urine analysis, culture and sensitivity. However, chronic infections can be difficult to diagnose and treat. Indeed, one study from 1990 showed that no cause could be found in 25% of cases.[19]

The neurophysiology of arousal, plateau, ejaculation and resolution have been well described elsewhere and are outside the scope of this chapter.[3]

A sexual history should be taken especially to elicit any abuse, activities with partners and types of relationships, positions and associated sensory perceptions at arousal, ejaculation and orgasm. It is important to ascertain what meaning and significance the pain has for the patient. It may become apparent at this stage that psychological issues are pre-eminent and need psychological solutions (see Chapter 32).

## Pain of vas deferens and epididymis

In one postal survey, a third of patients who underwent vasectomy complained of chronic testicular pain. Only 5% sought further medical intervention. On ultrasound investigation, epididymal cysts were found commonly in both symptomatic and asymptomatic patients.[20] The surgical removal of sperm granulomas, when present, has been reported as effective – but they are rare.

Chronic epididymis can occasionally follow an acute infection, and it can be refractory to antibiotic treatment. It has been treated effectively by surgical excision. However, it may be satisfactorily managed along the general management lines indicated. A new treatment, pulsed radiofrequency, to the dorsal root ganglia at T12 and L1 is showing promise but is still being evaluated. It presents as a beneficial treatment that does not damage nerves but acts by neuromodulation of the cell bodies in the dorsal root ganglia.

## Penile pain

Penile pain is extremely rare. Sometimes the underlying cause is obvious (paraphimosis, priapism, Peyronie's disease, herpes genitalis) and needs treating in its own right. It is not reported in men complaining of impotence. The author has experience of one case of a middle-aged single man complaining of pain in the glans who had been extensively investigated by an urologist and nothing found. It responded well to gabapentin and reassurance.

## Perineal pain

Perineal pain derives its nerve supply from the pudendal nerve (S2–4) and branches of the genitofemoral and ilioinguinal nerves anteriorly and the anococcygeal nerves posteriorly. Pudendal nerve entrapment has been reported, which can be confirmed by pudendal nerve blocks.[21] Tension myalgias can occur in the levator ani muscles that produce pain in the rectum, pelvis and low back. This can be exacerbated by poor posture, infection, trauma and emotional tension.

Pain in the anorectal area may be constant or paroxysmal. Proctalgia fugax was first described in 1917[22] and is characterized by periods of intense pain around the anal sphincter and the anorectal ring. It is more common in men and tends to have resolved by late middle age. Many treatments have been tried with little consistent success. They include calcium antagonists like diltiazem, antispasmodics, nitroglycerine and salbutamol. As there is a high incidence of irritable bowel syndrome in these patients[23] the newer treatments such as alosetron and tegaserod might be worth trying. Stress management and muscle relaxation techniques should also be included in the overall management of this condition.

Lastly, meningiomas or meningeal cysts can be a rare cause of perineal pain. The patient may require MRI of the thoracolumbarsacral spine to confirm the diagnosis if suspected.

## Conclusions

Patients presenting with urogenital pain frequently have a complex mixture of somatic, visceral and psychological problems. Treating them takes time, patience and sensitivity. Problems may have begun as a simple physical problem but due to diffidence, fear or denial, can develop into complex behavioural, cognitive and somatic problems that require considerable unravelling. Some patients will already have been extensively investigated, with little or nothing to show for it but the conviction that something is terribly wrong and that nobody can or will tell them. Trust between patient and doctor has to be earned, on both sides, for the professional relationship to bear fruit. But, if you can help your patient, their genuine gratitude is a reward in itself.

# References

1. Rowland DL, Greenleat W, Mas M, Myers L, Davidson JM. Penile and finger sensory thresholds in young, aging and diabetic males. *Arch Sex Behav* **18**: 1–12 1989
2. Xin ZC, Chung WS, Choi YD, Seong DH, Choi YJ, Choi HK. Penile sensitivity in patients with primary premature ejaculation [Comment]. *J Urol* **156**: 979–981, 1996
3. Baranowski AP, Mallinson C and Johnson NS. A review of urogenital pain. *Pain Rev* **6**: 53–84, 1999
4. Lane RM. A critical review of selective serotonin reuptake inhibitor-related sexual dysfunction; incidence, possible aetiology and implications for management. *J Psychopharmacol* **11**: 72–82, 1997
5. Lenz AC, Stephens J, Hines J, McNicholas TA. A case of carbamazepine related ejaculatory failure. *Br J Urol* **79**: 485, 1997
6. Giamberardino MA, de Bigontina P, Martegiani C, Vecchiet L. Effects of extracorporeal shock-wave lithotripsy on referred hyperalgesia from renal/ureteral calculosis. *Pain* **56**: 77–83, 1994
7. Bultitude MI, Young, Bultitude MF J, Allan JDD. Loin pain haematuria syndrome: distress resolved by pain relief. *Pain* **76**: 209–213, 1998
8. Allan J, Bultitude MI, Bultitude MF, Wall PD and McMahon SB. The effect of capsaicin on renal pain signalling systems in humans and Wistar rats. *J Physiol* **505**: 39P, 1997
9. Ratliff Tl, Klutke CG, McDougall EM. The etiology of interstitial cystitis. *Urol Clin N Am* **21**: 21–30, 1994
10. Elbadawi A. Interstitial cystitis: a critique of current concepts with a new proposal for pathologic diagnosis and pathogenesis. *Urology* **49**: 14–40, 1997
11. Miller JL, Rothman I, Bavendam TG, Berger RE. Prostatodynia and interstitial cystitis: one and the same? *Urology* **45**: 587–589, 1995
12. Berger RE, Miller JE, Rothman I, Krieger JN, Muller CH. Bladder petechiae after cystoscopy and hydrodistension in men diagnosed with prostate pain. *J Urol* **159**: 83–85, 1998
13. Parsons CL, Albo M. Intravesicval potassium sensitivity in patients with prostatitis. *J Urol* **168**: 1054–1057, 2002
14. Drach GW, Fair WR, Meares EM, Stamey TA. Classification of benign diseases associated with prostatic pain: prostatitis or prostatodynia? *J Urol* **120**: 266, 1978
15. Orland SM, Hanno PM, Wein AJ. Prostatitis, prostatosis and prostodynia. *Urology* **25**: 439–459, 1985
16. Barbalias GA, Nikiforidis G, Liatsikos EN. Alpha-blockers for the treatment of chronic prostatitis in combination with antibiotics. *Journal of Urology* **161(1)**: 230–231, 1999
17. Nickel JC, Sorenson R. Transurethral microwave thermotherapy of nonbacterial prostatitis and prostatodynia: an initial experience. *Urology* **44**: 458–460, 1994
18. Levine LA, Matkov TG. Microsurgical denervation of the spermatic cord as a primary surgical treatment of orchialgia. *J Urol* **165**: 1927–1929, 2001
19. Davis BE, Noble MJ, Weigel JW. Analysis and management of chronic testicular pain. *J Urol* **143**: 936–939, 1990
20. McMahon AJ, Buckley J, Taylor A, et al. Chronic testicular pain following vasectomy. *Br J Urol* **69**: 188–191, 1992
21. Bensignor MF, Labat JJ, Robert R, Ducrot P. Diagnostic and therapeutic pudendal nerve blocks for patients with perineal non-malignant pain. Abstract, *8th World Congress on Pain* 1996, p. 56
22. MacLennan A. Rectal crises of non-tabetic origin. *Glasgow Med J* **88**: 129, 1917
23. Thompson WG, Heaton KW. Proctalgia fugax. *R Coll Physicians Lond* **14**: 247–248, 1980

# 15 Pelvic Pain

*Beverly J Collett*

Pelvic pain is a significant and perplexing problem in current medical practice. The pathophysiology is poorly understood, and there is often little correlation between the severity of the patient's pain complaints and the degree of tissue pathology. Patients with pelvic and perineal pain have often consulted many doctors, had numerous investigations and undergone surgery with no benefit.

This chapter will focus on pelvic pain in women. A recent comprehensive review has described the clinical presentation and treatment strategies for vulvar and perineal pain in women and in men.[1]

## Incidence

Chronic pelvic pain has been reported to be responsible for 10% of outpatient gynaecological consultations and approximately 30% of laparoscopies. It is listed as the indication for 10–12% of the hysterectomies performed in the US, accounting for approximately 70 000 procedures annually. A recent population-based study in the US found a 3-month prevalence of 15% in 5263 women aged between 18 and 50 years.[2] In the UK, an annual prevalence in primary care of 38/1000 was found in women aged between 15 and 73 years, a rate comparable to that of asthma and back pain.[3] The personal cost to the affected woman in terms of years of suffering and disability, sexual dysfunction, marital discord and loss of employment can be calculated less easily.

## Neuroanatomy

Figure 15.1 demonstrates the innervation of the female genital organs.

Somatic branches of the pudendal nerve, derived from the second, 3rd and 4th sacral root ganglia (S2–S4), innervate the perineum, anus and lower vagina. Painful visceral stimuli from the upper vagina, cervix, body of the uterus, medial fallopian tubes, broad ligament, upper bladder, caecum, appendix and terminal large bowel travel in the thoracolumbar sympathetics. Impulses pass via the uterovaginal and inferior hypogastric plexuses to the hypogastric nerves, through the superior hypogastric plexus (or presacral nerve) to the lumbar and lower thoracic sympathetic chain, entering the spinal cord at T12, L1 and L2.

The afferent pathway from the ovary travels along the ovarian artery, enters the main sympathetic chain at the 4th lumbar sympathetic ganglion and ascends with the sympathetic chain to enter the spinal cord in the lower thoracic segments. The outer two-thirds of the fallopian tubes and the upper ureter have similar innervation.

The superior hypogastric plexus does not, therefore, contain any fibres from the ovary or outer fallopian tube, and so resection of the superior hypogastric plexus (presacral neurectomy) relieves only central (uterine) pain and does not diminish pain of adnexal origin.

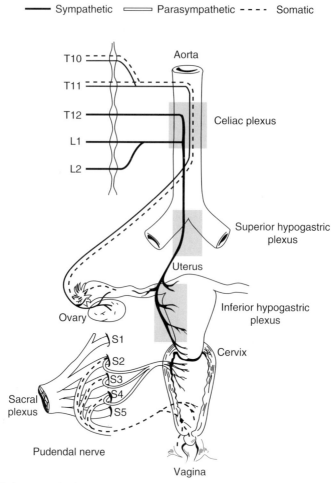

——— Sympathetic   ⇐⇒ Parasympathetic   - - - -   Somatic

**Figure 15.1** Pathways involved in gynaecological pain (From Cousins MJ, Wilson PR. Gynecologic pain. In: Coppleson M, ed, *Gynaecologic Oncology*. Edinburgh: Churchill Livingstone, 1981, pp. 1013–1043)

Mixed somatic nerves, originating in the ventral branches of the first and second spinal lumbar segments (L1 and L2), innervate the lower abdominal wall and anterior aspect of the vulva, including the clitoris and urethra. The dorsal rami derived from L1 and L2 innervate the lower back, often a region of referred gynaecological pain.

Viscerosensory axons are almost entirely thinly myelinated Aδ or unmyelinated C fibres. The receptors exhibit chemosensitivity, thermosensitivity and/or mechanosensitivity. Current research indicates that there are two physiological classes of nociceptive viscerosensory receptors: high-threshold receptors that respond to mechanical stimuli within the noxious range, and low-threshold receptors that respond to innocuous and noxious stimuli. Data suggests that the viscera also contains spinal nociceptive afferent fibres that are normally considered 'silent' but are sensitized by inflammation.[4]

## Visceral hyperalgesia

Viscera are relatively insensitive to painful stimuli that are considered painful to somatic structures, such as cutting, pinching and burning. Studies have shown that pain can be induced in visceral organs by:

- Distension or abnormal muscle contraction (e.g. uterine contraction in childbirth)
- Sudden stretching of the capsule of solid organs (e.g. rupture of a follicular cyst)
- Hypoxia or necrosis of viscera (e.g. torted ovarian cyst or fibroid)
- Production of pain-producing substances (e.g. prostaglandins in dysmenorrhoea or endometriosis)
- Chemical irritation of visceral nerve endings (e.g. with sebaceous fluid from ruptured cystic teratoma)
- Inflammation (e.g. salpingo-oophoritis).

Inflammatory stimuli, in particular, can trigger pain and can render the viscus hypersensitive, such that pain can now be evoked in the viscus by a stimulus that was previously non-painful, or by a lower intensity of stimulus.

Secondly, hypersensitivity of somatic tissues in the areas of referred pain from viscera results from prolonged or repeated internal painful processes. This hypersensitivity is localized mainly in the muscles.[5] The most accepted hypothesis regarding the mechanisms involved in this process attributes the phenomenon to a process of central sensitization that takes place in the central nervous system (CNS) and is triggered by massive afferent visceral barrage upon convergent viscerosomatic neurons. Viscerosomatic convergence has been well demonstrated by electrophysiological studies on animals and N-methyl-D-aspartate (NMDA) receptors have been postulated to play a pivotal role.[5,6] Somatic hyperalgesia is a persistent phenomenon that outlasts not only the spontaneous pain but often also the presence of the primary visceral focus.

Thirdly, the concept of viscero-visceral hyperalgesia has been postulated, in which pain in one visceral organ can be increased by a painful process in another internal organ. This phenomenon usually involves viscera with partially overlapping innervation.[5] Clarification of the pathophysiology of the hyperalgesic mechanisms from viscera is fundamental to the development of clinical therapeutic strategies.

## Acute cyclical pelvic pain

Recurrent self-limited acute cyclical pain may occur in relation to the menstrual cycle. Mittelschmerz is pain associated with the rupture of the ovarian follicle at the time of ovulation. Primary dysmenorrhoea, menstrual pain not associated with underlying pelvic structural abnormalities, occurs in 50% of adult women and in 15% of women may be severe and disabling. Pain is associated with intense myometrial contractions, secondary to excess prostaglandins, that give rise to hypoxic conditions. Primary dysmenorrhoea is successfully relieved by non-steroidal anti-inflammatory drugs (NSAIDs) in 70–80% of patients and by oral contraceptive pills in an additional 10%. Presacral neurectomy removes the main afferent innervation of the uterus. However, this invasive intervention is not without its risks and complications.

Secondary dysmenorrhoea is defined as menstrual pain that originates from organic pelvic pathology. The intra-uterine contraceptive device, submucosal fibroids, and adenomyosis (internal endometriosis) and endometriosis can all cause secondary dysmenorrhoea.

**151**

# Chronic pelvic pain

## Definition

A number of definitions of chronic pelvic pain (CPP) have been used in the literature. In this chapter, the term chronic pelvic pain is used to mean pain in the lower abdomen or pelvis of at least 6 months duration, occurring continuously or intermittently and not associated exclusively with menstruation or sexual intercourse.

It is distinguished from dysmenorrhoea (pain occurring during menstruation) and dyspareunia (pain occurring during sexual intercourse), although it may continue throughout the period or it may be exacerbated by intercourse.

## Major causes of chronic pelvic pain

The prevalence and type of pathology seen at laparoscopy for CPP varies greatly from study to study (Table 15.1). It is not easy to draw conclusions from this data as different definitions have been used for chronic pelvic pain, many studies are retrospective and some authors have a particular interest in a pathology and, hence, their results have inbuilt bias. However, it appears that approximately two-thirds of women with chronic pelvic pain have laparoscopically-detectable pathology, most commonly endometriosis or adhesions, and approximately one-third have a normal laparoscopy.[15]

### Endometriosis

Endometriosis, the presence of ectopic tissue that possesses the histological structure and function of the uterine mucosa, is a poorly understood condition with a variable clinical presentation. The most common sites of implantation are the ovaries, the pouch of Douglas, the uterosacral ligaments and the pelvic peritoneum. Endometriotic tissue can also deposit on the gut, bladder, ureter, vagina, vulva and in scar tissue. More distal spread, such as to the lungs, can occur.

Endometriosis presents with a variety of appearances that may make visual diagnosis difficult and inaccurate. In a study of 142 patients diagnosed by laparoscopic findings as having endometriosis, 110 had biopsies taken and in only 60% did histological findings confirm the diagnosis.[16] The role of endometriosis in chronic pelvic pain is also debated. Although endometriosis can be asymptomatic, the prevalence of endometriosis in women laparoscoped for chronic pelvic pain is higher than most estimates for the general population. However, there is no correlation between the severity of endometriosis and pain symptomatology.

Endometriosis potentially involves several mechanisms that can cause pain. The ectopic endometrium behaves like normally-sited endometrium, in that it develops throughout the

| Table 15.1 Laparoscopic findings in women with chronic pelvic pain (CPP) | | | | |
|---|---|---|---|---|
| Study | Number | Endometriosis | Adhesions | No pathology |
| Liston[7] | 134 | 6 (5%) | 21 (16%) | 102 (76%) |
| Lundberg[8] | 95 | 13 (14%) | 29 (31%) | 37 (39%) |
| Beard[9] | 35 | 3 (17%) | 6 (33%) | 17 (49%) |
| Cunanan[10] | 1194 | 43 (4%) | 229 (19%) | 355 (30%) |
| Kresch[11] | 100 | 32 (32%) | 38 (38%) | 17 (17%) |
| Rapkin[12] | 100 | 37 (37%) | 26 (26%) | 36 (36%) |
| Vercellini[13] | 126 | 41 (33%) | 31 (25%) | 47 (37%) |
| Mahmood[14] | 156 | 24 (15%) | 43 (28%) | 89 (51%) |

menstrual cycle and local bleeding occurs at the time of menstruation. Prostaglandins, chemical mediators of pain and inflammation, are released. Fibrosis and adhesion formation may lead to tissues becoming bound down so that coitus and physiological movement, such as ovarian distension at ovulation, causes traction and pain.

The most common indications for the treatment of endometriosis are pain and infertility. Asymptomatic endometriosis does not need to be treated. Treatment for pain needs to be individualized depending on the patient's age, desire for the preservation of fertility, severity of pain and the site of endometriotic deposits. Anti-prostaglandin agents and analgesics are used for patients who wish fertility to be maintained. Hormonal therapy is effective in relieving pain in a majority of women. However, pain generally recurs after discontinuation of medication and side-effects preclude long term use. Surgical treatment can be conservative or radical. Conservative surgery attempting to resect or vaporize all visible endometriotic deposits can be performed at laparoscopy. Deneverating procedures (such as presacral neurectomy or uterosacral ligament resection) cannot be recommended based on the evidence available. Hysterectomy may be helpful in some patients.

## Adhesions

Adhesions are found in some women with pelvic pain, but their relationship to pain is uncertain. In a prospective study, Mahmood reported that women with adhesions complain of pelvic pain, deep dyspareunia and pain after intercourse significantly more frequently than women with a normal pelvis.[14] Conversely, Rapkin reviewed retrospectively 100 consecutive laparoscopies for pelvic pain and compared them with 88 undertaken for infertility, in which group only 4 patients complained of pain. A total of 26% in the pain group and 39% in the infertility group were found to have adhesions. There was no significant difference in either location or density of adhesions.[12]

Steege reported that preoperative ratings of dyspareunia and pain during daily activities did not correlate with the severity of adhesions found at laparoscopy.[17] In his study, lysis of adhesions improved both pain and dyspareunia in some patients. Patients in the study were categorized into those with, what the authors termed, 'chronic pain syndrome' and those without. 'Chronic pain syndrome' was diagnosed in women with a least four of the following:

- Pain of 6 or more months duration
- Incomplete relief by previous treatments (e.g. analgesics, prior operation)
- Impaired physical function
- At least one vegetative sign of depression
- Altered family role.

Patients with 'chronic pain syndrome' had a poorer response to treatment than those without this syndrome. This study concluded that lysis of adhesions was useful, but that additional psychological evaluation and appropriate treatment should be incorporated into patient management.

Other gynaecological conditions, such as ovarian remnant syndrome, fibroids, ovarian cysts, pelvic congestion syndrome and chronic pelvic inflammatory disease may be the cause of pain in some patients. However, it is important to appreciate that pathology does not always cause pain. Trimbos prospectively recorded the laparoscopic findings in 200 asymptomatic, healthy women undergoing sterilization.[18] Of these, 148 (74%) women had a normal laparoscopy, but distinct pathological findings were seen in 52 (26%). Adhesions were present in 28 patients (14%), endometriosis in 5 (3%) and uterine fibromyomas in 10 (5%). Nearly half of the adhesions were graded moderate or severe, and 68% involved the colon or omentum. Thus gynaecological pathology may play a role in the genesis of chronic pelvic pain in some women, but not in all. The importance of these organic disorders relative to affective, cognitive and psychosocial factors will vary from case to case.

**153**

# Laparoscopic conscious pain mapping

Laparoscopic conscious pain mapping is a diagnostic laparoscopy under local anaesthesia with or without sedation, performed with the goal of discovering sources of pain in the patient with chronic pelvic pain. It has been suggested that laparoscopy under local anaesthesia can lead to the identification of subtle or atypical areas of disease that may have been overlooked if the procedure had been performed under general anaesthesia.

At present, the role for this technique is being evaluated. There is some evidence that patients with CPP have generalized visceral hypersensitivity to probing in all areas of the pelvis when compared with patients being evaluated for fertility. Another concern is that tenderness elicited by probing or traction is in response to a mechanical stimulus and, hence, may not be physiological. It remains to be seen whether the source of pain, as identified at laparoscopy under local anaesthesia, is responsible for the symptom.

# Pathology

## Gastrointestinal

It is sometimes difficult to determine if lower abdominal pain is of gynaecological or gastrointestinal origin, as the cervix, uterus and its adnexa share the same afferent visceral pathways to the spinal cord as afferent impulses from the lower ileum, colon and rectum. Therefore, a full gastrointestinal history should be taken in patients with pelvic pain. Diagnoses to be considered include irritable bowel syndrome (IBS), inflammatory bowel disease (Crohn's disease, ulcerative colitis), diverticular disease and endometriosis affecting the bowel.

Irritable bowel syndrome (IBS) is a common cause of lower abdominal and pelvic pain. It is a functional disease, meaning that pain and changes in bowel habit arise from abnormal behaviour of the bowel or abnormal perception of physiological events, rather than any structural abnormality. It affects 10–20% of the population. It can be diagnosed from the history using the Rome criteria, which can be found at *www.romecriteria.org* (Table 15.2). Various non-colonic symptoms have been associated with IBS, including dypareunia, dysmenorrhoea, backache and urinary frequency and urgency.

## Urological

Chronic pelvic pain of urological origin may arise from the kidney, ureter, bladder or urethra. The principal urological causes of chronic pelvic pain are interstitial cystitis and urethral syndrome.

Interstitial cystitis is an inflammatory condition of unknown aetiology, characterized by pain and symptoms such as urgency, frequency and nocturia. Typically, pain increases as the bladder fills, and it is relieved by micturition. It may be recreated by pressure over the bladder base in vaginal examination. Chronic urethral syndrome is characterized by irritative symp-

| **Table 15.2**   Irritable bowel syndrome: Rome criteria (www.romecriteria.org) |
|---|
| At least 12 weeks, in the preceding 12 months, of abdominal discomfort or pain that has two out of three features: |
| 1. Relieved with defecation; and/or |
| 2. Onset associated with a change in frequency of stool; and/or |
| 3. Onset associated with a change in appearance of stool. |

toms, as well as post-void fullness and incontinence. Pressure over the bladder base may also recreate the pelvic pain. It has been postulated that urethral syndrome and interstitial cystitis are early and later variations of the same disease.

## Musculoskeletal

Musculoskeletal dysfunctions and myofascial syndromes have been clearly demonstrated as important primary and secondary factors in the aetiology of chronic pelvic pain, and they have been comprehensively reviewed.[19,20] Musculoskeletal problems identified as primary causative factors in chronic pelvic pain appear to occur most commonly in response to chronic repetitive stress and strain, associated with faulty posture and poor body mechanics. Direct trauma has been reported following accidents, surgery and childbirth.

Many musculoskeletal structures of the back and pelvis share a common segmental innervation with urogenital organs and pain referred from these structures can mimic pain of a gynaecological or urological origin. The severity of musculoskeletal pain can vary throughout the menstrual cycle as a consequence of hormonal changes, and this can compound diagnostic confusion. Pain arising from pelvic organs can be referred to dermatomes supplied by somatic afferent fibres of the same spinal segment. Pain arising from the ovaries (segmental innervation T10–T11) can be referred to the lower abdomen and back. Pain arising from the uterus and cervix can be referred to the lower abdominal wall supplied by T12 and also to the lower lumbar and upper sacral area. Pain from the bladder (T11–T12, S2–S4) can be referred to the suprapubic, thoracolumbar and sacrococcygeal region. The hyperalgesia accompanying referred pain can initiate the onset of true pain in the overlying muscle, fascia and cutaneous tissue within that dermatome.

Education, posture advice, therapeutic exercise, stretching, manual myofascial release techniques, muscle re-training and mobilization may all be helpful in the management of the patient with chronic pelvic pain.

## Nerve entrapment pain

When nerves become trapped in scar tissue they may give rise to pain at or beneath the scar or in the distribution of the nerve. It has been postulated that nerves may also become trapped at the edge of the rectus muscle as they penetrate the fascia. Myofascial pain accounted for 30% of somatic diagnoses in 122 women with pelvic pain and negative laparoscopy.[21] In two-thirds of these women, it appeared to be related to a previous surgical incision. Painful ilioinguinal and/or iliohypogastric nerve entrapment has been described following surgery in the lower abdomen. The diagnostic triad of nerve entrapment after operation comprises:

- Typical burning or shooting pain near the incision that radiates to the area supplied by the nerve
- Evidence of impaired sensory perception of the nerve
- Pain relieved at least on a temporary basis by infiltration with local anaesthetic.

Physiotherapy and desensitization techniques may benefit some patients. Tricyclic antidepressants and anticonvulsants are often prescribed. Local anaesthetic and steroid injections into the tender scar may be helpful.

# Psychological factors

Early studies postulated that women with pelvic pain and no obvious pathology had common psychological traits. Most had experienced an insecure family life during childhood and were felt to display an inability to function as women, either sexually or maternally. Emotional immaturity and strong dependency needs were also common. The onset of the pain could, in many cases, be temporally related to a stressful life event. However, these early studies can be subjected to methodological criticism, as the absence of pelvic pathology was not confirmed by laparoscopy or laparotomy. More recently, several investigators have reported that women who have pelvic pain with positive and negative laparoscopic findings exhibit similar psychological profiles. Renaer reported inflated scores on the MMPI for hypochondriasis, depression and hysteria in patients with pelvic pain, with and without clear organic cause, when compared with a pain-free control group.[22] Castelnuovo-Tedesco found no difference in psychiatric pathology between patients with chronic pelvic pain who have pelvic pathology and those who do not.[23] Women with chronic pelvic pain, regardless of the presence or absence of pathology, have significantly higher prevalence rates of lifetime and current major depressive illness, lifetime drug abuse, phobic behaviour and adult sexual dysfunction than a pain-free control group.

Many studies have shown an increased incidence of childhood and adult sexual abuse in patients with chronic pelvic pain.[24-29] Somatization disorder in adult women has been shown to be associated with sexual abuse in childhood.[30] Previous sexual abuse is also more common in women with functional bowel disease.[31] Physical abuse in childhood has also been shown to be more common in pelvic pain patients.[32] Whilst there is evidence of an association between sexual abuse and chronic pelvic pain, this does imply causality. However, an awareness of this possible association is important in the assessment and management of the polysymptomatic patient with CPP.

## Management

Chronic pelvic pain can be a diagnostic and therapeutic dilemma, and it has proved difficult to manage using a uniprofessional model. Women with pelvic pain in whom no clear diagnosis is present, or where diagnoses overlap, need to be given clear explanations that do not undermine the legitimacy of their own experience of pain or convey a message of dismissal. The multidisciplinary team can undertake assessment and treatment using a broader psychosocial concept of the pain experience. Integrated approaches using somatic and behavioural therapies have been shown to reduce pain and other symptoms and improve functional ability.[33] This approach will not be needed, and may not be practical, for all patients. However, early identification of those patients who may benefit from such an approach may be helpful and may provide the opportunity to work simultaneously with the many contributing factors often present. Further research is needed to identify which are the essential elements of interdisciplinary approaches to secure optimum outcome for the individual patient.

## References

1. Wesselmann U, Burnett AL, Heinberg LJ. The urogenital and rectal pain syndromes. *Pain* **73**: 269–294, 1997
2. Mathias SD, Kuppermann M, Liberman RF, Lipschutz RC, Steege JF. Chronic pelvic pain: Prevalence, health-related quality of life, and economic correlates. *Obstet Gynecol* **87**: 321–327, 1996
3. Zondervan KT, Yudkin PL, Vessey MP, Dawes MG, Barlow DH, Kennedy SH. The prevalence of chronic pelvic pain in women in the United Kingdom: a systematic review. *Br J Obstet Gynaecol* **105**: 93–99, 1998
4. McMahon SB, Koltzenberg M. *Silent afferents and visceral pain. Pharmacological approaches to the treatment of chronic pain: new concepts and critical issues. Progress in pain research and management, vol 1.* Seattle: IASP Press, 1994, pp. 11–30.

5. Giamberardino MA. Visceral hyperalgesia. In: Devor M, Rowbotham MC, Wiesenfeld-Hallin Z, eds. *Proceedings of the 9th World Congress on Pain*. Seattle: IASP Press, 2000, pp. 523–550

6. Cervero F. Mechanisms of visceral pain: past and present. In: Gebhart GF, ed. *Visceral Pain. Progress in Pain Research and Management, vol 5*. Seattle: IASP Press, 1995, pp. 25–40

7. Liston WA, Bradford WP, Downie J, Kerr MG. Laparoscopy in a general gynecologic unit. *Am J Obstet Gynecol* 105: 1088–1098, 1969

8. Lundberg WI, Wall JE, Mathers JR. Laparoscopy in evaluation of pelvic pain *Obstet Gynecol* 42: 872–876, 1978

9. Beard RW, Belsley EM, Lieberman BA, Wilkinson JCM. Pelvic pain in women. *Am J Obstet Gynecol* 128: 566–570, 1977

10. Cunanan RG, Courey NG, Lippes J. Laparoscopic findings in patients with pelvic pain. *Am J Obstet Gynecol* 146: 589–599, 1983

11. Kresch AJ, Seifer DB, Sachs LB, Barrese I. Laparoscopy in 100 women with chronic pelvic pain. *Obstet Gynecol* 64: 672–674, 1984

12. Rapkin AJ. Adhesions and pelvic pain: A retrospective study. *Obstet Gynecol* 68: 13–15, 1986

13. Vercellini P. Fedele L, Molteni P, Arcaini L, Bianchi S, Candiani GB. Laparoscopy in the diagnosis of gynecologic chronic pelvic pain. *Int J Gynecol Obstet* 165: 73–79, 1990

14. Mahmood TA, Templeton AA, Thomson L, Fraser C. Menstrual symptoms in women with endometriosis. *Br J Obstet Gynaecol* 98: 558–563, 1991

15. Howard F. The role of laparoscopy in chronic pelvic pain: promise and pitfalls. *Obstet Gynceol Survey* 48: 357–387, 1993

16. Cornillie FJ, Oosterlynck D, Lauweryns JM, Koninckx PR. Deeply infiltrating pelvic endometriosis: Histology and clinical significance. *Fertil Steril* 53: 978–983, 1990

17. Steege JF, Stout AL. Resolution of chronic pelvic pain after laparoscopic lysis of adhesions. *Am J Obstet Gynecol* 165: 278–281, 1991

18. Trimbos JB, Trimbos-Kemper GCM, Peters AAW, van der Does CD, van Hall EV. Findings in 200 consecutive asymptomatic women having a laparoscopic sterilization *Arch Gynecol Obstet* 247: 121–124, 1990

19. King Baker P. Musculoskeletal problems. In: Steege JF, Metzger DA, Levy BS, eds. *Chronic Pelvic Pain: An Integrated Approach*. Philadelphia: WB Saunders, 1998, pp. 215–240

20. Costello K. Myofascial syndromes. In: Stege JF, Metzger DA, Levy BS, eds. *Chronic pelvic pain: An Integrated Approach*. Philadelphia: WB Saunders, 1998, pp. 251–266

21. Reiter RC. Occult somatic pathology in women with chronic pelvic pain. *Clin Obstet Gynecol* 33: 154–160, 1990

22. Renacr M, Vertommen H, Nijs P, Wagemans L, van Hemelrijck T. Psychological aspects of chronic pelvic pain in women. *Am J Obstet Gynecol* 134: 75–80, 1979

23. Castelnuovo-Tedesco P, Krout BM. Psychosomatic aspects of chronic pelvic pain. *Psychol Med* 1: 109–126, 1970

24. Harrop-Griffiths, J, Katon W, Walker E. The association between chronic pelvic pain, psychiatric diagnosis and childhood sexual abuse. *Obstet Gynecol* 71: 589–594, 1988

25. Walker E, Katon W, Harrop-Griffiths J, Holm L, Russo J, Hickok L. Relationship of chronic pelvic pain to psychiatric diagnosis and childhood sexual abuse. *Am J Psychiat* 145: 75–80, 1988

26. Reiter RC, Gambone JC. Demographic and historic variables in women with idiopathic chronic pelvic pain. *Obstet Gynecol* 75: 428–432, 1990

27. Peters AAW, van Dorst E, JellisB, van Zuuren E, Hermans J, Trimbos JB. A randomized clinical trial to compare two different approaches in women with chronic pelvic pain. *Obstet Gynecol* 77: 740–744, 1991

28. Toomey T, Hernandez JT, Gittelman DF, Hulka JF. Relationship of sexual and physical abuse to pain and psychological assessment variables in chronic pelvic pain patients. *Pain* 53: 105–109, 1993

29. Collett BJ, Cordle CJ, Stewart CR, Jagger C. A comparative study of women with chronic pelvic pain, chronic nonpelvic pain and those with no history of pain attending general practitioners. *Br J Obstet Gynaecol* 105: 87–92, 1998

30. Morrison J. Childhood sexual histories of women with somatization disorder. *Am J Psychiat* 146: 239–241, 1989

31. Drossman DA, Leserman J, Nachman G, et al. Sexual and physical abuse in women with functional or organic gastrointestinal disorders. *Ann Int Med* 113: 828–833, 1990

32. Rapkin AJ, Kames L, Darke LL, Stampler FM, Naliboff BD. History of physical and sexual abuse in women with chronic pelvic pain. *Obstet Gynecol* **76**: 92–96, 1990
33. Kames LD, Rapkin AJ, Naliboff BD, Afifi S, Ferrer-Brechner T. Effectiveness of an interdisciplinary program for the treatment of chronic pelvic pain. *Pain* **41**: 41–46, 1990

# 16 Back Pain: Surgeon's View

## John O'Dowd

The role of surgery in the management of degenerative lumbar spine disease, causing either nerve root pain or low back pain, has become much more clearly defined in the last decade. There has been a simultaneous explosion of interest in interventional treatments for managing both leg and back pain and, many of these treatments have been introduced into routine clinical use without an appropriate evidence base to support them. The life cycle of these new techniques starts with an enthusiastic description by the inventor surgeon and then intense marketing by the manufacturer or producer. There is then a phase of widespread clinical use with sporadic reports of problems and then, ultimately, the technique is subject to a prospective randomized control trial and is shown to be either no better than the pre-existing gold standard treatments, or associated with poor clinical results or a higher complication rate and the new technique fades into disuse. This review will focus on treatments with an established evidence base. However, there are now well-recognized guidelines for the management of acute and chronic leg pain in patients with degenerative spondylosis, and there is an emerging evidence base to support long-standing surgical treatments for the management of low back pain.

## Epidemiology

There is no significant evidence to suggest that there has been an increase in the incidence or prevalence of lumbar spondylosis as measured in population radiology or pathology studies. It is well recognized, however, that there has been an exponential increase in reported levels of disability and compensation for occupational and other types of back injury. Management of degenerative lumbar conditions is increasingly a very large financial load on a health care system already at breaking point. There is a complex cultural interplay, such that it would seem that in advanced western civilizations many patients are able to substitute poor wages from menial occupations with some degree of income generation from the benefits and support that they receive for their disability. In one part of Florida, compensation payments for occupational back injury are increased by 50% if the occupational back injury requires surgery and doubled if the surgery has a poor outcome.[1]

## Leg pain

### Intervertebral disc herniation

Disc herniation remains by far the most common cause of pain in the distribution of a nerve root, typically L4, L5 or S1 in the leg in adults under the age of 60 years. Widespread use of magnetic resonance imaging (MRI) and a concomitant use of minimal-access techniques for removing the disc has led to the need for an increased degree of precision in defining the type and size of disc herniation.

Nuclear material that has migrated to the periphery of the disc and causes a focal bulge in the annulus fibrosus is termed a protrusion. If this same material migrates through the annulus fibrosus, then this is termed disc extrusion and may be sub- or transligamentous (posterior longitudinal ligament). If the same disc material migrates free into the spinal canal, this is termed disc sequestration. All of these may produce significant nerve root pain. Recent work has confirmed the natural history and the results from intervention such as surgery for the large disc herniations and, particularly, sequestrations are rather better than the natural history and interventional treatments for small disc protrusion. The disc herniation may be at the level of the disc or above or below the disc, and, in the transverse plane, the disc herniation may be central, paracentral, posterolateral, foraminal or extra foraminal.

## Clinical presentation

The combination of nerve root pain in a dermatomal distribution associated with neurological symptoms and, on examination, restriction of straight leg raising, commonly associated with sensory and reflex changes and less commonly with motor changes, is almost pathognomonic of an acute disc herniation. The differential diagnosis includes nerve root canal stenosis and alternative, extremely rare, pathologies such as nerve root tumours. The investigation of choice is MRI, which will confirm the nature of the pathology and its exact location. It is worth noting that population studies have shown that the background incidence of disc herniation in the asymptomatic population is 20%.[2] Although an X-ray is not essential for making diagnosis, because of a 20% incidence of segmentation anomalies, X-rays are advised strongly before interventional procedures such as microdiscectomy.

## Treatment

The natural history of disc herniation is excellent, with 90–95% of patients settling spontaneously. It is unlikely that any treatments in this phase actually modify the natural history of the condition, but non-operative treatments, including non-steroidal anti-inflammatory drugs (NSAIDs) and injected epidural steroids and local anaesthetic, can certainly relieve symptoms in any patient whose disc is settling spontaneously. It is well recognized that physical resolution of the disc herniation is not required for resolution of symptoms, which implies that an inflammatory component is actually producing the pain. Recent work with the infusion of a monoclonal antibody that blocks the activity of tumour necrosis factor $\alpha$ (TNF-$\alpha$), suggests that the inflammatory process is the final common pathway for production of pain, and this non-surgical approach may, following a formal prospective trial, lead to a non-interventional treatment for managing this common condition.[3]

A small number of patients with acute sciatica from lumbar disc herniation will require surgical treatment. Patients who have leg pain beyond 6–12 weeks, which is showing no signs of improvement and who are fully informed of the potential risks and complications of the procedure, are candidates for disc excision. In addition, progressive motor weakness in the distribution of one nerve root or an acute cauda equina presentation remain indications for discectomy, although the evidence that emergency decompression for managing cauda equina syndrome makes any difference to the neurological outcome is very limited. Over the last two decades, there has been a plethora of alternative interventional treatments for managing disc herniation, but few have achieved the level of success of the classical open discectomy. Techniques such as the automated percutaneous lumbar discectomy are greeted with initial enthusiasm, but, when subject to randomized controlled trials,[4] they have been shown to have far inferior results to discectomy. The established and generally accepted gold standard is open discectomy, which, when performed through a small incision without magnification, has become known as minimal intervention fenestration. Most surgeons performing significant numbers of discectomies will also use a microscope, and the only evidence based difference that this makes to the surgery is better illumination. Nonetheless, microdiscectomy allows cauterization of fine epidural blood vessels and, in most people's hands, a smaller incision, and it is likely that this combination of effects will lead to a reduced complication rate and possibly a reduction in the incidence of symptomatic, epidural scarring. Historically, discectomy involved laminectomy to access the spine and then a wide clearance of the disc space. This has been demonstrated to correlate with an increase in the radiological progression of the degenerative process; the modern alternative after either a minimal intervention fenestration or microdiscectomy approach will be to remove the disc fragments causing the nerve root compression (fragmentectomy) and to probe the disc space for any residual large unstable disc fragment. The main complications of discectomy are a 4 or 5% incidence of epidural scarring, which becomes symptomatic and can lead to the so-called 'failed back syndrome'. There is a small (3%) incidence of further disc herniation and, with modern microdiscectomy techniques, this may be very early – within the first 4–6 months following the surgery. This means that if patients have recurrence of pre-existing nerve root pain following discectomy surgery, a recurrent disc herniation should be assumed until excluded by contrast enhanced MRI.

# Spinal stenosis

Spinal stenosis is due to an increase in volume of all the elements involved in the pathology of lumbar spondylosis, decreasing the cross-sectional area of the spinal canal and/or root canals leading to symptoms either due to central canal stenosis affecting the cauda equina or, more commonly, nerve root canal stenosis affecting the nerve root in its transit from the main dural sleeve, past the disc and underneath the facet joint and then on out into the foraminal zone as a nerve root exits the spinal canal.

### Clinical features

Nerve root canal stenosis is typically a monoradicular pain in a classical distribution of a dermatome in the leg, brought on by exercise or posture. This is in contradistinction to central canal stenosis, which has rather more poorly defined and vague symptoms of weakness or tiredness in the lower limbs, not necessarily in a dermatomal distribution but also with exercise. With the latter diagnosis, which can be confused with vascular claudication, there can be neurological signs in the lower limbs, but root tension signs are generally negative. As for disc herniation, MRI remains the investigation of choice for identifying the site of neurological compression, but it is essential to scan every level of the motion segment. Three or four transverse slices restricted to the disc/facet joint level are not adequate and pathology may be missed. Computed tomography (CT) in isolation can show the bony compressive elements but is much less effective at showing either the state of the nerve root or the soft tissue compressive elements, although in patients who cannot tolerate MRI, CT-myelography is one alternative imaging medium for visualizing the stenotic spine. Plain X-rays are important in managing patients with stenosis as there may commonly be an associated degenerative spondylolisthesis or degenerative scoliosis. Both of these patterns of instability are more marked on an upright X-ray and, sometimes, may not be clearly visible on a supine MRI scan.

### Treatment

If there is no radiological evidence of instability, such as spondylolisthesis or degenerative scoliosis in a patient who has a leg-pain predominant clinical picture, spinal stenosis can be treated by surgical decompression. It is recognized that the medium-term natural history of spinal stenosis is generally good, and all patients should have a full non-operative programme before considering surgery. This may include epidural injections, selective nerve root blocks and a posture restoring and trunk stabilizing physiotherapy programme. It is rare to require surgery for progressive neurological deficit, and most patients will need to make a quality of life decision based upon their perception of the severity of their symptoms. Most spinal stenosis is addressed through a segmental spinal decompression with preservation of the midline structures, including supraspinous ligament and spinous processes. After performing a wide laminotomy at each level, the dural sleeve and nerve roots can be decompressed by undercutting facet joints and performing extensive flavectomy. It is generally worth exploring a symptomatic nerve root both at the disc space and sub-facet region where it is the traversing root, and at the motion segment below where the same nerve is the exiting root in the foraminal zone. The results of spinal stenosis surgery are mixed and although, on balance, the majority of patients will have some symptomatic improvement, it is rare to become asymptomatic following decompressive surgery. Disappointingly, a large percentage of patients will have persistent symptoms despite adequate decompression.

# Back pain

Surgical management of back pain remains a very controversial area in spinal surgery. Until 2001, there was no high quality randomized control trial data to support the use of any form of surgery for the management of any form of degenerative condition producing low back pain. The Cochrane collaboration group[5] who reviewed the evidence for the Cochrane database in 1999 found no randomized control trials of surgery against natural history, placebo or non-operative treatment, and most of the randomized trials that were found compared different types of surgical technique and were of poor quality. It was generally thought that with established instability, such as degenerative spondylolisthesis or degenerative scoliosis in the presence of a back pain predominant clinical picture, a stabilization surgery was appropriate. Recent evidences cast doubt even upon this basic premise.

However, the Swedish Lumbar Spine Study Group[6] reported last year the results of a multicentre randomized controlled trial, comparing lumbar fusion with non-surgical treatment for chronic low back pain. Whilst accepting the various criticisms of this study, particularly regarding the non-surgical group, which received uncontrolled further physiotherapy input, the study still has significant power looking at this particular area, and it has to be said that the non-operative arm of this trial is probably more intense and effective compared with treatments accessible to patients in the UK. This paper demonstrated very significant differences between the surgical and non-surgical groups with a high level of power. The surgical group were better in relation to back pain reduction, disability reduction, depressive symptom reduction and return to work. There was however, a 17% early surgical complication rate, which was not sustained in the non-operative group.

Christensen reported the 5-year results of 129 patients who had been entered into a randomized control trial of different types of surgical intervention in Denmark.[7] Whilst demonstrating a higher complication rate in instrumented fusion over non-instrumented fusion and no essential outcome differences between the two techniques, this study demonstrated overall the impact of this type of surgery on patients with back pain. Such patients should, on average, expect a significant improvement following the initial surgery, and this improvement continues to the 5-year follow-up, such that at 5 years 40% of the patients were working and 70% of the patients felt that it was worth having been through the surgery. It is currently much more difficult to be dogmatic about surgical technique, but these two studies have demonstrated that straight forward posterolateral fusion (Figure 16.1) achieves acceptably good results and generally provokes a satisfactory or excellent response on patients undergoing the intervention. A meta-analysis performed in 1997 suggested that of all of the surgical techniques for fusing the spine, the use of posterolateral fusion combined with pedicle fixation and a posterior approach past the dura to achieve interbody fusion (PLIF)[8] (Figure 16.2) achieved the highest fusion rates (94%) and clinical success rates (87%). Unfortunately, use of PLIF is associated with a significantly higher incidence of epidural scarring and nerve root injury, and it should probably be reserved for patients who are having simultaneous nerve root decom-

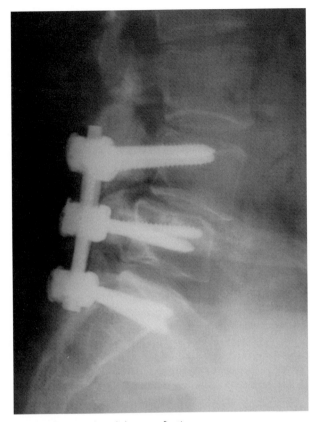

**Figure 16.1** Posterolateral fusion with pedicle screw fixation.

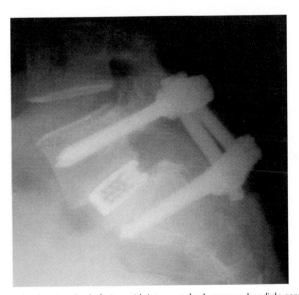

**Figure 16.2** Posterior lumbar interbody fusion with intervertebral cages and pedicle screw fixation.

pression. Review of an innovative cage technique for achieving interbody spinal fusion[9] demonstrated that, although on average most patients had a reduction of pain following this type of spinal fusion, there was a residual level of 70% preoperative pain and 70% preoperative disability at a 2-year follow-up. Certainly the message from all the recent published studies is that back pain is not cured by spinal fusion, but rather is reduced.

There is now a long list of emerging interventional techniques for managing back-pain predominant patients with lumbar spondylosis in addition to fusion techniques, but none of these techniques have been subject to randomized control trials to date and so should be considered as experimental. These interventions include:

- Intradiscal electrocoagulation therapy (IDET)
- Vertebroplasty
- Graf ligament stabilization
- Dynesys stabilization
- Disc replacement
- Nucleus replacement
- Intervertebral cages
- Use of growth factor sponges as opposed to bone graft for fusion.

Disc replacement (Figure 16.3) illustrates the type of problem seen with release of implants into the market place before fully randomized control trials are available. The advantage of disc replacement appears to be preservation of some movement at the operated motion segment, and there is some evidence that this reduces the rate of radiological deterioration at the adjacent segment. Disc replacement, however, requires a major anterior approach and there are significant hazards associated with this, including a risk of vascular injury, and the risk of retrograde ejaculation in young male patients, from injury of the presacral nervous plexus. The longest established disc replacement has been around to allow a follow-up of over 10-years, and the results appeared to be in the range of 70 to 80% improvement at 2 years.[10] There would appear, therefore, to be no clinical advantage over spinal fusion, which is now an evi-

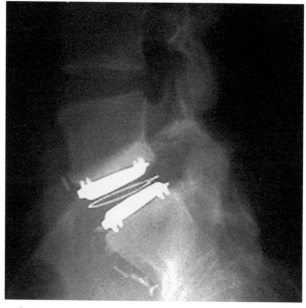

**Figure 16.3**  Disc replacement.

dence based treatment. However, there has been a very substantial investment by the manufacturing industry into disc replacement, and there are currently six prostheses available in the market place for clinical use, despite the absence of high quality trial data to support their use. A recent orthopaedic industry analysis demonstrated the global market potential for disc replacement to be $2.5 billion and it is the largest single contributor to the expansion in growth of the spine market worldwide. It is very difficult to identify an altruistic driver for change for the genuine benefit of patients. This degree of shareholder expectation has been generated in the implants already openly available for clinical use.

## Surgical decision making

Patients who have an axial back-pain predominant clinical presentation and who, as judged by themselves and their primary care advisors, have tried an appropriate and extensive range of non-operative treatments might be considered for spinal surgery to manage the back pain. It seems appropriate that the starting point for the decision-making process is the pathological diagnosis, which is made with the combination of the clinical picture, results of X-ray, MRI and CT and the use of isotope bone scanning. At this stage, before patient expectations are raised too much, the suitability for surgery should be assessed. This would include measurement of physical health and the use of psychometric testing to help in identifying illness behaviour; direct questions should be used to identify issues of secondary gain. The impact of the patient's condition should be measured, which should include formal assessment of pain, disability and quality of life. It is well-recognized that senior clinicians involved in the surgical decision-making process are poor at assessing overall patient psychological function.[11] Finally, the patients pain source should be identified over and above the static radiology. Apart from the clinical picture, this often involves spinal probing, including the use of facet joint injections, annular probing and discography and selective nerve root blocks. At the end of this process, if a fully informed patient understands the risks and complications of surgery and the likely success rate, and they are convinced that they have tried all alternative options and are equally convinced that their perception of their level of pain and disability warrants it, then they can be considered for spinal fusion or one of the more modern alternatives to treat their back pain. Such patients, however, will require intensive postoperative assistance and further rehabilitation and physiotherapy. One of the advantages of modern spinal instrumentation, such as pedicle screw fixation, is that it allows early return to work: some patients can expect to return to light duties within 2–4 weeks of surgery. Whilst accepting that in the long term it seems unlikely that surgery will remain a valid option for managing degenerative spinal disease, particularly with the advent of growth factor manipulation and genetic modification early in the degenerative process, in the short to medium term future, there does appear to be an established niche for use of posterolateral fusion in managing axial lumbar back pain.

# References

1. Personal communication from Prof. Glen Rechtine
2. Powell MC, Wilson M, Szypryt P, Symonds EM, Worthington BS et al. Prevalence of lumbar disc degeneration observed by magnetic resonance in symptomless women. *Lancet* **13**: 1366–1367, 1986
3. Karpinnen J, Korhomen T, Malmivaara A et al. Tumour necrosis factor-alpha monoclonal antibody, infliximab used to manage severe sciatica. *Spine* **28**: 750–753, 2003
4. Chatterjee S, Foy PM, Findlay GF. Report of a controlled clinical trial comparing automated percutaneous lumbar discectomy and microdiscectomy in the treatment of contained lumbar disc herniation. *Spine* **15**: 734–738, 1995
5. Gibson JNA, Grant IC, Waddell G. The Cochrane review of surgery for lumbar disc prolapse and degenerative lumbar spondylosis. *Spine* **17**: 1820–1832, 1999

6. Fritzell P, Hagg O, Wessberg P, Nordwall A and the Swedish Lumbar Spine Study Group et al. Volvo award winner in clinical studies: Lumbar fusion versus nonsurgical treatment for chronic low back pain. A multicentre randomised controlled trial from the Swedish Lumbar Spine Study Group. *Spine* **26**: 2521–2534, 2001

7. Christensen FB, Hansen ES, Laursen M, Thomson K, Bunger CE et al. Long term functional outcome of pedicle screw instrumented instrumentation as a support for posterolateral spinal fusion. Randomised clinical study with 5 year follow up. *Spine* **27**: 1269–1277, 2002

8. Boos N, Webb J. Pedicle screw fixation in spinal disorders: a European view. *Eur Spine J* **6**: 2–18, 1997

9. O'Dowd J. Laparoscopic lumbar spine surgery. *Eur Spine J* **9**: S3–7, 2000

10. Zeegers WS, Bohnen LM, Laaper M, Verhaigen MJ et al. Artificial disc replacement with the modular type SB Charite III: 2 year results in 50 prospectively studied patients. *Eur Spine J* **8**: 210–217, 1999

11. Grevitt M, Pande K, O'Dowd J. Do first impressions count? A comparison of subjective and psychologic assessment of spinal patients. *Eur Spine J* **7**: 218–223, 1998

# 17 Back Pain: Medical Approach

## Martin G Ridley and John Coppin

Low back pain (LBP) remains an increasing source of disability and loss of time from work and the commonest musculoskeletal reason for consulting doctors. It has an estimated lifetime prevalence of 59%.[1] Approximately 10% of back pain episodes lead to consultation with a General Practitioner, but 90% of patients will have improved at 1 month.[1] However, it is now clear from epidemiological evidence, that recurrences are common, and up to 70% of patients with back pain will have three or more episodes in their lifetime. The emerging pattern is that back pain is a chronic disorder, with continuing symptoms in a significant majority, although not disabling most of the time, but with a tendency to recurrence.[2] The prevalence and severity of low back pain has not changed over a number of years, but the trend for back problems to cause chronic disability continues to rise. In the UK in 1993, there were over 100 million days lost from work through LBP. The economic cost of LBP is massive, and recent reports suggest that the direct health care cost of LBP in 1998 was £1632 million.[3] It is evident, therefore, from increasing invalidity payments and health care utilization, that traditional biomedical management of LBP is not effective. Over the last 15 years, a wealth of evidence-based guidelines for the efficacy of treatment and management of acute back pain (up to 3 months duration) have emerged.[4–8] The intention of these guidelines is to help identify those patients with potentially serious spinal pathology who require the biomedical approach, but also to try and identify those patients who are at increased risk of chronic disability, in whom a modified biopsychosocial approach, provided at an early stage, may help prevent the development of chronic disability. If the management of LBP is to improve, and its effect on the health economy to reduce, it requires clinicians and patients to adopt a paradigm shift from regarding back pain as a traditional biomedical issue to one where an integrated biopsychosocial approach is the norm.[9]

## Aetiology

In the context of the pain clinic, the aetiology of chronic LBP is rather different from the full spectrum of disease (Table 17.1), which needs to be considered when seeing a patient with new back pain. Most pain clinic patients with LBP will either have non-specific mechanical back pain or post-disc surgery low back pain with varying degrees of associated leg pain. There is an evolving further group of patients with the consequences of spinal osteoporosis. Many patients with so-called mechanical back pain will have little or no radiologically demonstrable pathology. Such age-related X-ray changes as exist will be combinations of varying degrees of lumbar disc degeneration and/or facet joint arthritis. As will probably be only too apparent, the aetiology of chronic LBP remains as much a question of pain as of the back. It includes those factors that are so important in all chronic pain: psychological distress, the destructive combination of fear and avoidance of provocative activity, coping difficulties, depression and the development of the sick role. Whatever can be achieved in purely nociceptive terms, with specific treatment, will only be successful in the longer term if combined with a thorough assessment and management of these other factors. It is important to remember, whatever the

| Table 17.1 Causes of low back pain with/without leg pain |
|---|
| Non-specific mechanical back pain |
| Facet joint syndrome ± facet joint arthritis |
| Lumbar disc degeneration (lumbar spondylosis) |
| Lumbar disc prolapse |
| Spondylolisthesis |
| Spinal stenosis |
| Osteoporosis |
| Sero-negative spondyl arthritis (including ankylosing spondylitis) |
| Vertebral infection |
| Disc space infection |
| Malignancy – secondary myeloma and primary |
| Paget's disease, referred – visceral, pancreatic/pelvic etc |

possible aetiology in anatomical terms, that what the patient believes to be cause of his or her pain is even more important. Inappropriate or misplaced health beliefs are one of several significant factors that determine the likelihood of chronicity in chronic pain in general and in back pain in particular.[6] It is, unfortunately, all too easy for a patient to have acquired conflicting explanations for the physical basis of their problem from the various practitioners, both orthodox and heterodox, that they consult. Once the patient reaches the pain clinic, it is important that these beliefs are explored and that any further explanations given are consistent, simple and in language readily understood. They should emphasize function rather than anatomy, so that they can be rationally incorporated into a positive approach towards a rehabilitation programme.

# Clinical Assessment

## Diagnostic triage

Diagnostic triage has become clarified and should be applied to patients presenting with new episodes of back pain. In our unit, in common with others, we have developed a system that allows specialist physiotherapists to provide the initial assessment of patients in secondary care, supported by appropriate algorithms for the use of radiological and haematological investigations. The physiotherapist works closely with their colleague consultants in orthopaedics/ rheumatology and pain relief, which ensures appropriate re-direction of patients as required.[10] The purpose of diagnostic triage is to identify serious pathology or any specific diseases that require conventional medical management. 'Red flag' symptoms and signs are carefully evaluated (Table 17.2). Although the identification of such red flags is important, they remain a rather crude and insensitive method of identifying potentially serious pathology.[11]

## Clinical assessment in the pain relief clinic

It is important that the initial consultation in the pain clinic of a patient with chronic LBP is given a realistic allocation of time, since patients often have long multifaceted histories. This consultation is an important first step in the reassurance and re-education that are such an important part of patient management – a principle that is common to the management of most chronic conditions. The consequent development of a rapport between doctor and patient may go a long way to open up the path to better understanding. Time spent at this point will be saved many times over.[12]

**Table 17.2** Red flags – possible serious spinal pathology[5]

Age of onset: <20 or >55 years
Violent trauma, e.g. fall from a height, RTA
Constant, progressive, non-mechanical pain
Thoracic pain
PMH – carcinoma
Systemic steroids
Drug abuse, HIV infection
Systemically unwell
Weight loss
Persistent severe restriction of lumbar flexion
Widespread neurological deficit
Structural deformity

HIV, human immunodeficiency virus; PMH, past medical history; RTA, road traffic accident
**Note:** If there are suspicious clinical features or if pain has not settled in 6 weeks, an ESR and plain X-ray should be considered in the above situations.

The history should establish:

- Characteristics of pain, including using pain diagram[13] and McGill Pain Questionnaire[14]
- Patients' beliefs about their LBP (Table 17.3)
- Previous treatment in chronological order
- Functional impact of condition on daily life
- Functional impact and condition at work (sadly most will not be at work)
- Whether litigation is involved.

**Table 17.3** Psycho-social yellow flags. Summary of the Quick Reference Guide in Acute Low Back Pain

There is good agreement that the following factors are important and consistently predict poor outcomes:

- Presence of a belief that back pain is harmful or potentially severely disabling
- Fear-avoidance behaviour and reduced activity levels
- Tendency to low mood and withdrawal from social interaction
- An expectation of passive treatment, rather than a belief that active participation will help.

To assess the above factors, the following questions are suggested, appropriately phrased:

- Have you had time off work in the past with back pain?
- What do you understand to be the cause of your back pain?
- What are you expecting will help you?
- How is your employer responding to your back pain? Your co-workers? Your family?
- What are you doing to cope with back pain?
- Do you think you will return to work? When?

From Kendall, Linton and Maine[6]
**Note:** The key goal with this guide is to identify risk factors that increase the probability of long-term disability and work loss in association with back pain. The assessment can be used to target effective early management to try and prevent the onset of these problems.

| Table 17.4    Risk factors for chronicity |
|---|
| Previous history of low back pain |
| Total work loss (due to low back pain) in past 12 months |
| Radiating leg pain |
| Reduced straight leg raising |
| Signs of nerve root involvement |
| Reduced trunk muscle strength and endurance |
| Poor physical fitness |
| Poor self-rated health |
| Heavy smoking |
| Psychological distress and depressive symptoms |
| Disproportionate illness behaviour |
| Low job satisfaction |
| Personal problems – alcohol, marital, financial |
| Adversarial medicolegal proceedings |

Reproduced from the Clinical Standards Advisory Group Report, 1994.[5]

**Note:** Low educational attainment and heavy physical occupation slightly increase the risk of low back pain and chronicity, but markedly increase the difficulty of rehabilitation/re-training.

At this point, it is perhaps worth noting the risk factors for chronicity in back pain (Table 17.4).

## Examination

This should include assessment of:

- Pain behaviour
- Spinal signs
- Neurology, including nerve root tension/dural tension signs
- Vascular assessment
- Exclude peripheral joint disease (e.g. hips).

### Pain behaviour

Assessment of pain behaviour begins as the patient enters the consultation room and continues while taking the history, but, specifically, includes noting the presence/absence of signs that indicate emotional distress and illness behaviour. Waddell in particular, has drawn attention to these signs, and a useful assessment can be made to gauge them more objectively.[15]

More recently Main has outlined a simple classification system to help identify distress and predict risk for chronicity and/or poor outcome in LBP.[16]

### Spinal signs

Assessment of spinal signs begins with inspection – looking specifically for deformity, most commonly scoliosis, which can either be structural or due to muscle spasm and pelvic tilt. With the patient standing, movements of the lumbar spine can be assessed, making allowance for age. Lumbar spinal flexion can be measured by the modified Schober test. Percussion to assess vertebral tenderness can be useful for localizing vertebral pathology. Palpation for muscle spasm/tenderness and trigger points can also be performed, but it can usefully be re-assessed with the patient on the couch.

## Neurology

Assessment of neurology starts with the patient standing as minor S1 weakness, in particular, can otherwise be missed. Standing and walking on tiptoe tests the S1 nerve root, walking on heels, the L5 root. On the couch, quadriceps strength tests L4. Nerve root tension signs should now be addressed. Straight leg raising (SLR) assesses dural tension in the lower lumbar nerve roots L5 and S1. It requires the patient to be relaxed and involves passive elevation of the leg by the examiner. It is often helpful as a preliminary to gain the patient's cooperation and good muscle relaxation to flex the hip and knee passively first, then elevating the straightened leg. The test is positive if it produces buttock or leg pain, but not just back pain or mild tightness behind the knee, which is often due to shortening of the hamstrings, a frequent accompaniment of a chronic pain situation. Elicitation of leg pain/buttock pain on the symptomatic side when performing SLR on the contralateral leg (crossed positive sciatic nerve stretch) is powerful evidence of dural tension and frequently indicates an often large lumbar disc prolapse.

With the patient prone, high lumbar nerve root tension can be assessed using the femoral nerve stretch test. This tests dural tension in association with L3/L4 and sometimes L5 roots. Therefore, it is less frequently positive, since most lumbar nerve root entrapment syndromes affect L5 or S1, but it should be borne in mind in patients with atypical leg pain, possibly indicating a higher lumbar disc lesion. The patient lies prone and the symptomatic leg is passively flexed at the knee. A positive test produces anterior thigh pain. Again, reproduction of back pain alone is not indicative of dural tension.

Finally, elicitation of deep tendon reflexes and sensory examination complete the neurological examination. The ankle reflex is usually subserved by S1, but can include L5. The knee reflex is subserved by L3 or L4, but occasionally includes elements of L5. In the sensory examination, it is important to ascertain whether there is true dermatomal loss, including the saddle area. Whole leg anaesthesia tells the clinician more about the patient's illness behaviour than his or her neuropathology.

# Differential diagnosis

At the initial assessment, the referring diagnosis should be reconsidered and positively re-confirmed if appropriate (see Diagnostic triage section). Conditions that can lead to confusion with chronic LBP, even at this stage, include:

- Sero-negative spondylo-arthritis, typified by ankylosing spondylitis (AS) – typically, patients with AS should have experienced their first symptoms before the age of 40 years. They will usually have suffered continuous symptoms for several months at a time; early morning and post-immobility stiffness should be prominent features, with relative relief by exercise. They may experience marked night pain. There is usually a good response to anti-inflammatory drugs, but sometimes side-effects, or concern about using the drugs in the right way, will have precluded an inadequate trial of therapy. The presence of human leukocyte antigen HLA-B27 supports, but is not absolute confirmation of, the diagnosis. Similarly, the absence of HLA-B27 does not totally exclude the diagnosis. HLA-B27 is carried by 98% of patients with classical AS, but only 60–80% of patients with other sero-negative spondylo-arthritides, and by 8–10% of the healthy Caucasian population.
- Metabolic bone disease – not infrequently, osteoporotic vertebral collapse will have occurred without typical acute pain and limitation; therefore, the patient with multiple sequential osteoporotic collapses can present to the pain clinic with more chronic pain without the diagnosis having previously been made. Osteomalacia causes spinal and more generalized musculoskeletal pain and needs to be considered in the relevant at-risk population, especially females originating from the Indian sub-continent. Serum alkaline phosphatase should be elevated.

- Infections – tuberculosis and brucellosis are the two chronic indolent infections that can elude diagnosis for some months and, hence, may find their way to the pain clinic. Both are likely to be associated with systemic symptoms, including weight loss. They need particularly to be considered in the relevant at-risk populations – those working with animals for brucellosis, and the immuno-suppressed, alcoholics or immigrants for tuberculosis. Measurement of ESR and CRP will be helpful.
- Tumours – these are unlikely to remain undiagnosed prior to referral to a pain clinic. Unremitting localized pain should arouse suspicion. Severe limitation of spinal movement needs an explanation and appropriate investigation before it can be assumed to be related to the consequences of persistent fear/avoidance of movement.
- Myeloma, in particular, can have an indolent course and cause diagnostic problems, especially in those lacking a serum protein band on electrophoresis and only excreting light chains in the urine. Bone scanning will frequently be negative, since myeloma deposits do not excite an osteoblastic reaction around them, hence appearing as cool spots or normal tracer intensity, rather than the hot spots so typical of metastatic bony secondaries from carcinomas.

Clearly associated leg pain widens the differential diagnosis, which will then include potentially surgically correctable lumbar nerve root entrapment syndromes. These require careful clinical assessment combined with review of the relevant scans: mostly now magnetic resonance imaging (MRI), but, occasionally, computed tomography (CT). Sometimes consideration needs to be given to re-investigation if the clinical evidence of nerve root entrapment is strong. This re-assessment can usefully be undertaken in a Combined Clinic with the relevant orthopaedic and rheumatological colleagues.

## Management

We need to consider:

- Injection treatment (See Chapter 18)
- Drug treatment
- Transcutaneous nerve stimulation (TENS)
- Physical treatment.

### Drug treatment

Non-steroidal anti-inflammatory drugs (NSAIDs) are likely to have been used extensively before the patient comes to the pain clinic. However, their full potential should be explored before they are abandoned as unhelpful in an individual case. They are often helpful for night pain and morning stiffness, and a slow release preparation is often the most logical form of treatment. Use of the newer, relatively cyclooxygenase-2 (COX-2) selective anti-inflammatories should be considered in patients over 65 years of age, because of such patients' intrinsically greater risk of gastrointestinal (GI) side-effects. However, before prescribing an anti-inflammatory to any patient, consideration should be given to the relative risks of such treatment: the risk of GI side-effects is increased in the presence of increasing age and significant co-morbidity, particularly cardiovascular. This increased risk is compounded by the fact that many such patients will be on low-dose aspirin because of the prevalence of cardiovascular disease. There is also some uncertainty regarding the cardiovascular risks with COX-2 selective drugs. These factors are in addition to the risks associated with a prior history of peptic ulcer disease or definite GI haemorrhage. There is evidence of some advantage for the use of the relatively COX-2 selective drugs in patients without significant co-morbidity, but there is no such advantage in patients with significant co-morbidity or other major risk factors for complications of therapy, and, in these patients if a decision is made to give an anti-inflammatory drug, a conventional non-steroidal drug should be given with full gastric protection with proton pump inhibitors.[17]

Tricyclic anti-depressants in low to medium dosages have a definite effect in chronic pain, which is independent of their anti-depressant action.[18] They are also useful in patients with radicular pain. Patients can be reassured about their lack of addictive potential and the specific reason for their prescription.

Gabapentin has an increasing role in the management of neuropathic pain, and it is worth considering in patients with radicular pain.

## Transcutaneous nerve stimulation

Transcutaneous nerve stimulation is a form of symptomatic relief that is commonly used in pain clinics. The machines have become more affordable recently and, after a trial period, patients often purchase their own. The benefits of TENS include symptomatic relief without the risk of overdose or complications. There are few contraindications. Unlike other physical modalities that enforce a passive role (such as heat or ice) or therapy dependence (such as acupuncture or manipulation), TENS provides analgesia whilst the patient is active. This may be used in an attempt to enhance capacity during rehabilitation. When used successfully, the chronic pain patient is encouraged by gaining control over their symptoms. Along with many other physical modalities there is little evidence that TENS provides lasting benefits or is sufficiently powerful to alter the natural history of back pain.

## Physical treatment

Physical de-conditioning is an important factor in the chronic pain cycle. Pain problems frequently cause a reduction in activity and behavioural changes, leading to immobility, physical impairment and disability. Patients with chronic pain may require assistance with a broad spectrum of physical and psychological needs. Physiotherapists play a major role in providing physical treatments for chronic low back pain and are increasingly aware of the relevance of potential psychosocial barriers to recovery. By the time patients reach the pain clinic setting, it is likely they have had a number of courses of physiotherapy, possibly with some exposure to complimentary approaches such as chiropractic or osteopathy. The physiotherapist is often the best judge of whether further physical treatments will be of benefit to the patient. An in-depth appraisal of previous treatments and their effect will guide as to whether further physical treatments are indicated.

Physical treatments are provided by a number of different methods. Individual treatments of manual therapy and specific exercises may be still beneficial as, not infrequently, patients develop chronic pain problems but somehow miss straightforward and basic treatment approaches. Depending on local arrangements, the physiotherapist may have extended their traditional scope of practice to employ methods such as acupuncture, trigger point injections or relaxation techniques. Individual treatments may be used as an adjunct to, or follow, specific pain clinic procedures (see Chapter 1). Physical treatment may also be part of treatment programmes. Two such commonly used programmes are pain management programmes and functional restoration programmes. The nomenclature can often confuse. Main and Benjamin have made a useful comparison of approaches[19] (Tables 17.5 and 17.6).

As previously stated, the treatment needs of patients vary. These needs are likely to change as the time passes. It seems that the crucial time for development of chronicity is approximately 6 weeks following onset.[5] Traditional biomedical models of back care can lead to fragmentation of management between primary and secondary care at this stage. When primary

**Table 17.5** A comparison of philosophy of care

|  | General medical approach | Back schools | Functional restoration programmes | Pain management programmes |
|---|---|---|---|---|
| Education | None | Major | Moderate/major | Major |
| Patient involvement in: |  |  |  |  |
|   Treatment | None | Major | Major | Major |
|   Decision making | None | Minor | Minor | Major |
| Emphasis on self-help | None | Major | Major | Major |
| Emphasis on return to work | Minor | Minor | Major | Minor |

From Main & Benjamin 1995[19], with permission from Oxford University Press

care individual treatment fails, patients should be offered an opportunity to engage in group-based rehabilitation programmes. Whereas traditional functional restoration programmes are typically aimed at established chronic back problems with a focus on return to work and attempts to normalize back function, back rehabilitation groups can be based on cognitive-behavioural principles and be implemented at an earlier stage. Using a biopsychosocial approach combined with simple questionnaires (see Table 17.3) allows a greater degree of accuracy for predicting who, from the vast numbers with acute back pain, will go on to develop chronic problems. It is beneficial to anticipate a poor response to individual treatment and arrange more intensive multidisciplinary rehabilitation at an early stage. Although there is little evidence for this approach preventing chronicity, it reinforces key messages such as keeping active, use of medication, pacing activity and the meaning of pain at an early stage. In an ideal world, this message will be repeated throughout their episode of care.

## Psychosocial management

The background stresses and strain, which aggravate and potentiate patient's distress in LBP, may be difficult to clarify, and it may take some time before the pain team is able to explore this aspect usefully. Once the patient's confidence has been gained, as the physical aspects of management begin to be addressed, they are then better able to accept the involvement of other members of the pain team, including the psychologist. The importance of addressing pain in all its aspects should be emphasized. Reassurance, regarding the acceptance of the real-

**Table 17.6** A comparison of treatment goals (from Main & Benjamin 1995,[19] with permission from Oxford University Press)

|  | General medical approach | Back schools | Functional restoration programmes | Pain management programmes |
|---|---|---|---|---|
| Pain reduction | Major | Minor | Minor | Minor |
| Increase mobility | Minor | Moderate | Major | Major |
| Increase strength | Minor | Minor | Major | Minor |
| Reduce distress | None | Minor | None/minor | Major |
| Reduce invalidism | None | Minor | Moderate | Major |
| Give coping skills | None | Moderate | Minor | Major |

ity of the patient's pain, often needs to be repeatedly reinforced. Behavioural methods of treatment are useful in those with marked illness behaviour and the psychologist can help by guiding other therapists, as well as the patient, in applying these. To be successful, all these treatments need to be applied as part of a team approach, often most usefully with patients in groups, where patients gain insight and confidence by shared experiences. Whether this is equally successful when done on an outpatient or inpatient basis probably relates more to the local logistics of organization, but studies have shown a greater benefit for inpatient based rehabilitation regimes.[20]

Most rehabilitation programmes provide a combination of physical re-education, aerobic conditioning and cognitive behavioural therapy. Such approaches positively influence pain and pain behaviour and can reduce the rate of subsequent medical intervention.[21,22] The ability of such programmes to restore patients in the workplace is more variable. It may be that the rather poor apparent effect on this outcome, relates to the fact that many programmes are instituted at a late point in the natural history of the patient's chronic pain problem. Patients who have been disabled with back pain for a year stand only a 30% chance of returning to work, and those that have been disabled for up to 2 years, 10%. Clearly, if rehabilitation programmes are to influence these statistics, the sooner they can be instituted the better.

# References

1. Coste J, Delecoeuillerie G, Cohen de Lara, Le Parc JM, Paolaggi JB. Clinical course and prognostic factors in acute low back pain: an inception cohort study in primary care practice. *Br Med J* **308:** 577–580, 1994
2. Department of Health Statistics Division. The prevalence of back pain in Great Britain in 1998. London: Government Statistical Service, 1999
3. Maniadakis N, Gray A. The economic burden of back pain in the UK. *Pain* **84:** 95–103, 2000
4. Agency for Health Care Police and Research. Management guidelines for acute low back pain. Rockville MD: US Department of Health and Human Services, 1994
5. Clinical Standards Advisory Group. Report on back pain. London: HMSO, 1994
6. Kendall NAS, Linton SJ, Maine CJ. Guide to assessing psycho-social yellow flags in acute low back pain: risk factors for long term disability and work loss. Wellington NZ: Accident Rehabilitation & Compensation Insurance Corporation of New Zealand and the National Health Committee, 1997
7. Royal College of General Practitioners. Clinical guidelines for the management of acute low back pain. London: RCGP, 1996
8. Spitzer WO, LeBlanc FE, Dupuis M, et al. Scientific approach to the assessment and management of activity-related spinal disorders. (Report of the Quebec Task Force on Spinal Disorders) *Spine* **12:** 1–5, 1987
9. Waddell G. The Back Pain Revolution. Edinburgh: Churchill Livingstone, 1998
10. Daker-White G, Carr AJ, Harvey I, et al. A randomised controlled trial. Shifting boundaries of doctors and physiotherapists in orthopaedic out-patient departments. *J Epidemiol Common Health* **53:** 643–650, 1999
11. Wipf JF, Deyo RA. Low Back Pain. *Med Clin N Am* **79:** 231–246, 1995
12. Price J, Leaver L. ABC of psychological medicine: beginning treatment. *Br Med J* **325:** 33–35, 2002
13. Ransford AO, Cairns D, Mooney V. The pain drawing as an aid in the psychological evaluation of patients with lower back pain. *Spine* **1:** 127–134, 1976
14. Melzack R. The McGill pain questionnaire: major properties and storing methods. *Pain* 1: 277–299, 1975
15. Waddell G. A new clinical model for the treatment of low back pain. *Spine* **12:** 632–644, 1987
16. Main CJ, Wood PLR, Hollis S, Spanswick CC, Wadell G. The Distress and Risk Assessment Method. A simple patient classification to identify distress and evaluate risk of poor outcome. *Spine* **17:** 42–45, 1992
17. National Institute for Clinical Excellence. Guidance on the use of COX II selective inhibitors, celecoxib, rofecoxib, meloxicam and etodolac for osteoarthritis and rheumatoid arthritis. London: NICE, 2001

18. Ward NG. Tricyclic anti-depressants for chronic low back pain: mechanisms of action and predictors of response. *Spine* **11**: 661–665, 1986

19. Main CJ, Benjamin S. Psychological treatment and the health care system. Is there a need for a paradigm shift? In: Mayou R, Bass C, Sharpe M, eds. *Treatment of functional somatic symptoms*. Oxford: Oxford University Press, pp. 214–230, 1995

20. Harkapaa, Mellin G. Jarvikoski A. et al. A controlled study on the outcome of in-patient and out-patient treatment of low back pain, disability and compliance. *Second J Rehab Med* **22**: 181–188, 1990

21. Kroenke K. Swindle R. Cognitive behavioural therapy for somatization and symptom syndromes: a critical review of controlled clinical trials. *Psychother Psychosom* **69**: 205–215, 2000

22. Van Tuller MW, Stelo RWJG, Vlaeyeu JWS, Lindon SJ, Morley SJ, Assendelft WJJ. Behavioural treatment of chronic low back pain (Cochrane Review) In: *The Cochrane Library*. Oxford: Update software, Issue 4, 2000

# 18 Back Pain: Interventional Approach

*Simon J Dolin*

Low back pain is initially dealt with as outlined in Chapter 17. If pain persists and continues to adversely affect the patient's quality of life, or ability to function, there are a number of interventional techniques that can be considered. The interventional perspective aims to find the structure(s) within the lumbar spine that is acting as primary pain site, and then consider ways of diminishing pain from that site.

The lumbar spine has four main sites for pain generation:

- Lumbar facet joint
- Lumbar disc
- Muscle groups around the spine and posterior pelvis
- Nerve roots that traverse the lumbar spine.

## Lumbar facet joint as an origin of pain

The lumbar facet joints (zygapophysial joints) are posterior stabilizing joints that limit the spine in extension and rotation. There are two joints, one on each side, at every vertebrae from L5 up to C1, with inferior and superior articulating surfaces. The facet joints are supplied by sensory nerves from ipsilateral dorsal nerve roots, both segmentally and non-segmentally.[1] The primary dorsal rami supplies a medial branch to adjacent joints. The medial branch also supplies some muscle groups, in particular multifidis.

Defining a 'facet joint syndrome' remains problematic. There is no clear agreement on what aspects of history and examination characterize the facet joint as the origin of low back pain.[2] In essence, the only way to determine whether the facet joint is contributing to a patients back pain is if they have pain relief on injecting the joint itself or its nerve supply (the medial branch). A number of clinical factors have been shown to be predictive of a positive response to local anaesthetic facet joint injection but do not define diagnostic criteria.[3] Lumbar facet joints are thought to cause pain in 15–40% of patients with chronic low back pain, as judged by response rates to local anaesthetic injections.[4]

Lumbar facet joints do develop osteoarthritic changes with age. They develop osteoarthritic changes following on from disc degeneration. It may well be the disc degeneration that is the primary event in development of back pain with ageing and facet joint changes are a consequence.[5] There are anatomical variations in the orientation of facet joints, some of which are associated with osteoarthritis.[6] Following trauma, subtle changes have been demonstrated in lumbar facet joints, including capsular tears, damage to subchondral bone and small fractures, none of which may be apparent on radiography. All of this supports the importance of the lumbar facet joint as a pain generator in low back pain.

### Lumbar facet joint injection (see Chapter 34)

Lumbar facet joint injections are commonly performed for treatment for low back pain. The principle is the same as injecting any other joint (e.g. shoulder or knee) in that injection of

**177**

local anaesthetic and depot steroid often gives a good clinical result in terms of decreased pain and increased function. Older patients with proven osteoarthritis on imaging may be suitable candidates, although other practitioners will perform the injection on any patients with persistent mechanical back pain. Morbidity is minimal. Initial pain relief may provide a good opportunity for follow-on back rehabilitation.

### Evidence base

Proving efficacy remains a problem. A Cochrane Systematic Review, in 2002, identified only three well-designed trials, which demonstrated neither short- nor long-term efficacy.[8] The authors concluded that the amount of useful information was scarce, and that potential beneficial effects could have been missed because of small sample sizes, varying follow-up times, high improvement rates in control groups, and lack of diagnostic accuracy in defining a 'facet joint syndrome'. They concluded that facet joint injections have been shown to be neither effective, nor ineffective.

## Radiofrequency lumbar facet denervation (see Chapter 34)

Following positive diagnostic facet joint or medial branch blocks with local anaesthetic, longer-term treatment of facet joint pain can be achieved by percutaneous thermocoagulation of the medial branch using a radiofrequency (RF) current. The technique has been in use since 1974, and it remains fairly widely practiced in pain clinics to this day. The RF current heats the surrounding tissue and inactivates the medial branch of the segmental nerve. The nerve itself, with its cell body and dorsal root ganglion, survives intact, and it is only the terminal branch that is affected. Duration of action is uncertain, but probably very long. Regeneration of the nerve branch may occur. Long-term outcome studies do show benefits still present after 1 year. Morbidity is minimal, and the procedure can be repeated, if needed. The medial branch also supplies the multifidus muscle, and the lesion will affect it's innervation. Multifidus is a very long muscle (from sacrum to cervical vertebrae) and having 2 or 3 segments denervated does not appear to affect spinal function, in practice. Initial pain relief following facet denervation may afford a good opportunity to follow on with a back rehabilitation programme.

### Evidence base

There are many uncontrolled outcome studies, including some prospective ones, demonstrating long-term benefits, in the range of 60% of patients demonstrating 90% relief at 1 year, and 87% of patients obtaining at least 60% relief.[9] There are a limited number of randomized controlled trials, showing improvement at 6 and 12 months.[10,11] One trial showed only short-term improvement.[12] The only systematic review of randomized controlled trials concluded that there was moderate evidence that lumbar facet denervation was more effective for chronic low back pain than placebo.[13]

## Lumbar disc as an origin of pain

Lumbar disc space narrowing on plain radiographs and disc degeneration by magnetic resonance imagery (MRI) are frequently found in patients with low back pain. This appears to be part of the ageing process, although it can be a result of repetitive axial loading as a result of heavy lifting or in athletes. The lumbar disc is made up of a central nucleus and an outer annulus. The outer third of the annulus is richly innervated, including pain fibres from segmental nerves, and this may be even more extensive in degenerated discs.[14] Magnetic resonance imagery of degenerated discs often shows tears extending from the nucleus to the outer parts of the annulus. Nociceptive nerve endings grow into the inner annulus and become sensitized by biochemical degradation products. This lowers the pain threshold for mechanical stimulation during normal loading of the lumbar disc. This phenomenon is known as internal disc disruption, a term adopted by the International Association for the Study of Pain (IASP) in its taxonomy. Fissures can also occur in discs that appear to be normal from plain radiographs and MRI. Pain coming from the disc itself is known as discogenic pain, and this is different from nerve root pain caused by disc prolapse. Discogenic pain is thought to account for 30–50% of low back pain.[15] There are no clinical features that are pathognomonic of discogenic pain, and the only real test available is provocative discography. This is a situation analogous to facet joint syndrome and diagnostic facet joint blocks.

## Lumbar discography (see Chapter 34)

Discography is a physiological test that explicitly determines whether a disc is painful. It involves artificially pressurizing the disc by injection of small volumes of fluid, usually radio-opaque contrast material. The key feature of discography is the patient's response to disc stimulation. It is rarely painful in asymptomatic individuals, but is frequently painful in patients with low back pain. For discography to be positive, stimulation of the disc must reproduce the patient's pain, irrespective of the morphology of the disc. It is helpful, also, to perform discography on adjacent disc(s) without pain reproduction. Leak of contrast from the disc, which can be seen during the injection using real-time fluoroscopy may give additional evidence about annular tears. Some practitioners follow on with computed tomography (CT) scanning to confirm contrast in fissures in the annulus. Generally, loss of disc height on plain radiograph and abnormal signal intensity on MRI are highly predictive of symptomatic tears extending into or beyond the annulus.[16] There is, however, continuing debate about the value of discography, but it seems to have won fairly wide acceptance as a useful investigational technique.[17]

## Annuloplasty for discogenic pain (see Chapter 34)

Recent developments in the field of discogenic pain have been techniques for heating the posterior annulus of the disc, in an attempt to inactive nociceptors. Primary indication is low back pain of discogenic origin, confirmed by imaging and discography, and not responsive to conservative treatments.

One newly introduced treatment is intradiscal electrothermal annuloplasty (IDET), which involves placing a catheter within the nucleus of the disc, using a percutaneous approach, and a standard disc puncture technique, under fluoroscopic control. The catheter (30 cm long with 6 cm active resistant tip) curls around inside the nucleus to lie across the posterior junction between nucleus and annulus at the offending portion of the annulus. Using a direct current, the tip of the catheter is heated to 85–90°C, rising gradually for 13 minutes and maintaining for 4 minutes. A gentle progressive exercise regimen may be suitable to follow-on. Early results show good clinical improvement rates of 23–76%, depending on stringency of criteria.

Another technology involves introduction of an RF electrode into the lamellae of the posterior annulus (Disctrode). This uses RF current and aims to heat the annulus to temperatures between 42–48°C, for similar times to IDET. These two annuloplasty techniques have not been compared.

The role of annuloplasty will be determined over coming years. It is potentially a very important technique because it offers the promise of minimally-invasive treatment for discogenic pain. The only other treatment currently available is spinal fusion.

### Evidence base

This is a new technique with little published data available. In a prospective uncontrolled outcome study over 12 months good improvements were recorded for pain intensity and measures of function.[18] A recent controlled trial compared IDET with physical rehabilitation, using a 12 month outcome, and concluded that annuloplasty can eliminate or dramatically reduce the pain of internal disc disruption in a substantial proportion of patients and appears to be superior to conventional conservative care.[19]

## Muscle groups as origin of back pain

Assessment and treatment of muscle pain is covered in Chapters 8 and 17.

## Nerve roots of origin of back pain

Pathologies affecting nerve roots are likely to present as leg pain and are covered in Chapter 16.

## References

1. Suseki K, Takahashi Y, Takahashi K, Chiba T, et al. Innervation of lumbar facet joints. Origins and functions. *Spine* 22: 447–485, 1997
2. Schwarzer A, Derby R, Aprill C, Fortin J, Kine G, Bogduk N. Pain from lumbar zygapophysial joints: a test of two models. *J Spinal Disorders* 7: 331–336, 1994
3. Revel M, Poiraudeau S, Aulely G, Payan, et al. Capacity of the clinical picture to characterize low back pain relieved by facet joint anesthesia. Proposed criteria to identify patients with painful facet joints. *Spine* 23: 1972–1976, 1998
4. Manchikanti L. Facet joint pain and the role of neurological blockade in its management. *Curr Rev Pain* 3: 248–358, 1999
5. Moore R, Crotti T, Osti O, Fraser R, Veron-Roberts B. Osteoarthritis of the fact joints resulting from annular rim lesions in sheep lumbar discs. *Spine* 24: 519–525, 1999
6. Fujiwara A, Tamai K, An H, Lim T, et al. Orientation and osteoarthritis of the lumbar facet joint. *Clin Orthopaed Rel Res* 385: 888–894, 2001
7. Taylor J, Twomey L, Corker M. Bone and soft tissue injuries in post-mortem lumbar spines. *Paraplegia* 28: 119–129, 1990
8. Nelemans P, Bie R, Vet H, Sturmans F. Injection therapy for subacute and chronic benign low back pain. *Cochrane Database of Systematic Reviews.* Issue 1, 2002.
9. Dreyfuss P, Halbrook B, Pauza K, Joshi A, McLarty J, Bogduk N. Efficacy and validity of radiofrequency neurotomy for chronic lumbar zygapophysial joint pain. *Spine* 25: 1270–1277, 2000
10. Gallagher J, Petriccione D, Wedley J, et al. Radiofrequency facet joint denervation in the treatment of low back pain: a prospective controlled double-blind study to assess its efficacy. *Pain Clin* 7: 193–198, 1994
11. Van Kleef M, Barendse G, Kessels A, Voets H, Weber W. Randomized trial of radiofrequency lumbar facet denervation for chronic low back pain. *Spine* 24: 1937–1942, 1999
12. Leclaire R, Fortin L, Lambert R, Bergeron Y, Rossignol M. Radiofrequency facet joint denervation in the treatment of low back pain: a placebo-controlled clinical trail to assess efficacy. *Spine* 26: 1411–1416, 2001
13. Geurts J, van Wijk R, Stolker R, Groen G. Efficacy of radiofrequency procedures for the treatment of spinal pain: a systematic review of randomized clinical trials. *Reg Anesth Pain Med* 26: 394–400, 2001
14. Coppes M, Marani E, Thomeer R, Groen G. Innervation of painful lumbar discs. *Spine* 22: 2342–2349, 1997
15. Schwarzer A, Aprill C, Derby R, Fortin J, Kine G, Bogduk N. The prevalence and clinical features of Internal Disc Disruption in patients with chronic low back pain. *Spine* 20: 1878–1883, 1995

16. Millette P, Fontaine S, Lepanto L, Cardnal E, Breton G. Differentiating lumbar disc protrusions, disc bulges, and discs with normal contour but abnormal signal intensity. Magnetic resonance imaging with discordant correlations. *Spine* **24**: 44–53, 1999
17. Bogduk N, Modic M. Controversy: Lumbar Discography. *Spine* **21**: 402–404, 1996
18. Saal JA, Saal JS. Intradiscal electrothermal treatment for chronic discogenic low back pain: A prospective outcome study with minimum 1 year follow-up. *Spine* **25**: 2622–2627, 2000
19. Karasek K, Bogduk N. Twelve-month follow-up of a controlled trial of intradiscal thermal annuloplasty for back pain due to internal disc disruption. *Spine* **25**: 2601–2607, 2000

# 19 Coccygodynia

*Nicholas L Padfield*

Coccygodynia is a distressing condition affecting 1% of all back pain sufferers, and it is five times more common in women than men. This prevalence in females is thought to be due to the greater prominence of the 'cuckoo-shaped' part of the axial skeleton. This condition has been described from the 1600s but was first labelled by Simpson in 1859.

The pain can involve the adjoining myotomes, producing the characteristic ache in the levator ani muscle and gluteal muscles as well as pain in the anococcygeal, sacrotuberal and sacrospinal ligaments.

## Aetiology

Coccygodynia can arise in a number of ways:

- Trauma from a fall (e.g. as a result of a slip going down stairs, from a horse or when skiing) can result in direct injury to the sacrococcygeal synchondrosis or surrounding tissues. These can also be similarly damaged by a kick during contact sports, from an injury on a trampoline when struck by the bar or springs that surround the jumping pad.
- Childbirth causes abnormal movement of the coccyx during labour and delivery. As a result of the hormonal changes during the third trimester of pregnancy, the pelvic ligaments become more elastic in preparation for the distension of the pelvic brim to come during labour and delivery. Thus the increased mobility of the synchondrosis between the sacrum and the coccyx allows the fused or unfused 3–5 segment of the coccyx more flexion and extension, which in turn results in stretching and a permanent change in the resting tension of the ligaments and muscles surrounding and attaching to the coccyx.
- Repetitive trauma can result in stretching of the surrounding ligaments and muscles causing the joint to be repeatedly forced out of its normal position. This can lead to inflammation of these tissues resulting in pain and soreness when the patient sits or strains at stool. Therefore, it is a common occupational problem in those that ride horses or motorbikes regularly.
- A typical characteristic of the condition is its inability to heal because of continued movement resulting in further damage and perpetuation of the cycle. (It is consequently a particular problem in rowers or cyclists or those that spend a lot of time in the car for a living.) This has implications for lifestyle changes as part of pain management.
- Other less common causes of the condition include piriformis pain/syndrome, where the piriformis muscle causes an abnormal entrapment of the sciatic nerve at the greater sciatic notch. It characteristically causes pain in the buttock but can radiate to the thigh or more distally to resemble radicular pain. It is provoked by prolonged hip flexion, adduction and internal rotation and there is typical tenderness around the buttock and sciatic notch.[1] Pudendal nerve injury or neuropathic pain secondary to repeated injury to the nerves, pilonidal cyst formation, meningeal cysts, obesity as a result of excessive pressure on the coccyx when sitting and a bursitis-like condition that can arise in slim patients

who have little fat padding over the buttocks, which allows the tip of the coccyx to rub against the subcutaneous tissues causing friction.
- Up to a third of all cases of coccygodynia no direct cause can be found.

## History and examination

- A history of sudden trauma, pregnancy, sports where a repetitive injury to the area is likely or an occupation where prolonged sitting occurs, especially in awkward postures, may immediately indicate the likely cause.
- Onset, provoking factors, radiation of pain, response to analgesics, surgery or pain relieving interventions to date may indicate other organic causes as already mentioned. Body language and behaviour and the use of primarily affective descriptors may indicate psychological stress leading to the major portion of the disability.
- On-going litigation needs to be discovered, especially if there is pain behaviour or secondary gain suspected, as this will have a major impact on the outcome of treatment and may in itself determine treatment strategy.

Examination may reveal:

- Abnormal anatomy following a mal-united fracture, abnormal mobility of the joint on rectal examination
- Adverse neural tension in the obturator, sciatic or femoral nerves, and excessive pain provoked by hip flexion or internal rotation
- Hypersensitivity and allodynia over the area
- Myofascial trigger areas in the glutei indicating a more widespread problem and the need for a full musculoskeletal examination
- Scar from a previous coccygectomy and the patient complains bitterly about phantom pain.

If the coccyx is not directly exquisitely tender then other pathology should be sought, such as herniated disc, rectal or gynaecological tumours compressing/invading the sacrococcygeal nerve supply. Therefore, rectal and vaginal examination should be part of a normal examination for this condition – it is, after all, the only way the mobility of the coccyx can be determined.

It is important to get a history of all interventions. The results of epidural steroids, the results of cryotherapy or radiofrequency lesioning and the response to non-steroidal analgesics, tricyclic antidepressants and gabapentin will give the pain clinician a good idea of the impact the condition has on the patient and may determine the treatment strategy. Patients themselves may volunteer what they do in order to cope, for example, the employment of a C-shaped cushion to relieve direct pressure on the coccyx. The presence of effective coping strategies lessens the likelihood of depression.

## Investigation

Lateral X-rays of the coccyx reveal four distinct types of coccygodynia:

- Type 1 (68%) a – the tip of the coccyx is slightly curved forward.
- Type 2 – the coccyx is curved forward with the tip almost pointing straight forward.
- Type 3 – the coccyx is sharply angled forward.
- Type 4 – there is actual subluxation of either the sacrococcygeal joints or the intercoccygeal joints.

It has recently been suggested that a dynamic sitting view should be taken as the coccyx can move 22° when a person goes from sitting to standing. Subtle subluxations of the coccyx may only be detected with these combined views.[2]

As with most joint injuries involving fibrous tissue, connective tissue or cartilage radiographs and even magnetic resonance imaging (MRI) rarely throw up any significant pathology. The use of such sophisticated imaging is only worthwhile when there is a strong suspicion of coccygodynia. However, in one recent dynamic radiographic prospective study 208 consecutive patients were assessed standing and in the painful sitting position. In addition to the known posterior luxation of the joint, two new lesions, anterior subluxation and the presence of spicules, were demonstrated. Furthermore, obesity made posterior subluxation significantly more likely whilst spicules were more likely to occur in thin patients. A history of trauma of less than 1 month before the onset of coccydynia made instability of the joint more likely.[3]

## Treatment

Treatment will depend on whether this is a recent onset of pain following a specific trauma or it has become a chronic condition where many interventions have already been undertaken. The management needs of patients will, therefore, vary enormously and have to be tailored specifically for the individual patient. They fall into the following categories: surgery, medication, physiotherapy and exercises, pain interventions and psychological therapy.

### Surgery

A clearly fractured and mal-united coccyx has been considered the indication for refracture and manipulation under anaesthesia. The outcomes, unfortunately, are extremely varied, and the patient not uncommonly develops neuropathic pain as well as the incident pain (i.e. provoked by movement) already experienced. Coccygectomy was initially reported to have 70% success rate,[4] but a more critical analysis of the results would challenge this and urge caution before embarking on blanket coccygectomy for this condition. When sacrococcygeal rhizotomy was employed for perineal pain, arising either from non-malignant coccydynia or malignant pain, the non-malignant group only achieved a 22% improvement. What the study did not report was the incidence of intractable neuropathic pain arising as a result of this intervention![5] Coccygectomy can lead to bowel herniation, which can prove refractory treatment even by mesh grafting and, in one case report, bilateral gluteus maximus flaps were required to repair the defect.[6] It is practised less frequently now and surgery is, at best, only undertaken reluctantly these days because of the significant risks of developing neuropathic pain or even phantom pain in the area. One study of 37 patients was designed to validate an objective criterion for patient selection. Out of the 37 patients, 23 patients at 2-year follow-up were deemed by independent assessment to be excellent, 11, were good and only 3 were poor.[7] Whilst this hardly qualifies as more than class 3 evidence, it is a good start to critically appraise a technique that has suffered inconsistent efficacy in the past from inappropriate patient selection.

It is always important to advise the patient that surgery is more likely to be effective if combined with other physical measures, such as a support cushion and exercises, and that it may take from 6 months to 1 year for the patient to experience relief.

### Medical

Anti-inflammatory drugs are frequency prescribed in the early stages, and can prove beneficial if combined with appropriate rest or avoidance of the provoking stimulus. For example, if coccygodynia has developed following a prolonged period of horse riding, the patient should desist for a period to allow the acute inflammation to settle. This may be combined with a support cushion when sitting. If the pain is running a chronic course, and it is likely to be neurogenic, then tricyclic antidepressants may prove helpful and even the addition of gabapentin, which needs to be titrated to an effective dose. Sadly, the chronic cases can prove refractory to such treatment, or such unpleasant side-effects from treatment are experienced that the patients stop their medication. It is important to be completely honest with the patient about the likelihood of success, as compliance with further drug treatment can be a problem.

## Interventional treatment

Epidural steroids administered through the sacral hiatus can occasionally ease the acute situation but rarely confer any lasting benefit in the chronic one. Local steroid injections around the inflamed ligaments can be helpful, and their appropriateness will depend on the accuracy of diagnosis and of locating the pain generators. Some authors even report success rates of 60%.[8]

Cryotherapy of the sacrococcygeal nerves, the pudendal nerves had been used repeatedly in some patients with good effect.[9] However, this is not the universal experience and, commonly, it only provides a 'pain holiday' with diminishing returns on subsequent treatments as fibrosis around the frozen nerves develops.

Radiofrequency (RF) thermocoagulation of the sacrococcygeal nerves had also been undertaken. But, all too often, neuropathic pain develops within a few months.

Pulsed RF is a relatively untested novel treatment where pulses of very high frequency radio waves, 500 MHz, are applied in short bursts for up to 8 minutes to the sacrococcygeal nerves. This is achieved by inserting Teflon insulated (apart from the exposed metallic tip) needles through the sacral hiatus under fluoroscopic control. Electrical stimulation is then applied at 100 Hz and 2–3 Hz to test the sensory and motor location of the needle tips. Once a satisfactory position is found, the treatment is then begun. The output from the RF generator should just be detectable by the patient, in the author's experience, and not unpleasant. The temperature should never rise above 41°C; it usually rises to between 39–40°C. At the end of the procedure, the patient should experience a tingly numbness in place of the previously experienced pain if the treatment is going to be effective. A lot of clinical studies need to be undertaken by different centres to evaluate this particular form of treatment, but early results are looking encouraging, and enthusiasts will point out that it adds another non-destructive form of interventional treatment. Peripheral nerve stimulation, retrograde passage of electrodes through L5, has been tried. It is technically challenging and not every back will permit the percutaneous insertion and fine positioning needed to achieve this. Appropriate patient selection is paramount. An open, honest approach to the likelihood of achieving not only satisfactory placement but analgesic paraesthesia will ensure you do not make a rod for your back in managing these difficult patients.

## Physiotherapy

If there are trigger areas or poor posture because of differences in muscle tone in the glutei and piriformis levator ani muscles then stretch exercises and acupuncture may be beneficial. Lifestyle changes to avoid repetitive provoking factors may have to be insisted upon if all other measures fail to control the pain.

## Psychological

It is not uncommon for patients to become depressed when coccygodynia has been intractable and no treating physician/therapist has provided any significant help. It is, by all accounts, a very difficult pain to live with, as it can be constant, intense and very restricting because so many daily activities will aggravate it. If, as a result, patients have developed significantly inappropriate fears and beliefs about the pain, its nature and the prognosis, then cognitive behavioural therapy may ease some of their suffering even though it will not affect the sensation of the pain per se. The development of coping strategies, if these were rudimentary or non-existent, may prove to be the most valuable help a patient receives. Relaxation techniques and techniques to manage negative thoughts can all be helpful. The goal should always be to make the unbearable bearable. An honest admission that medication and other physical therapies are unlikely to produce any significant reduction or change in the physical sensation of the pain, whilst unpalatable at the time, leaves the path open to pain management and, hopefully, the retention of trust between patient and therapist.

## Summary

Success or failure of management will be determined by the sympathy and communication skills of the pain clinician. Many modalities of treatment may need to be simultaneously applied to ease the distress of this condition. It can be one of the greatest challenges of the pain clinician to orchestrate medical treatments, interventions and cognitive behavioural therapy. But, if you can help your patient, they will express their sincerest gratitude.

## References

1. Barton PM. Piriformis syndrome: a rational approach to management. *Pain* **47**: 345–352, 1991
2. Maigne JY, Tamalet B. Standardised radiological protocol for the study of common coccydynia and characteristics of the lesions observed in the sitting position. Clinical elements differentiating luxation, hypermobility, and normal mobility. *Spine* **21**: 2588–2593, 1996
3. Maigne J-Y, Dousounain L, Chatelier G. Causes and mechanisms of common coccydynia: Role of body mass index and coccygeal trauma. *Spine* **25**: 3072–3079, 2000
4. Eng JB, Rymaszewski L, Jepson K. Coccygectomy. *J Roy Coll Surg Edinburgh* **33**: 202–203, 1988
5. Saris SC, Silver JM, Vieira JFS, Nashold Jr BS. Sacrococcygeal rhizotomy for perineal pain. *Neurosurgery* **19**: 789–793, 1986
6. Zook NL, Zook EG. Repair of a long-standing coccygeal hernia and open wound. *Plastic Reconstr Surg* **100**: 96–99, 1997
7. Maigne J-Y, Lagauche D, Doursounian L. Instability of the coccyx in coccydynia. *J Bone Joint Surg* **82**: 1038–1041, 2000
8. Wray CC, Easom S, Hoskinson J. Coccydynia. Aetiology and treatment. *J Bone Joint Surg* **73**: 335–338, 1991
9. Evans PJD, Lloyd JW, Jack TM. Cryoanalgesia for intractable perineal pain. *J Roy Soc Med* **74**: 804–808, 1981

# 20 Postspinal Surgery Pain

## Jonathan Richardson

Lumbar spinal surgery is a powerful weapon for good or ill and needs to be wielded with the utmost care. Correct patient selection, knowledge of the level involved, choice of surgical procedure and its flawless execution are pivotal. The most important overall outcome determinate is surgeon education. Appropriate referral patterns are essential. In countries where patients self refer to spinal surgeons an in-built surgical intervention bias is evident.

Surgeons are not alone in failing these patients. Suboptimal outcomes occur with physical therapy, pharmacotherapy and pain interventions. What makes the failed back surgery syndrome such a responsibility is that its consequences are so severe. It amounts to a personal, physical, psychological, social, economic and societal disaster.

Nothing to do with this subject is easy: all the practitioner's skill will be tested. There are many pitfalls and the challenges and rewards in this field are formidable.

### Definition

Postspinal surgery pain is frequently referred to as the failed back surgery syndrome (FBSS). It can be defined as 'lumbar spinal pain of unknown origin either persisting despite surgical intervention or appearing after surgical intervention for spinal pain originally in the same topographical location'.[1]

Put another way, it is a surgical end-stage after one or several operative interventions on the lumbar neuroaxis, indicated to relieve lower back pain, radicular pain or the combination of both without positive effect.[2]

Many different conditions are covered by these definitions.

## Incidence

Measuring the incidence of FBSS is not easy. One estimate is that between 10 and 40% of operations fail to relieve pain,[3] but surgical outcome depends upon the reporter. In a rheumatologist's review of six studies, 30–50% of patients had residual low back pain at 1 year and 25% were still unable to work.[4] In a neurologists retrospective study of 371 patients, 70% continued with permanent low back pain, which was severe in 23%. Residual nerve root pain was present in 45%.[5]

The type of surgery is irrelevant to the production of epidural fibrosis and the incidence of chronic pain,[6] with the exception of spinal fusion when successful outcomes appear to be higher.[7] A microsurgical approach might be expected to produce better results because of a smaller incision, reduced weakening of the posterior wall of the spine and generally lower revision rates compared with percutaneous disc surgery. However, there are higher risks of inadequate surgical decompression and neurological damage.[8]

Major variations in outcomes and rates of surgery between developed countries illustrate the unclear crossover between conservative and surgical treatments. The greatest chance of success is with clear nerve root compression on imaging that correlates with the patient's clinical symptoms and signs. Back pain alone, particularly if it has been present for over 6 months, has poor correlation with good outcome.

# Aetiology

There are many potential reasons for a poor surgical outcome. Practically useful is the division of patients into immediate postoperative failures, usually due to poor patient selection, a new source of impingement or a faulty technique and those whose symptoms relapse (Table 20.1).[9]

## Epidural fibrosis

Epidural scar tissue arises as a result of a chronic chemical radiculitis, neurogenic inflammation and, probably, an autoimmune response following leakage of nucleus pulposus.[10] Venous stasis in the epidural vessels and impaired fibrinolysis are contributory.[11] Surgery undoubtedly results in the most florid epidural fibrotic changes, but its presence with lumbar radiculopathies associated with disc disease is almost universal.[12,13] Crude imaging estimates of the amount of fibrosis versus symptoms invariably fails, as does the relationship of the amount of fibrosis to the extent of the surgical procedure.[14]

Pain generation in the presence of fibrosis is a complex process. Some authors apportion 8–14% of FBSS patients to scar tissue,[14] while others reject that pain is produced by fibrosis, using as evidence the grossly similar anatomical mass of scar between symptomatic and asymptomatic patients. This argument ignores the potential pathophysiological effects of nerve root tethering and compression.

## Generation of nerve root pain

Paraesthesiae may arise through nerve root compression but, for the production of pain, inflammation of nerve roots is also required. The mechanisms involved include vascular, neu-

| Table 20.1 | Differential diagnosis according to time of presentation | |
|---|---|---|
| Immediate failure (continuation of radicular pain) | Recurrence of radiculopathic pain | Persistent low back pain |
| Wrong diagnosis e.g. zygapophysial joint pain,[a] tumour | Wrong diagnosis e.g. zygapophysial joint pain,[a] tumour | Wrong diagnosis e.g. zygapophysial joint, sacroiliac joint pain, tumour |
| Immediate re-prolapse | Re-prolapse or new prolapse | Disc degeneration, annular tear or discitis |
| Incorrect level | Formation of scar tissue (epidurally, intrathecally) | Epidural abscess, osteomyelitis |
| Persistent compression, incomplete surgery | Spinal, lateral recess or foraminal stenosis | Paraspinal muscle pain |
| Neurological injury | Meningeal cyst | Pseudomeningocoele |
| Textiloma[b] | Textiloma | Textiloma |
| Segmental spinal instability | Segmental spinal instability | Segmental spinal instability |

[a]Synovial cytokines can leak from zygapophysial joints to produce radicular symptoms
[b]Retained surgical sponge.

rotoxic, immunological and inflammatory reactions arising from the leakage of nucleus pulposus into the epidural space. Nerve root (especially dorsal root) blood supply is relatively poor and approximately 75% of its nutrition depends upon a flow of cerebrospinal fluid (CSF).[15] In disease states, especially with adhesive arachnoiditis, nutrition of the nerve root becomes critical. Mechanical constriction of vessels through fibrous constriction or tethering leads to intraneural oedema, encouraged by rapid thrombus formation in intraneural capillaries following contact with nucleus pulposus.[16] Impairment in intraneural blood flow is probably the final common pathway leading to abnormalities in nerve conduction and pain generation.[17]

## Psychological factors

Failure to recognize abnormal pain behaviour before operation is a great mistake.[18] Fear of pain leads to avoidance of activity in order not to provoke further discomfort. Patients can be separated along a spectrum into 'pain confronters', those who after a period of rest challenge their back pain through gradually increased activity and 'pain avoiders', those who for long periods shun activity to avoid pain. Fear avoidance is a maladaptive process, which has no value in injury recovery, even in the subacute phase following injury.[19] A high level of pain avoidance equates with a poor prognosis for recovery regarding pain levels, physical impairment, depressive symptoms and inability to return to work.[19]

The role of compensation or litigation as it affects outcomes (return to pain or return to work) is highly negative. Seventy one percent of patients examined by orthopaedic experts appointed by the Workman's Compensation Board in the United States undergoing a first operation had not returned to work 4 years after operation (out of 600 claimants). This figure rose to 95% in the multiple operations group (out of 400 claimants). In every case, this was due to ongoing pain, never due to neurological deficits.[20]

Table 20.2 lists features associated with a poor prognosis.

# Clinical assessment

In practical terms (in the lumbar region) the clinician is usually faced with a patient with radicular pain and persistent low back pain.

A list of differential diagnoses (see Table 20.1) and the time to relapse should be correlated. A careful clinical history is the most useful diagnostic tool available to the clinician.

| Table 20.2 Some outcome predictors | |
|---|---|
| Good outcome | Poor outcome |
| Positive straight leg raising test | Litigation |
| Positive collateral straight leg raising test | Compensation claim |
| Clear impingement on imaging | MMPI hysteria, hypochondria |
| Sensory and motor loss | Psychological factors |
| Predominant nerve root pain | Predominant low back pain |
| Pain in the entire nerve root distribution | Injury in the workplace |
| Short duration of symptoms | Sick leave >3 months |
| Concordance of imaging and clinical findings | Unemployed >6 months |

Modified from Goupille.[9]
MMPI, Minnesota multiphasic personality inventory

## Diagnosis

Establishing the source of the pain is not always straightforward. Projection of non-nociceptive as well as nociceptive information onto wide dynamic range neurones in the spinal cord leads to referral of pain to other areas.[21] Referral patterns tend to involve previously injured painful areas, a phenomenon known as 'habit preference'.[22] The referral pattern may not be obvious (e.g. in the case of referred pain from any lumbar intervertebral disc to the groin) due to false localizing signs.[23] Expansion of painful areas due to central sensitization (wind-up) leads to further diagnostic difficulties due to expansion into adjacent dermatomal areas.

Referral patterns – e.g. from the zygapophysial (Z) and sacroiliac (SI) joint – overlap. Z joint pain may not have been the original diagnosis, but it is very common and may have arisen postoperatively, encouraged by a loss of disc height. It is suggested by pain on extension, not flexion, ipsilateral pain on lateral flexion combined with extension, a lack of radicular features and tenderness over these joints. Pain can be referred to the posterior thigh (as is the case with SI and hip joint pain), but a simple distinction between radicular pain and referred pain is that only the former is below the knee. The patient's response to medial branch blocks of the dorsal primary rami is diagnostic.[24]

Sacroiliac joint pain never gives rise to pain above the ilium, it is non-radicular, usually unilateral and is suggested by pain on manoeuvres that strain the joint. Like pain from intervertebral discs, it too may falsely project onto the groin.

Hip pain, likewise, does not radiate superiorly. It is detected fairly readily with movements that put the hip through a wide range of movement.

A retroperitoneal tumour is suggested by relentless pain progression, pain at rest and at night, night sweats, malaise and weight loss. The differential diagnosis includes infection – e.g. osteomyelitis and tuberculosis of the spine.

An epidural abscess or haematoma should be considered in the early postoperative period.

The incidence of mechanical, discogenic pain following disc surgery is probably common. It is suggested by low backache on standing and sitting, exacerbated by coughing, sneezing and flexion. The differential diagnosis is between a meningeal cyst and a pseudomeningocoele, which is a cyst containing CSF, but without a meningeal lining. Magnetic resonance imaging will distinguish between the two and will also show annular tears in discs. Diagnostic discography is indicated if definitive treatment is to be considered.

Spinal instability should be considered in the differential diagnosis of low back pain.

An immediate re-prolapse is indicated by recurrence of symptoms in the postoperative period. The differential diagnosis is an epidural haematoma.

Muscular pain is common. Muscular spasm may be secondary to pain per se or else may be due (e.g. in the case of iliopsoas) to the leakage of nucleus pulposus from an adjacent disc.

In the subacute phase, a recurrence of radicular pain involves distinguishing between a further disc prolapse and epidural fibrosis. There are no distinguishing clinical features, although less restriction of movement, less pain with coughing and an ability to straight-leg raise greater than 30° are said to make a recurrent disc less likely than fibrosis.[25]

A canal stenosis can also give rise to radicular symptoms, which may have an element of neurogenic claudication.

Diagnosis is an art as well as a science. The aphorism 'listen to the patient and he will tell you the diagnosis' holds true. An active and ordered form of listening is required. The clinician must carefully examine case after case. A thorough understanding of physical signs, especially neurological signs, and how to accurately illicit and interpret them is fundamental.

# Investigations

## Imaging techniques

High quality MRI is almost essential. It will demonstrate central canal, lateral recess and neural foramen narrowing, the state of the intervertebral disc, evidence of continuing bone infection and abnormal epidural space masses – e.g. disc herniation, scar, abscess and a posterior joint synovial cyst. Gadolinium enhancement, with repeat scanning within 2 minutes of injection, can distinguish epidural scar tissue from a disc fragment in all cases.[3] Scar tissue in general is more vascularized than a disc herniation, which often has a central non-enhancing area.

Computed tomography (CT) is the investigation of choice for bony abnormalities – e.g. osteophytes, spinal stenosis or calcified disc fragment. Myelography, using water-soluble, non-ionic contrast medium, may still be indicated for possible postoperative instability, using flexion-extension imaging.

Time after surgery makes a major difference to the images obtained. Ninety-two percent of patients scanned within the first week have a mass lesion the same size as their original herniation.[26] This figure falls to 40% and 32% at 1–2 months and 1 year after surgery, respectively.[26] Interpretation of early postoperative images is, therefore, difficult.

Thickening of nerve roots seen by CT or MRI, possibly due to oedema, does not necessarily relate to chronic pain, whereas dural sac compression does.

Table 20.3 summarizes aetiology versus the appropriate investigation.[27]

## Spinal endoscopy

The major drawback of all imaging techniques is that they cannot distinguish symptomatically relevant anatomical abnormalities from ubiquitous postoperative changes. The exception is

**Table 20.3** Postoperative complications with their appropriate investigation

| Postoperative complication | Investigation of choice |
| --- | --- |
| Haemorrhage | MRI |
| Recurrent disc herniation | Non-Gadolinium enhancement on MRI |
| Infection | Biochemical markers of inflammation, radionucleotide scanning, MRI |
| Sterile arachnoiditis | CT myelography, MRI, spinal endoscopy |
| Pseudomeningocoele | MRI |
| Spinal stenosis | CT or MRI<br>For neural foramen stenosis – MRI |
| Radiculitis | Spinal endoscopy<br>If >8 months postoperative Gadolinium enhancement on MRI |
| Segmental instability | Flexion and extension MRI<br>?Myelography |
| Efficacy of fusion | Not fully mineralized until 9 months.<br>MRI marrow continuity. Dynamic X-rays |
| Musculoligamentous degeneration | Fast spin MRI |
| Textiloma | Often impregnated with barium.<br>X-ray, CT. MRI confusing. |

Adapted from Jinkins JR and Van Goethem JWM.[27]
CT, computed tomography; MRI, magnetic resonance imaging.

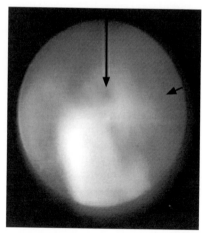

**Figure 20.1** An abnormal S1 nerve root in a patient unable to straight leg raise. The nerve root (left of picture) exits the dura (on the right). A sling of scar tissue is seen around its origin.

spinal endoscopy. Non-inflamed healthy nerve roots with a transmitted marked pulsation are non-tender when gently contacted, whereas inflamed (pain generating) roots, with redness and oedema are markedly tender to touch.[12,13] The author uses the technique for identification of nerve roots involved in pain generation (Figure 20.1). Magnetic resonance imaging and spinal endoscopy appear to be mutually informative and together offer greater accuracy of diagnosis (Table 20.4).

## Management

The primary goal is pain relief of a dynamic nature. If the resumption of activity can be facilitated, the patient can start to rebuild his or her life and psychosocial behavioural factors frequently will start to reverse.[24] A graded rehabilitation programme will be required to rebuild muscle power and endurance and encourage the psychological fortitude required to confront symptoms, deconditioning and disabilities.

**Table 20.4** Suggested comparison of spinal endoscopy with magnetic resonance imaging (MRI)

|  | Spinal endoscopy | MRI |
|---|---|---|
| Nerve root anatomy | − (close up views only possible) | ++ |
| Nerve root vascularity | ++ | − |
| Nerve root inflammation | ++ | +/− |
| Nerve root sensitivity | ++ | − |
| Diagnostic localization of pain | ++ | − |
| Identification of fibrous tissue | ++ | + |
| Disc prolapse identification | − | ++ |
| Assessment of spinal canal size | − | ++ |
| Exclusion of serious pathology | + (biopsy possible) | ++ |
| Therapeutic aspects | ++ | − |

++, very helpful; +, helpful; −, not helpful

It is clinically useful to separate back pain from leg pain. In broad terms, low back pain involves nociceptor mechanisms (NB. L4, L5 and S1 have no cutaneous low-back representation) and lower leg pain involves neuropathic mechanisms (see Table 20.1).

## Pharmacotherapy

Nociceptive low back pain usually requires treatment with systemic analgesics. Controlled release opiates are frequently needed due to its severity, but these drugs are disappointing for pain on movement. The author's ladder roughly reads: paracetamol, codeine, tramadol, controlled release morphine, oxycodone or fentanyl with fast onset additional opiate (e.g. oramorph or oral fentanyl) occasionally prescribed for breakthrough pain. Transdermal buprenorphine is an interesting potentially useful new development.

Non-steroidal anti-inflammatory drugs (NSAIDs), through their effect on nociceptors may help with pain on movement, but efficacy is often incomplete. Knowledge of a number of these drugs is useful. Cyclooxygenase 2 (COX-2) drugs make long term prescribing safer. Glucosamine, a herbal therapy, can be effective.[28]

Neuropathic analgesics will be required for radiculopathic pain. Prescribing should be along the lines of individual effectiveness combined with tolerance. In practice, this comes down to single or combined drug regimens involving one or two classes of agent: tricyclic antidepressants, anticonvulsants and antiarrhythmics. The newer anticonvulsant gabapentin, almost uniquely licensed for use in neuropathic pain, is effective in many patients, although tolerance can be a problem. For assembly of one's own armamentarium the reader is referred to McQuay and Moore.[28]

All systemic analgesics can impair cerebration and, as FBSS affects many patients in the working-age population, this effect may be intolerable. Alternative analgesic strategies become more attractive in this situation. Topical treatments (eg NSAID gels) are useful for nociceptive pain, while capsaicin cream is helpful for this as well as neuropathic pain.[28] Transcutaneous electrical nerve stimulation (TENS) is cheap, innocuous, and many patients find it helpful. Heat, acupuncture, manipulation and massage may help individual patients. Abdominal and back extensor muscle strengthening and nerve stretch exercises can be effective in motivated individuals.

## Low back pain interventions

Z joint pain should be diagnosed and effectively treated through medial branch blocks of the dorsal primary rami followed by radiofrequency lesioning.[24,29]

SI joint pain can be diagnosed and treated with intra-articular steroids and sometimes with radiofrequency lesioning.

Surgical re-referral will be needed for missed diagnoses, such as spinal instability, severe spinal stenosis with spinal cord claudication, pseudomeningocoele, hip pain, any possibility of a retroperitoneal tumour and chronic spinal infection (osteomyelitis, discitis, tuberculosis, etc.).

Muscular pain should be treated with physiotherapy advice regarding posture and exercises, possibly with muscle relaxants, such as baclofen or diazepam in the short term. Spasm in particular muscle groups (e.g. iliopsoas) can be successfully managed with botulinum toxin injection, although it must be remembered that it is often secondary to another event, such as an unstable leaking disc.

Mechanical, discogenic pain may occur at the operated level or adjacent levels encouraged through excessive movement (especially following fusion) in frequently already degenerate motion segments. Magnetic resonance provides excellent images, but provocative discography is needed to make the diagnosis. Intradiscal steroids may be helpful. Intradiscal electrothermal annuloplasty is a highly promising technique for the effective probably long-term treatment of this condition.[30]

## Radiculopathic pain interventions

Epidural steroids are effective in the long term (3–12 months) for some patients with chronic sciatica.[28] In patients with chronic radicular pain, there may be a failure of injectate to reach the nerve root because of scar tissue, and there is probably increased vascular uptake by granulation tissue. These are almost universal findings although the worst examples occur following surgery.[12,13] Steroid targeting needs to be provided in these cases.

### Spinal endoscopy

Specific nerve root involvement in pain generation diagnosed through spinal endoscopy can subsequently become the focus of endoscopic adhesiolysis (neuroplasty) (Figures 20.1–20.3). It is possible that adhesiolysis reduces pain generation through improvement in nerve root nutrition by removal of obstruction to blood supply and CSF flow.[12,13] Dilution or 'washing-out' of phospholipase A2 and synovial cytokines, which are known to leak from damaged intervertebral discs and Z joints, may also contribute to an improvement in symptoms. Spinal endoscopy allows for the highly accurate placement of epidural medication, along with the effective prior formation of a pocket for the steroid solution (Figures 20.2 & 20.3). Results so far in terms of pain relief, improvement in physical function, side-effects and complications are encouraging, but accurate scientific assessment is awaited.

Steerable catheters without the facility of direct vision can be used for targeted medication delivery (e.g. Racz catheter). Diagnostic localization is inferior and, in the presence of copious scar tissue, there may be a possibility for accidental intrathecal delivery of steroid.

A further, simple method of targeted steroid delivery is through transforaminal injection (Figure 20.4). This technique is of great practical value to the clinician, with some patients experiencing long term pain improvements.[31] Radiofrequency lesioning of dorsal root ganglia is generally disappointing.[32]

Further methods of adhesiolysis include the successful use of hyaluronidase and hypertonic saline.

### The role of surgery

Surgical re-exploration for radiculopathic pain may be counter productive,[9] except in the presence of a disc fragment when success rates of 70–80% have been reported.[33] Repeat surgery for epidural fibrosis has failure rates of 50–80% with risks of dura mater and nerve root damage increasing with the number of operations.[9]

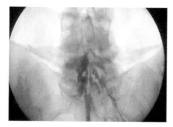

**Figure 20.2**  A pre-spinal endoscopic neuroplasty epidurogram of a patient with right sided S1 nerve root pain.

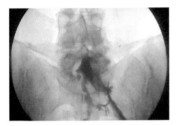

**Figure 20.3**   In the same patient as in Figure 20.2, the postoperative epidurogram appearances show much better contrast medium filling of the S1 nerve root.

## Spinal cord stimulation

Spinal cord stimulation should be considered for the most severely affected patients with this syndrome. High-quality analgesia can be obtained of a dynamic nature. Intractable radiculopathic pain is the main indicator, although some improvement in the low back pain component is common-place. Repeat surgery has been compared with spinal cord stimulation and has been found to be highly inferior.[34] Funding for these devices remains a constant practical difficulty, while facilities for repeat surgery are unquestioningly provided. Analgesic usage reduction goes someway to reduction in costs. A high level of expertise is required particularly for patient selection, but also for avoidance of stimulator related complications.

Fully implantable programmable intrathecal drug delivery systems are useful in the most intractable pain cases.

## Pain rehabilitation programmes

Abnormal fear-avoidance beliefs should be addressed as early as possible, probably through graded physical exercise exposure, combined with cognitive-behavioural therapy.[35]

Key objectives of chronic pain rehabilitation programmes are to improve the physical and psychological functioning of patients thereby enabling less dependency, a reduction in distress caused by chronic pain, an improvement in the knowledge and skills of the patient to enable them to manage their own pain, optimization of medication usage and help with family beliefs and manipulation. Such programmes involve multidisciplinary cooperation. This approach is excellent at helping patients and their families cope with pain. Overall, a combination of medication optimization, interventions to reduce pain and a psychosocial behavioural approach is ideal.

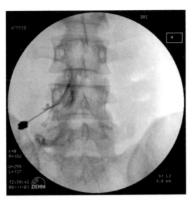

**Figure 20.4**   Targeting epidural medication. X-ray contrast appearance of an L4 transforaminal nerve root block. Note the unilateral epidural spread. An earlier L5 block has been performed.

# Conclusion

Generation of chronic pain after back surgery is a complex process. Attempts to treat the multiple processes involved through repeat surgery is destined to failure in many cases. An accurate diagnosis is required and multimodal, often multidisciplinary solutions should be sought. Realistic goals need to be set, and achievement of a pain free state is frequently elusive. Prevention is all important.

# References

1. Merskey H, Bogduk N. Lumbar spinal or radicular pain after failed spinal surgery XXVI-10. In: *Classification of Chronic Pain. 2nd Ed.* Seattle: IASP press, 1994
2. Follet KA, Dirkes BA. Etiology and evaluation of the failed back surgery syndrome. *Neurosurg Quart* **3**: 40–59, 1993
3. Shafaie FF, Blundschuh C, Jinkins JR. The posttherapeutic lumbosacral spine. In: Jinkins JR, ed. *Posttherapeutic Neurodiagnostic Imaging.* Philadelphia: Lippincott-Raven, 1997, pp. 223–243
4. Lequesne M, Lamotte J. Les suites douloureuses à distance de la lombo-sciatique discale opérée vues par le rhumatologique. *Rev Chir Orthop* **68**: 226–229, 1982
5. Dvorak J, Geuchat MH, Valach L. The outcome of surgery for lumbar disc herniation. I. A 4–17 years follow-up with emphasis on somatic aspects. *Spine* **13**: 1418–1422, 1988
6. Silvers HR. Microsurgical versus standard lumbar discectomy. *Neurosurgery* **22**: 837–841, 1988
7. Fritsch EW, Heisel J, Rupp S. The failed back surgery syndrome: reasons, intraoperative findings and long term results: a report of 182 operative treatments. *Spine* **21**: 626–633, 1996
8. Barrios C, Ahmed M, Arrotegui J, Björnsson A, Gillström P. Microsurgery versus standard removal of the herniated lumbar disc. *Acta Orthop Scand* **61**: 399–403, 1990
9. Goupille P. Causes of failed back surgery syndrome. *Rev Rhum Engl Ed* **63**: 235–239, 1996
10. Olmarker K, Rydevik B, Nordborg C. Autologous nucleus pulposus induces neurophysiologic and histologic changes in porcine cauda equina nerve roots. *Spine* **18**: 1425–1432, 1993
11. Cooper RG, Mitchell WS, Illingworth KJ, Forbes WS, Gillespie JE, Jayson MIV. The role of epidural fibrinolysis in the persistence of postlaminectomy back pain. *Spine* **16**: 1044–1048, 1991
12. Richardson J, McGurgan P Cheema S, Prashad R. Gupta S. Spinal endoscopy in chronic low-back pain with radiculopathy. A prospective case series. *Anaesthesia* **56**: 447–484, 2001
13. Geurts JW, Kallewaard JW, Richardson J, Groen GJ. Targeted methylprednisolone/ hyaluronidase/ clonidine injection after diagnostic epiduroscopy for chronic sciatica: a prospective, 1-year follow-up study. *Anesth Pain Med* **27**: 343–352, 2002
14. Anertz M, Jönsson B Strömqvist B, Holtås S. No relationship between epidural fibrosis and sciatica in the postdiscectomy syndrome. A study with contrast enhanced magnetic resonance imaging in symptomatic and asymptomatic patients. *Spine* **20**: 449, 1995
15. Rydevik B, Holm S, Brown MD, Lundborg G. Diffusion from the CSF as a nutritional pathway for spinal nerve roots. *Acta Physiol Scand* **138**: 247–248, 1990
16. Olmarker K, Myers RR. Pathogenesis of sciatic pain: role of herniated nucleus pulposus, and deformation of spinal nerve root and dorsal root ganglion. *Pain* **78**: 99–105, 1998
17. Kayama S, Konno S, Olmarker K, Yabuki S, Kikuchi S. Incision of the annulus fibrosus induces nerve root morphologic, vascular and functional changes. An experimental study. *Spine* **21**: 2539–2543, 1996
18. Dhar S, Porter RW. Failed lumbar spinal surgery. *Int Orthop* **16**: 152–156, 1992
19. Fritz JM, George SZ, Delitto A. The role of fear-avoidance beliefs in acute low back pain: relationships with current and future disability and work status. *Pain* **94**: 7–15, 2001
20. Berger E. Late postoperative results in 1000 work related lumbar spine conditions. *Surg Neurol* **54**: 101–108, 2000
21. Gilette RG, Kramis RC, Roberts WJ. Characterization of spinal somatosensory neurons having receptive fields in lumbar tissues of cats. *Pain* **54**: 85–98, 1993
22. Reynolds OE, Hutchins HC. Referral of pain to dental area after sinus maxillary stimulation. *Am J Physiol* **152**: 658–662, 1948

23. Yukawa Y, Kato F, Kajino G, Nakamura S, Nitta H. Groin pain associated with lower lumbar disc herniation. *Spine* **22:** 1736–1740, 1997
24. Wallis BJ, Lord SM, Bogduk N. Resolution of psychological distress of whiplash patients following treatment by radiofrequency neurotomy: a randomised, double-blind, placebo-controlled trial. *Pain* **73:** 15–22, 1997
25. Jönsson B, Strömqvist B. Repeat decompression of lumbar nerve roots: a prospective two-year evaluation. *J Bone Joint Surg Br* **75:** 894, 1993
26. Tullberg T, Rydberg J, Isacson J. Radiographic changes after lumbar discectomy. Sequential enhanced computerised tomography in relation to clinical observations. *Spine* **18:** 843, 1993
27. Jinkins JR, Van Goethem JWM. The postsurgical lumbosacral spine. *Radiol Clin N Am* **39:** 1–29, 2001
28. McQuay HJ, Moore RA. *An Evidence-Based Resource for Pain Relief.* Oxford: Oxford University Press, 1998
29. Dreyfuss P, Halbrook B, Pauza K, Joshi A, McLarty J, Bogduk N. Efficacy and validity of radiofrequency neurotomy for chronic lumbar zygapophysial joint pain. *Spine* **25:** 1270–1277, 2000
30. Karasek M, Bogduk N. Twelve month follow-up of a controlled trial of intradiscal thermal annuloplasty for back pain due to internal disc disruption. *Spine* **25:** 2601–2607, 2000
31. Vijay V, Bhat A, Lutz G, Cammisa F. Transforaminal epidural steroid injections in lumbosacral radiculopathy: a prospective randomized study. *Spine* **27:** 11–15, 2002
32. Geurts JW, Van Wijk RM, Stolker RJ, Groen GJ. Efficacy of radiofrequency procedures for the treatment of spinal pain: a systematic review of randomized clinical trials. *Regional Anesthesia and Pain Medicine.* **26**: 394–400, 2001
33. Cauchoix J, Ficat C, Girard B. Repeat surgery after disc excision. *Spine* **3:** 256–259, 1978
34. North RB, Kidd DH, Lee MS, Piantodosi S. A prospective, randomized study of spinal cord stimulation versus reoperation for failed back surgery syndrome: initial results. *Stereotact Funct Neurosurg* **62:** 267–272, 1994
35. Crombez G, Vlaeyen JW, Heuts PH, Lysens R. Pain-related fear is more disabling than fear itself: evidence on the role of pain-related fear in chronic back pain disability. *Pain* **80:** 329–339, 1999

# 21 Peripheral Vascular Disease

## Nicholas L Padfield

Pain arising from peripheral vascular disease arises not only from the condition itself but also, more often, from the resulting problems of amputation surgery such as stump pain or phantom pain. Stripping of varicose veins when done in a traumatic way with large strippers used to cause a lot of pain, which was largely unnoticed by any medical attendants because of damage to the saphenous nerve. Fortunately, this has been recognized by more enlightened surgeons, who now only strip to just below the knee and not down to the medial malleolus.

For practical purposes, pain arising from vascular disease should be differentiated into that which arises from the arteries themselves, the microvessels (arterioles, capillaries and venules) and the veins. It is important to consider pathological processes, as these will need to be controlled optimally.

Table 21.1 lists the common causes of pain with vascular disease.

## Atherosclerosis

Atherosclerosis is by far the most, common source of referral. Its development is insidious starting with the fatty streak through fibrous plaque. The advanced state produces pain from ischaemia to direct pressure effects from aneurismal dilatation. It usually develops into a clinical condition requiring medical attention in the fifth and sixth decades of life. Vascular insufficiency of the lower extremities can result from occlusive lesions at any of several sites, from the aortoiliac segment to the femoral, popliteal and/or tibial vessels. Progressive occlusion of these arteries causes intermittent claudication in the affected gastrocnemius muscle. Rest pain, ischaemia ulceration, and gangrene usually signify severe distal or multifocal occlusion and seldom result from single isolated aortoiliac occlusion.[1] There is often associated hypertension, diabetes mellitus and high cigarette consumption. Patients frequently come from less privileged socioeconomic groups and they may also be malnourished – so that healing may be impaired.

Leriche's syndrome is due to isolated aortoiliac occlusive disease, which produces a characteristic clinical picture of intermittent claudication of the back, buttocks and thigh or calf muscles, impotence and atrophy of the limbs and pallor of the skin of the legs and feet. In rare cases, where the atheroma involves abdominal vessels, the patient suffers from abdominal angina – discussed in Chapter 13.

### Arteritis

Thromboangiitis obliterans (Burger's disease) is an obstructive arterial disease caused by segmental inflammation and proliferative lesions of the medium and small arteries and veins of the limbs.[2]

The symptoms result from impairment of arterial blood supply to the tissues and, to some extent, from local venous insufficiency. The symptoms are:

| **Table 21.1** Causes of pain in peripheral vascular disease |
| --- |
| Atherosclerosis |
| Arteritis |
| Giant cell arteritis |
| Raynaud's phenomenon |
| Erythromelalgia |
| Pain due to dysfunction of microvessels |
| Venous pain |

- Rest pain when severe ischaemia of tissues has developed
- Pain from ulcerations and gangrene
- Pain from ischaemic neuropathy, which must be considered an important component.

### Takayasu's syndrome

Takayasu's syndrome (aortic arch syndrome) is due to arteritis and arteriolitis of the vessels of the upper part of the body as far as the arterioles of the eye. It is prevalent in adolescent girls and young women. In a prodromic phase about two-thirds of the patients complain of malaise, fever, limb-girdle stiffness and arthralgia; this prodromic phase is similar to that seen in giant cell arteritis, rheumatic diseases and systemic lupus erythematosus. In many instances, this is soon followed by local pain over the affected arteries, erythema nodosum and erythema induratum. In some cases, it evolves into angina pectoris or myocardial infarction.

### Giant cell arteritis

Giant cell arteritis is an inflammatory condition of medium and small arteries, characteristically the branches of the internal carotid, particularly the temporal artery. It occurs in patients older than 55 years, women more than men, and presents as headache, which can be intense and unbearable. Untreated, the condition can rapidly lead to blindness. Intermittent claudication of the temporomandibular joint can occur. Giant cell arteritis is a systemic disease, and it can involve arteries in many locations.[3] The patient will often describe a 'flu'-like illness with severe malaise, fever and myalgia. The muscle pain becomes severe, involving mainly the neck and shoulder and pelvic girdle, but also the trunk and the distal limbs to a lesser degree. Intermittent claudication, myocardial infarctions and infarction of visceral organs have been reported.

## Raynaud's phenomenon

Raynaud's phenomenon and migratory superficial thrombophlebitis are common. It tends to be a disease of young men who smoke heavily. Sadly, despite mutilating surgery, the majority continue to smoke. They also tend to be malnourished and from lower socioeconomic groups.

Raynaud's phenomenon is characterized by episodes of intense pallor and pain in the fingers and toes (ischaemia phase) generally followed by rumor and cyanosis. The pain arises from sudden arteriolar constriction followed by a vasodilatation phase. It is classified as primary or secondary in association with other diseases. Treatment efficacy unfortunately wanes with time. It is centered on keeping the affected parts warm, and the use of calcium channel blockers and α-adrenergic blockers. Intravenous regional blocks of the affected limb with guanethidine have been very disappointing. The primary lesion appears to be genetic and involves abnormal activity of monoamine oxidase.

## Erythromelalgia

Erythromelalgia is a syndrome characterized by redness, increased temperature and pain in the limbs. The pain can be both deep and superficial and can be accompanied by oedema. Secondary erythromelalgia is commonly associated with myeloproliferative disorders, such as thrombocytosis and diabetes mellitus. It may be a part of the spectrum of conditions that comprise complex regional pain syndrome type 1.

# Pain genesis

Conditions leading to pain genesis:

- Ischaemia that leads to rest pain when it is severe; myalgic spots with the characteristics of trigger points are present in the limbs.[4] Dysfunction of the sympathetic nervous system resulting in changes in the permeability of the microvessels, tissue inbibation, vasomotor changes, release of active substances and direct modulation of sensory receptors.
- Ischaemia during muscular exercise because of a build up of lactic acid and other anaerobic metabolites because oxygen demand exceeds supply.
- Ischaemia and inflammation related to the rheumatic or metabolic disorder responsible for the ischaemia, e.g. thromboangiitis obliterans.
- Release of neurogenic inflammatory mediators such as histamine, 5-hydroxytryptamine (5-HT), kinins, substance P and calcitonin gene related peptide (CGRP). It is likely that nerve growth factors are involved in response to tissue damage caused by the ischaemia. This in turn can lead to a plethora of changes within the nervous system of pain signalling, and it may explain the extremely varied response seen to sympathetic blockade in the lower limbs when objective testing shows no change in limb perfusion but the patient can report significant pain relief.
- Venous insufficiency can be painful and is likely due to a combination of ischaemia, which in turn leads to release of inflammatory mediators, swelling and myofascial pain.

### Fontaine classification

- Stage 1 – Intermittent claudication
- Stage 2 – Intermittent claudication with trophic changes and/or skin discoloration
- Stage 3 – Ischaemic rest pain
- Stage 4 – Rest pain, ulcers and/or gangrene, where progress to amputation is inevitable.

# Investigation

The investigation has usually been undertaken by the referring surgeon or physician, and is likely to include:

- Arteriography
- Doppler ultrasonography
- Thermography
- Oximetry
- Galvanic responses
- Duplex scans
- Venography.

# Treatment

Because peripheral vascular disease may manifest in various ways, attention should be paid to the following measures, including some more specific measures for managing the arterial ischaemia rather than the pain itself. These include:

- Treating underlying medical cause where possible, controlling hypertension, diabetes, hyperlipidaemia, and rheumatic inflammatory condition
- Encouraging the patient to stop smoking
- Improving diet if appropriate
- Graded exercises
- Intravenous heparin and observation[5] in patients without motor disturbance or cyanosis
- Intravenous prostaglandin – one meta-analysis of placebo-controlled trials of Iloprost, a prostacyclin analogue, found 6 random clinical trials (RCTs) showed a significant beneficial effect over placebo on ulcer healing and pain relief, but surmised that the end points may have unblinded the patients and their observers. Meta-analysis of other pharmacotherapeutic agents concluded that patients with Fontaine stages 3 or 4 showed no significant benefit over placebo for any of the end points reported.[7]

When there is incipient gangrene, ulceration or rest pain, reconstructive surgery can be undertaken when the vessels are suitable for reconstruction. Such procedures would include:

- Angioplasty
- Vascular grafts
- Endoarterectomy.

Unfortunately there are frequent occasions when the vessels involved are non-reconstructable. The patient is then usually referred to the pain clinician. Before embarking on interventions, if the primary problem is a variety of autoimmune arteritis, the immune status of the patient must be optimized and ideally in remission. Usually, such patients are referred by rheumatologists who are monitoring and treating it accordingly.

Where pain is the predominant issue at consultation, and the above general measures have been optimized, the following drugs have been used with varied success

- Tricyclic antidepressants
- Gabapentin
- Calcium channel blockers
- Aspirin, clopidogrel
- Alpha antagonists
- Clonidine
- Gingko biloba extract.[6]

## Pain interventions

The pain interventions that the pain clinician will undertake are listed in the order in which they are most usually performed. Evidence of efficacy, if available, is included with each procedure.

### Lumbar sympathetic block

Lumbar sympathetic block with local anaesthetic and depot steroid, or even with phenol 6%, has been the mainstay of treatment for intermittent claudication when it was felt that surgery was not yet indicated.

## Operative sympathectomy

Operative sympathectomy had its advocates, where over a 5-year period studying 118 patients there was a 45% limb loss, occurring predominantly within 6 months of sympathectomy, but in the surviving limbs there was a 86% resolution of rest pain. The author concluded that lumbar sympathectomy coupled with local tissue management remained a valuable treatment option for the severely ischaemic limb not amenable to reconstructive surgery.[8] However, the effect on blood flow in the limb was minimal. Sometimes a 'steal' situation would arise when the actual blood flow down the ischaemic limb was reduced as it went preferentially to the dilated skin vessels. However, it was noticed that often, despite the altered haemodynamics, pain was improved. It is likely, in the light of recent work on the role of inflammatory mediators and neuromodulatory amines, that sympathetic blockade affects these in a beneficial way to produce reduction in pain experienced. However, there is very little good quality evidence that such measures will prevent the need for salvage arterial reconstruction or, at worst, serial amputation of the lower limb.

## Intravenous regional guanethidine block

Intravenous regional guanethidine blocks have been used for ischaemic limb pain. There use is to be deprecated, as the application of a tourniquet to a prosthetic graft has led to graft occlusion with disastrous results.

## Spinal cord stimulation

The employment of spinal cord stimulation (SCS) remains contentious. Practice varies either side of the Atlantic and within Europe itself.[9] It has been argued that the place for SCS is in a patient whose vessels are not suitable for grafting, as an alternative to amputation surgery when the ischaemia is likely to progress to gangrene. In the first half of the 1970s, early reports from the USA, with very small numbers of patients, showed that feelings of deadness or heaviness were replaced with feelings of warmth and lightness in multiple sclerosis patients,[10] and it was also reported to improve perfusion and pain beyond that obtained with sympathetic blockade.[11] The role of the sympathetic nervous system with SCS was studied in rats. The results indicated a major contribution of the sympathetic system to SCS-induced peripheral vasodilation and explains why the method can be clinically effective also after chemical or surgical sympathectomy. It is likely that sympathetic vasoconstrictor activity is depressed by stimulation-induced activation of spinal inhibitory mechanisms, and that this constitutes a major component of the vasodilatory effect of SCS in peripheral vascular disease.[12] In a Canadian study looking at 39 out of an initial 46 patients, if the transcutaneous $PO_2$, which was less than 30 mmHg pre-implantation, improved significantly then the outcome was deemed good and was associated with a significant increase in peak blood flow. If the transcutaneous $PO_2$ was less than 10 mmHg pre-implantation then the outcome was likely to be poor. The authors suggested SCS appeared to be a useful therapeutic modality for controlling pain and improving perfusion in a select group of patients with end-stage ischaemic vascular disease that was considered to be non-reconstructable.[13] Unfortunately, this enthusiastic report was not confirmed in one randomized controlled trial of 120 patients, where the conclusion was, in fact, that SCS in addition to the best medical care did not prevent amputation in patients with critical limb ischaemia.[14] However, in another randomized trial of 86 Fontaine stage 4 patients, where SCS was added to intravenous prostaglandin therapy in one group and withheld in the other, at 12-month follow-up the SCS group had 69% healing of foot ulcers compared with 17% in the non-SCS group. Foot transcutaneous $PO_2$ significantly increased in the SCS group, and those in the non-SCS group whose transcutaneous $PO_2$ rose to greater than 26 mmHg were able to heal their ulcers. In the prostaglandin infusion alone group these improvements in $tco_2$ were temporary.[15]

At a consensus meeting organized by ®Medtronic at the 9th International Association for the Study of Pain (IASP) congress in Vienna, it was concluded that the only patients that were likely to benefit from SCS were those whose ischaemia was not so bad that amputation was considered inevitable, but was not so good that conservative measures would suffice in preventing the need for reconstructive arterial surgery. Patients and physicians were then faced with a choice of reconstructive surgery or an implant with no clear guidelines. It certainly has not gained any popularity in the UK.

## Phantom and stump pain

One of the greatest challenges for the pain clinician is when the peripheral vascular disease process has resulted in amputation and patients experience problems with stump pain and phantom pain.

Stump pain tends to be nociceptive, and it is frequently the result of physical problems, such as a mal-fitting prosthesis, infection of the wound site, development of neuroma or skin excoriation and breakdown. Such problems are usually self evident and the solutions are straightforward. However, it is the development of 'phantom' sensations that can give the greatest challenges to the attending physician. In a recent systematic review looking at the evidence for the optimal management of acute and chronic phantom pain, 12 trials were identified. Of these, only three were randomized controlled studies with parallel groups and three were cross-over randomized trials. The use of epidural treatments, regional block treatments, transcutaneous nerve stimulation (TENS), calcitonin and ketamine were reported; the authors concluded that, although up to 70% of patients experience phantom limbs after amputation, there was little evidence from randomized trials to guide clinicians with treatment. They went on to say that the evidence for preemptive epidurals, early regional nerve blocks and mechanical vibratory stimulation provided inconsistent support for these treatments.[16]

Because the pathophysiology of post-amputation pain states is unclear, a randomized double-blind, active placebo-controlled trial was undertaken to examine the effects of intravenous lignocaine compared with morphine. The authors found that stump pain was diminished by both morphine and lignocaine while phantom pain was only diminished by morphine, and they concluded that the mechanisms and pharmacological sensitivity of stump and phantom pains are different.[17] In a report of four cases treated with methadone, an opiate with N-methyl-D-aspartate (NMDA) antagonist activity, the authors concluded that oral methadone may be of value in the treatment of phantom limb pain but, wisely, suggested that controlled trials would be appropriate to verify this observation.[18]

Lastly, whatever management is undertaken, it must not be forgotten that amputation causes an enormous economic and social burden on individuals and the community. In a recent study of the relationship between employment and pain and disability in an amputee population, the authors found that few amputees made use of the available services for general amputation-related problems, and even fewer services were utilized for phantom limb pain. Moreover, when these services were used, few were reported as helpful. Employment pre- and post-amputation diminished, and employment status was found to be related to the intensity of the phantom limb pain and prosthetic usage, with unemployed amputees reporting higher levels of pain and lower levels of prosthesis use.[19]

## References

1. Thompson JE, Garrett WV. Peripheral-arterial surgery. *N Engl J Med* **302**: 491, 1980
2. Konton HA. Vascular diseases of the limbs. In: Bennett JC and Plum F, eds. *Cecil Textbook of Medicine, 20th edn.* Philadelphia: WB Saunders, 1996, pp. 346–357

3. Fauci AS. The vasculitis syndromes. In: Fauci AS, Braunwald E, Isselbacher KJ eds. *Harrison's Principles of Internal Medicine*. New York: McGraw-Hill, 1998, pp. 1920–1922

4. Dorigo B, Bartoli V, Grisillo D, Beconi D. Fibrositic myofascial pain in intermittent claudication. Effect of anaesthetic block of trigger points on exercise tolerance. *Pain* 6: 183–190, 1979

5. Jivegard L, Bergqvist D, Holm J. When is urgent revascularisation unnecessary for acute lower limb ischaemia? *Eur J Vasc Endovasc Surg* 9: 448–453, 1995

6. Letzel H, Schoop W. [Gingko biloba extract Egb 761 and pentoxifylline in intermittent claudication. Secondary analysis of the clinical effectiveness] Gingko biloba extract Egb 761 und Pentoxifyllin bei Claudicatio intermittens. *Sekundaranalyse zur klinischen Wirksamkeit Vasa* 21: 403–410, 1992

7. Loosemore TM, Chalmers TC, Dormandy JA. A meta-analysis of randomized placebo control trials I. Fontaine stages III and IV peripheral occlusive arterial disease. *Intl Angiol* 13: 133–134, 1994

8. Baker DM, Lamerton AJ. Operative lumbar sympathectomy for severe lower limb ischaemia: still a valuable treatment option. *Ann Roy Coll Surg* 76: 50–53, 1994

9. Simpson BA. Neuromodulation in Europe-regulation, variation and trends. *Pain Rev* 5: 124–131, 1998

10. Cook AW, Weinstein SP. Chronic dorsal column stimulation in multiple sclerosis. Preliminary report. *NY State J Med* 73: 2868–2872, 1973

11. Cook AW, Oygar A, Baggenstos P, et al. Vascular disease of extremities: electrical stimulation of spinal cord and posterior roots. *NY State J Med* 76: 366–368, 1976

12. Linderoth B, Gunasekera L, Meyerson BA. Effects of sympathectomy on skin and muscle microcirculation during dorsal column stimulation: Animal studies. *Neurosurgery* 29: 874–879, 1991

13. Kumar K, Toth C, Nath RK, Verma AK, Burgess JJ. Improvement in limb circulation in peripheral vascular disease using epidural spinal cord stimulation: a prospective study. *J Neurosurg* 86: 662–669, 1997

14. Klomp HM, Spincemaille GH, Steyerberg EW, Habbema JD, van Urk H. Spinal-cord stimulation. I Critical limb ischaemia: a randomized trial ESES Study Group. *Lancet* 353: 1040–1044, 1999

15. Claeys LGY, Horsch S. Spinal cord stimulation (SCS) following intravenous prostaglandin E1 (PGE1) therapy in non-reconstructable peripheral vascular disease (PVD): Fontaine stage IV. *Pain Clin* 11: 235–243, 1999

16. Halbert J, Crotty M, Cameron ID. Evidence for the optimal management of acute and chronic phantom pain: a systematic review. *Clin J Pain* 18: 84–92, 2002

17. Wu CL, Tella P, Staats PS, et al. Analgesic effects of intravenous lidocaine and morphine on postamputation pain: a randomized double-blind, active placebo-controlled, crossover trial. *Anaesthesiology* 96: 841–848, 2002

18. Bergmans L, Snijdelaar DG, Katz J, Crul BJ. Methadone for phantom limb pain. *Clin J Pain* 18: 203–205, 2002

19. Whyte AS, Carroll LJ. A preliminary examination of the relationship between employment, pain and disability in an amputee population. *Disability Rehab* 24: 462–470, 2002

# 22 Postherpetic Neuralgia

*Simon J Dolin*

## Definition
Postherpetic neuralgia (PHN) is defined as the persistence of pain beyond 3 months after crusting of skin lesions of acute herpes zoster (shingles).

## Varicella zoster virus

- It is the smallest double-stranded DNA herpes virus.
- It produces two different diseases: varicella (chickenpox) generally in childhood, and herpes zoster (shingles) later in life.
- Varicella is uncommon in adults, but it can be a serious disease with high morbidity and mortality.
- A vaccine using a live attenuated virus has been developed, and its suitability for children and susceptible adults in currently under evaluation.
- The primary viral infection enters the dorsal root ganglion of the sensory nerve and establishes latency.
- Sub-clinical reactivation of the virus is thought to occur relatively often.
- The patient's cell-mediated immunity keeps the virus in check. This declines with age.
- It is possible, although not certain, that repeat vaccination may boost cell-mediated immunity.
- The incidence of acute herpes zoster (shingles) is age dependent. It has been estimated that the incidence is 1% per year by age 80 years.[1]
- Any decrease in cell-mediated immunity, such as by steroids, surgery, trauma, intercurrent illness or stress (such as death of a spouse), may initiate an attack of acute herpes zoster.

### Clinical spectrum of acute herpes zoster

- The preherpetic phase is characterized by radicular pain, pruritis and paraesthesiae.
- The typical skin rash of herpes zoster appears in a dermatomal pattern, usually about 4 days after onset of symptoms. The skin rash forms painful blisters, which then go on to crust over 1–2 weeks. Mostly, pain subsides after crusting.
- Postherpatic neuralgia is defined as pain persisting beyond 3 months after crusting.
- Acute herpes zoster pain is described as burning, itching, lancinating and electric shock-like. About 50% report allodynia to light touch.[2]

### Pathophysiology of acute herpes zoster

- Virus replicates in dorsal root ganglion.
- Virus spreads along sensory nerve to skin of relevant dermatome.

- Virus continues to replicate in skin and cerebrospinal fluid (CSF).
- There is direct neural, vascular and skin injury.
- Pathologic findings include acute haemorrhagic necrosis of dorsal root ganglion, and demyelination of peripheral nerves, both sensory and motor. Changes are often bilateral, with one side predominant.
- The pain is, in part, nociceptive due to inflammation and tissue destruction. Inflammation has been demonstrated to persist for months.
- The pain is also, in part, neuropathic from abnormal impulse generation from injured and dying nerves. The role of the sympathetic nervous system in maintaining pain remains unclear.

## Risk factors for development of PHN

- Initial severity of acute herpes zoster results in more severe nerve injury and likelihood of abnormal persistent pain state.[3]
- Age – the overall incidence of PHN after acute herpes zoster is about 10%, but this rises dramatically with age, so that about 80% will develop PHN after the age of 80 years.
- Coexisting neuropathy, such as diabetic neuropathy, may predispose to PHN.
- Various psychosocial risk factors include living alone, health belief, anxiety and depression.

## Prevention of PHN

- Antiviral therapy (acyclovir, famcyclovir) reduces the duration of zoster-associated pain, and reduces the incidence of PHN at 6 months.
- Oral corticosteroids added to antivirals reduce acute zoster-associated pain, but do not affect the incidence of PHN.
- A variety of nerve block techniques have been reported, in uncontrolled case series, to reduce acute zoster-associated pain and reduce PHN. A recent randomized controlled study reported that a 21-day infusion of epidural bupivacaine with epidural steroids reduced both acute zoster-associated pain and PHN compared with i.v. antivirals (PHN reduced from 34% to 6% at 1 year).[4]
- Tricyclic antidepressants, in particular low dose amitriptyline, taken during acute herpes zoster attack, prevented PHN.[5]

## Pathophysiology of PHN

- Dorsal root ganglia show extensive collagen replacement, and permanent neural loss.
- There is thinning of myelin sheaths, and collagen replacement of distal branches of peripheral nerves.
- Dorsal horn of spinal cord may show ipsilateral shrinkage over several segments.
- In skin – patches of severe nerve fibre loss adjoin areas of relatively well-preserved nerves. There is loss of cutaneous axons in contralateral, unaffected skin.
- There is evidence for both peripheral and central mechanisms for PHN, although a unifying theory is not attainable. Evidence is compelling for peripheral sensitization (increased firing of C nociceptors) as the driving mechanism is a subset of patients with little sensory loss. There is good indirect evidence that central mechanisms are dominant in subsets of patients with moderate-to-severe sensory loss, with preserved large diameter fibres forming abnormal patterns with dorsal horn nociceptor neurons. Most patients will have a mix of mechanisms, with varying kinds of pain and allodynia.[6]

# Treatment of PHN

## Drugs with proven efficacy

A variety of drug treatments have been proven effective in prospective controlled trials, but none have been directly compared. Allowing for differences in clinical trial methodology, these treatments are effective in about 50–60% of PHN patients. About 10% will achieve 'complete' relief with a single therapy, making poly-pharmacy commonplace. There are no formal studies to assess additivity or other drug interactions.

- Tricyclic antidepressants are the best established treatment. Numerous clinical trials have produced positive results. 'Number needed to treat' (NNT) for 50% pain relief with tricyclics in PHN is 2.3.[7] Commonly used drugs include amitriptyline 10–50 mg per day, dothiepin 25–75 mg per day and imipramine 25–75 mg per day. The most common side-effects are sedation and dry mouth. Constipation and urinary retention are less common problems. If the evening dose is taken early (9 p.m.), unpleasant sedative effects next morning are diminished. Tricyclics should be used with caution in patients with ischaemic heart disease. Several tricyclics, including amitriptyline and imipramine, are metabolized by a cytochrome-p450 enzyme that is lacking in 10% of the white population, which accounts for the observed pronounced pharmacokinetic variability with this drug.
- Gabapentin is an anticonvulsant with action at voltage-gated calcium channels. At doses up to 1800 mg per day, it has been shown to be an effective treatment for PHN, with an NNT for 50% pain relief of 3.2.[7,8] Side-effects include ataxia, slurred speech and sedation. Pregabalin, a close relative of gabapentin, is currently undergoing clinical trials for treatment of PHN.
- Oxycodone is an orally available opioid with proven efficacy for PHN at doses up to 60 mg per day, with an NNT for 50% pain relief of 2.5.[7,9] The debate about the role of opioids in neuropathic pain seems to have been settled in favour of this class of drugs having an important role in treatment. Side-effects are similar to other opioids, including sedation, nausea, vomiting and constipation.
- Capsaicin, topically applied at 0.075%, has been shown to be effective in PHN, but the efficacy is weak with an NNT for 50% pain relief of 5.3.[7] The quality of clinical trials is limited by problems with blinding due to the burning sensation the compound almost always elicits when applied to affected areas.[10]
- Topical local anaesthetics have proved to be a simple and effective treatment for PHN. Topical 5% lignocaine patches (Lidoderm) have few systemic side-effects, show efficacy within the first few applications, and are specifically approved for PHN in US.[11,12] Application site reactions (skin redness or rash) occurred in about 30% of patients. The patches can be cut to fit the area of the pain, and it also protects against the light tactile stimuli that so often provokes pain in PHN. EMLA cream has been reported to be beneficial in uncontrolled trials, but it is not often used.
- Intrathecal methylprednisolone and lignocaine injected on up to four occasions at weekly intervals has been reported to produce 70% pain reduction over 2 years, compared with a control group.[13] This is a greater effect than any trials of oral medication. There are concerns about possible risks of arachnoiditis with intrathecal steroids, and, although this technique has proven efficacy, uptake is likely to be slow at this stage.

## Drugs without proven efficacy

- Selective serotonin (5-HT) reuptake inhibitor (SSRI) antidepressants have not been evaluated in PHN, nor have tricyclic antidepressants with a selective inhibition of noradrenaline uptake (desipramine, nortriptyline and maprotiline). SSRIs have proved to be relatively ineffective in painful polyneuropathy.

- Anticonvulsants other than gabapentin have not been assessed for efficacy in PHN. Carbamazepine has been assessed in patients with PHN but only as part of a mixed neuropathic study.
- Other opioids have not been assessed for efficacy in PHN. Tramadol has been shown to be effective in diabetic neuropathy, but not formally tested in patients with PHN. Dextromethorphan has been assessed in PHN but was shown to be inactive.

## Invasive therapies

- Peripheral nerve and sympathetic blocks are not generally used in established PHN.
- Destructive lesions, such as cordotomy, are not recommended.
- There is insufficient prospective data on spinal cord stimulation or intrathecal drug delivery systems to justify their general use in PHN. These technologies are occasionally considered on a case-by-case basis.

# References

1. Lisegang T. Varicella zoster viral disease. *Mayo Clin Proc* **74**: 983–998, 1999
2. Haanpaa M, Laippala P, Numikko T. Pain and somatosensory dysfunction in acute herpes zoster. *Clin J Pain* **15**: 78–84, 1999
3. Dworkin R. Prevention of postherpetic neuralgia. *Lancet* **353**: 1636–1637, 1999
4. Pasquallucci A, Pasquallucci V, Galla F, De Angelis V, et al. Prevention of postherpetic neuralgia: acyclovir and prednisolone v epidural local anaesthetic and methylprednisolone. *Acta Anaesthesiol Scand* **44**: 910–918, 2000
5. Bowsher D. The effects of pre-emptive treatment of postherpetic neuralgia with amitriptyline: a randomised, double-blind, placebo-controlled trial. *J Pain Symptom Manage* **13**: 327–331, 1997
6. Nurmikko T. Postherpetic neuralgia – a model for neuropathic pain? In: Hansson P, Fields H, Hill R, Marchettini P, eds. *Neuropathic Pain: Pathophysiology and Treatment, Progress in Pain Research and Management, Vol 21*. Seattle: IASP Press, 2001, pp.151–167
7. Sindrup S, Jensen T. Efficacy of pharmacological treatments of neuropathic pain: an update and effect related to mechanism of drug action. *Pain* **83**: 389–400, 1999
8. Rowbotham M, Harden N, Stacey B, Bernstein P, Magnus-Miller L. Gabapentin for the treatment of postherpetic neuralgia: a randomized controlled trial. *J Am Med Assoc* **280**: 1837–1842, 1998
9. Watson C, Babul N. Efficacy of oxycodone in neuropathic pain: a randomised trial in postherpetic neuralgia. *Neurology* **50**: 1837–1841, 1998
10. Watson C, Tyler K, Bickers D, Millikan L, Smith S, Coleman E. A randomised vehicle-controlled trial of topical capsaicin in the treatment of postherpetic neuralgia. *Clin Ther* **15**: 510–526, 1993
11. Galer B, Rowbotham M, Perander J, Friedman E. Topical lidocaine patch relieves postherpetic neuralgia more effectively than a vehicle patch: results of an enriched enrollment study. *Pain* **80**: 635–645, 1999
12. Watson C. Topical local anaesthetics for neuropathic pain. In: Hansson P, Fields H, Hill R, Marchettini P, eds. *Neuropathic Pain: Pathophysiology and Treatments, Progress in Pain Research and Management, Vol 21*. Seattle: IASP Press, 2001, pp. 215–221
13. Kotani N, Kushikata T, Hashimoto H, Kimura M, et al. Intrathecal methylprednisolone for intractable postherpetic neuralgia. *N Engl J Med* **343**: 1514–1519, 2000

# 23 Trigeminal Neuralgia

*Simon J Dolin*

### Definition

Sudden, usually unilateral, severe brief stabbing recurrent pains in the distribution of one or more branches of the Vth cranial nerve (International Association for the Study of Pain; IASP)[1]

## Anatomy of trigeminal system

There are three divisions of the trigeminal (Vth cranial) nerve. The ophthalmic (V1) supplies sensation to upper face including eyes as far as vertex. The maxillary (V2) supplies sensation to middle face including upper teeth. The mandibular (V3) supplies sensation to the lower jaw, including anterior two-thirds of tongue. The ophthalmic division transits the skull via the superior orbital fissure; the maxillary via the foramen rotundum and the mandibular via the foramen ovale. All three divisions conduct pain from their area of distribution, although the mandibular division is most frequently involved in trigeminal neuralgia. All divisions come together at the trigeminal ganglion, also known as Gasserian ganglion, found in Meckel's cave on the floor of the middle cranial fossa of the skull.

From the Gasserian ganglion, sensory input is conducted to the trigeminal nuclear complex, which has components in the midbrain, pons, medulla, and even extends down to the upper cervical spinal cord. There are three sensory nuclei and one motor nucleus. The long attenuated spinal or descending nucleus descends as far as C4 to blend with substantia gelatinosa of the cervical spinal cord. The spinal nucleus is associated with pain conduction. The motor nucleus lies in the pons. Through reflex connections with the spinal sensory nuclei, it can produce activity of the muscles of mastication, such as clenching of the jaw and chattering of teeth, in response to noxious stimuli to the face.

Secondary fibres originating from the neurons of the elongated spinal nucleus cross the midline and ascend to the thalamus as the trigeminal thalamic tract. On the lateral aspect of the midbrain these fibres may be vulnerable to compromise by the firm edge of dura mater, such as by a meningioma or by trauma.

## Pathophysiology

Trigeminal neuralgia (TN) is a symptom indicative of pathology involving the Vth cranial nerve. Repeated observations from neurosurgeons indicate abnormal vascular cross-compression of the root entry zone of the trigeminal nerve.[2]

There is now compelling evidence that TN is caused by demyelination of trigeminal sensory fibres within either the nerve root or, less commonly, the brainstem. Most often, nerve root demyelination involves the proximal, central nervous system (CNS) part of the root, and results from compression by an overlying artery or vein. Other causes of TN in which

**213**

demyelination occur include multiple sclerosis and, probably, compressive space-occupying lesions in the posterior fossa. Examination of trigeminal nerve roots from patients with compression of the nerve root by an overlying blood vessel has revealed focal demyelination in the region of compression, with close apposition of demyelinated axons and an absence of intervening glia. Similar foci of nerve root demyelination and juxtaposition of axons have been demonstrated in multiple sclerosis patients with TN. Experimental studies indicate that this anatomical arrangement favours ectopic generation of spontaneous nerve impulses and their ephaptic conduction to adjacent fibres. Spontaneous nerve activity is likely to be increased by the deformity associated with pulsatile vascular indentation.[3]

## Clinical features

- Trigeminal neuralgia (tic douloureux) remains a clinical diagnosis.
- It presents as episodic, recurrent unilateral face pain. It is described as a sudden, high-intensity jab, or like an electric shock.
- It typically lasts only a few seconds, with repetitive bursts over a period of seconds to a few minutes, followed by a refractory period of a few minutes. Episodes may occur occasionally or many times per day. Episodes may occur frequently over several weeks to several months followed by prolonged pain-free intervals.
- It may occur in ophthalmic, maxillary or mandibular divisions, but most frequently occurs in the mandibular division in the region of lower lip and jaw. Involvement of the ophthalmic division is rare.
- Pain is frequently triggered by trivial stimulation of the face around the nose and mouth, such as touching the face, washing, shaving, chewing and talking. Avoidance of facial stimulation by the patient is helpful in differential diagnosis. Pain relief can sometimes occur by firm pressure by the hands around, but not touching the trigger point.
- Incidence per year has been reported as 2.7 in 100 000 men and 5 in 100 000 women. It occurs mostly after the 5th decade, but can occur in younger patients in association with multiple sclerosis and tumours.[4]
- Clinical examination of the face is nearly always normal. While sensory impairment has been documented using quantitative sensory testing,[5] this does not seem to be appreciated as sensory deficit by the patient.
- Routine imaging is generally not indicated,[6] although some centres that routinely do microvascular decompression will do so. Suspicion of underlying pathology, such as an abnormal neurological examination (diminished touch sensation or corneal reflex), and, in patients who do not respond to non-operative treatments, magnetic resonance imaging (MRI) of the cerebellopontine angle is recommended. The pathology to be excluded include meningioma and acoustic neuroma. Further imaging of optic nerves may be appropriate in younger patients if multiple sclerosis is suspected.

## Differential diagnosis (see Chapter 10)

- Tumours or multiple sclerosis (2–4% of patients with TN) will produce episodic lancinating pain of TN, but there may be a persistent pain in addition.[7] There may be facial sensory or other cranial nerve deficits. In younger patients (under 40 years old), especially with bilateral symptoms, multiple sclerosis should be considered.
- Lesions of upper cervical spinal cord can cause face pain but will usually have manifestations of spinal cord involvement.

- Glossopharyngeal neuralgia is similar to TN except that pain is located in the pharynx, tonsil and ear and is usually triggered by swallowing, yawning or eating.
- Atypical face pain describes face pain syndromes that cannot otherwise be classified. The pain is usually a constant, diffuse, aching pain lasting hours to days, without paroxysms or trigger zones, and most commonly seen in women aged 30–50 years.
- Postherpetic neuralgia does occur on the face, typically following painful rash and blistering of acute herpes zoster. The pain is intense, described as aching or burning, often with dysaesthesia and allodynia.

# Medical Treatment

Many patients will respond to medical therapy alone, although effectiveness may be limited by side-effects, in particular, sedation and ataxia in elderly patients. Titration of doses requires careful attention and combinations of drugs may be helpful.[8]

- Anticonvulsants are widely used to treat TN. No trials have compared different anticonvulsants.
- Carbamazepine, an anticonvulsant, remains the drug of first choice for TN. A number of placebo-controlled studies had a combined 'number needed to treat' (NNT) –95% confidence interval (CI) – for 50% pain relief of 2.5 (CI 2.0–3.4) for TN.[9] Clinical wisdom states that a good response to carbamazepine supports the diagnosis of TN. Starting dose should be 100 mg orally twice daily, increasing by 100–200 mg every 3–4 days until pain relief is achieved or side-effects develop. Maximum tolerated dose is in the range of 1000–2000 mg per day, in three or four divided doses, although it may be considerably less in elderly patients. A slow-release formulation is available. After symptoms have been controlled for several weeks, it is prudent to attempt reduction of the dose to minimum necessary. Carbamazepine can produce bone marrow suppression, liver and renal impairment, so these should be monitored in initial months of treatment. Main side-effects are sedation, dizziness, ataxia, nausea and vomiting, which may require reduction in dose or even discontinuation of the drug.
- Lamotrigine, an anticonvulsant, at doses of 50–400 mg per day has demonstrated efficacy in relieving pain in patients with TN refractory to other treatments, with an NNT of 2.1 (range 1.3–6.1).[10] Adverse effects are common, including dizziness, ataxia, constipation, nausea, somnolence and diplopia.
- Other anticonvulsants, gabapentin (up to 1800 mg per day) and phenytoin (300–600 mg per day) and clonazepam 1–3 mg per day, have been used in treatment of TN, but there are no clinical trials that have assessed their effectiveness directly, except as part of larger neuropathic pain studies, or as reports of small series of patients.
- New anticonvulsant drug oxcarbazepine, available in US, has been used to treat TN, with initially promising results.
- Baclofen, a GABA-B agonist, used to treat spasticity has also been used to treat TN, at doses of 40–80 mg per day. One small trial indicated effectiveness using a double blind cross-over design.[11]
- Tricyclic antidepressants are widely used to treat chronic neuropathic pain but have not been evaluated for TN, nor do they seem to be commonly used. The reasons for this are not clear.
- Opioids do not currently have a place in treatment of TN. Recent trials have indicated that opioids can be effective in treating neuropathic pain, but no studies have been done on patients with TN.

# Invasive Treatments

Unlike drug treatments, surgical interventions lack a rigorous evidence base, but this should not detract from the value in treatment of TN. The reasons for relative paucity of quality evidence are various – controlled studies are more difficult with surgical procedures, as placebos and blinding are difficult. Many pharmacological trials are driven by the requirements of registration bodies, which until recently have not constrained interventions. Nonetheless, large numbers of observational studies have been published. No formal comparisons have been done between techniques, and no single technique is recognized as being superior. At present, it seems that a wide variety of techniques have been tried and seem to be effective, but choice of technique varies from centre to centre.

- Radiofrequency (RF) trigeminal ganglion thermocoagulation (see Appendix) is a widely used technique for treatment of TN, when medical treatment has been ineffective or poorly tolerated. Under general anaesthesia or sedation, an insulated needle with a 5 mm exposed tip is introduced percutaneously and passed through the foramen ovale, which is usually clearly visible under fluoroscopy, to lie within the Gasserian ganglion. Using electrical stimulation it is possible to place the needle tip within the ganglion of the appropriate trigeminal division. The patient will need to be sufficiently cooperative during the stimulation phase. Radiofrequency current is then applied to heat the adjacent tissue to 75–80°C for 1–2 minutes. No controlled clinical trials have been reported but a number of large series of cases with many years experience have reported high success rates (more than 75%), with variable recurrence rates (up to 50%, depending on duration of follow-up). The procedure can be readily repeated when pain recurs, months or years later. It is also useful when TN is due to underlying pathology (e.g. multiple sclerosis). Mortality is negligible. Adverse events which occur in less than 10% of patients are dysaesthesia, corneal numbness and masseter weakness.[12]
- Glycerol rhizotomy – injection of 0.1–0.2 ml of glycerol into Meckel's cave, through a percutaneous needle placed as above. Placement can be confirmed by electrical stimulation or use of small volumes of contrast, with the patient in the sitting position. High success rates and low morbidity has been reported, although series tended to have relatively small numbers of patients.[13] This procedure has a relatively high recurrence rate. While routinely used in some centres, it is less widely used than RF thermocoagulation.
- Microvascular decompression of the trigeminal nerve involves a craniotomy via the posterior fossa. This presumes the demonstration of vascular compression by MRI. This technique has proved popular in neurosurgical centres, but no formal comparison has been done with other techniques. High long-term success rates (above 70%) have been reported. It is generally recommended for younger patients, as it is felt to be more long lasting, although recurrences have been reported in up to 30%.[14] Morbidity, including facial dysaesthesia, cerebellar injuries and hearing loss, and mortality are low.
- Peripheral neurectomy, usually using cryotherapy, is done directly to accessible branches of the trigeminal nerve, in particular the supraorbital, infraorbital and inferior alveolar nerves. There is a paucity of literature on the technique although it is commonly practiced within maxillofacial units. Published series, which are small in number, indicate relatively short-term relief. The procedure can be repeated, although scarring may reduce effectiveness in the longer term.
- Gamma knife – single high dose radiotherapy delivered with exquisite precision to a radiographically defined target, at the junction of trigeminal nerve and brain stem. This is a relatively new technique. Several series of relatively small numbers of patients report high rates of pain relief, with low rates of morbidity, mostly facial numbness.[14] This technique will be confined to a few centres with this technology.

- Balloon compression of the trigeminal ganglion is done by introduction of a balloon via the percutaneous route. The balloon is then inflated with small volumes 0.5–1 ml of contrast until it occupies Meckel's cave. Compression times vary from 1 to 6 minutes. Success rates and complication rates are not dissimilar to other techniques. This technique is not widely practiced.
- Stimulation of motor cortex – the mechanism of this is poorly understood. Only limited reports in patients with TN, but initial results are promising. Confined to a few neurosurgical centres.[16]

# References

1. Merskey H, Bogduk N. Classification of chronic pain. Descriptions of chronic pain syndromes and definitions of pain terms. Seattle: IASP Press, 1994: 59–71
2. Janetta PJ. Treatment of trigeminal neuralgia by suboccipital and transcranial operations. *Clin Neurosurg* **24**: 538–549, 1977
3. Love S, Coakham HB. Trigeminal neuralgia: pathology and pathogenesis. *Brain* **124**: 2347–2360, 2001
4. Bullitt E, Tew JM, Boyd J. Intracranial tumours in patients with facial pain. *J Neurosurg* **64**: 865–871, 1986
5. Bowsher D, Miles JB, Haggett CE, Eldridge PR. Trigeminal neuralgia: a quantitative sensory perception threshold study in patients who have not undergone previous invasive procedures. *J Neurosurg* **86**: 190–192, 1997
6. Darlow L, Brooks M, Quinn P. Magnetic resonance imaging in the diagnosis of trigeminal neuralgia. *J Oral Maxillofac Surg* **50**: 621–626, 1992
7. Cusick J. Atypical trigeminal neuralgia. *JAMA* **245**: 2328–2329, 1981
8. Zakrzewska J, Patsalos P. Drugs used in the management of trigeminal neuralgia. *Oral Surg Oral Med Oral Pathol* **74**: 439–450, 1992
9. Wiffen P, Collins S, McQuay H, Carroll D, Jadad A, Moore A. Anticonvulsant drugs for acute and chronic pain. *Cochrane Database of Systemic Reviews.* Issue 1, 2002.
10. Zakrzewska J, Chaudry Z, Nurmikko T, Patton D, Mullens E. Lamotrigine in refractory trigeminal neuralgia: results from a double-blind placebo controlled crossover trial. *Pain* **783**: 223–230, 1997
11. Fromm G. Baclofen as an adjuvant analgesic. *J Pain Symptom Manage* **9**: 500–509, 1994
12. Taha J, Tew J. Comparison of surgical treatments for trigeminal neuralgia: re-evaluation of radiofrequency rhizotomy. *Neurosurgery* **38**: 865–871, 1996
13. Slettebo H, Hirschberg H, Lindegaard K. Long-term results after percutaneous retrogasserian glycerol rhizotomy in patients with trigeminal neuralgia. *Acta Neurochirurgica* **122**: 230–235, 1993
14. McLaughlin M, Janetta P, Clyde B, Subach B, Comey C, Resnick D. Microvascular decompression of cranial nerves: lessons learned from 4400 operations. *J Neurosurg* **90**: 1–8, 1999
15. Brisman R. Gamma knife radiosurgery for primary management of trigeminal neuralgia. *J Neurosurg* **93**: 159–161, 2000
16. Linderoth B, Meyerson B. CNS stimulation for neuropathic pain. In: Hansson P, Fields H, Hill R, Marchettini P, eds. *Neuropathic Pain: Pathophysiology and Treatment. Progress in Pain Research and Management, Vol 21.* Seattle: IASP Press, 2001, pp. 223–249

# 24 Phantom Limb Pain

## Catherine F Stannard

There are a number of sensory sequelae of limb amputation. These include (painless) phantom limb, pain in the stump and phantom limb pain. Phantom sensations also occur after removal of other somatic structures (e.g. breast, teeth and visceral structures, such as the rectum or bladder) and after deafferentation injury, such as spinal cord or brachial plexus injury.

These phenomena were first described by the French military surgeon Ambroise Pare in the 16th century, and indeed it was the observation that pain could occur in a phantom limb that led to a challenge of the dualistic theory of pain processing proposed by Descartes (who was readily able to explain the phenomenon by explaining the theory of the 'false signal'), and providing an explanation for this phenomenon remains as much of a challenge for neuroscientists today. Weir Mitchell first coined the term phantom limb pain in 1871.

## Incidence

The incidence of painful phantom phenomena has been variously reported, ranging from 2–80%. Much of the data on incidence has been based on those requesting treatment for symptoms and, as these are considerably underreported, many of the earlier estimates of incidence are likely to be conservative. Probably about three quarters of amputees will experience painful phantom sensations, and about 10% of amputees will have severe pain. The incidence of these painful sensations diminishes with time, but the natural history of the condition is not clearly characterized. Non-painful phantom sensations are almost universal following amputation, with the patient describing the phantom as being similar in shape, size and (last remembered) position to the limb before amputation. These sensations usually change with time and, in particular, patients will describe 'telescoping' of the distal extremity (hand/foot) into the amputation stump, although in patients who have a painful phantom this occurs less often. Pain in the amputation stump also occurs commonly in the postoperative period, but it may persist in up to 10% of patients. The literature supports a strong correlation between stump and phantom limb pain both in adults and children.[1,2] There is no clear relationship between phantom limb pain and reason for amputation.[3]

## Clinical features

Phantom limb pain is a neuropathic pain, and patients will describe their pain in a manner consistent with this classification, typically shooting, crushing, burning and cramping. Symptoms are most frequently reported in the phantom foot or hand, and the extremity is often described as being in a clenched position. Symptoms may be continuous or intermittent (most usually the latter). The symptoms usually appear early in the post-amputation period. Severity of pain tends to vary, and typical precipitators are coexistent disease, use of prosthesis and environmental precipitators, such as change in weather. Stress is a common precipitator of symptoms, and this has experimental support in a descriptive study of stressful tasks compared with relaxing ones, in which the former increased stump reactivity and temperature.[4] There is evidence that patient's coping strategies also influence intensity of the phantom pain experience.[5]

Central nervous system reorganization following amputation may result in the patient describing unpleasant phantom sensations when touching distant body parts. Phantom sensations in upper limb amputees can be generated by light touch stimulus on the ipsilateral mandibular region. Such sensations can also be generated by stimulus of the ipsilateral chest wall and leg in both upper and lower limb amputees.

There is a considerable literature on the relationship between pain intensity and duration before amputation and phantom limb pain, and it is this putative relationship that has driven much of the research on prevention of the condition (see below). Most of the data relating pre- and post-amputation is in the form of (large) retrospective studies,[6,7] although more recent studies suggest that persisting painful phantom sensations may not be related to pre-amputation experience.[8] One interesting prospective study commented that patient's *recall* of their pre-amputation symptoms was at odds with the actual symptom severity recorded pre-operatively.[9] Patients who sustain traumatic amputations do not have an antecedent history of pain in the limb, although pain intensity at the time of the amputation is very high. It is noteworthy that painful phantom sensations can occur in children with congenital amputations.

# Mechanisms

There is still debate in the scientific literature about the pathophysiology of phantom limb pain. Both peripheral and central neural mechanisms are involved.

### Peripheral events contributing to painful phantom phenomena

A number of clinical observations suggest that peripheral events contribute to the phantom experience. The strong correlation between stump and phantom limb pain has been mentioned. Pressure on the stump can elicit or modify the phantom sensation, and infiltration of a stump neuroma may alleviate or abolish phantom limb pain in some cases. These findings may be explained by what we know of peripheral sequelae of nerve injury.

Amputation of a limb results in severing of the peripheral nerve axon with inevitable neuroma formation. The electrophysiological properties of such neuromata were described in the 1970s.[10] In particular, such neuromata generate abnormal spontaneous and evoked impulse activity. This is related to changes in the quantity and disposition of ion channel (particularly sodium channel) protein. Hyperexcitability is also seen in dorsal root ganglion cells (again related to changes in sodium channel expression) following axotomy.[11]

### Events in spinal cord and brain following amputation

The central terminations of injured primary afferents also demonstrate increased excitability with prolonged enhancement of responses to noxious stimuli and changes in the receptive fields of dorsal horn neurons. These changes are mediated by excitatory amino acids via the N-methyl-D-aspartate (NMDA) subclass of receptor and by neurokinins. Structural reorganization also occurs in the dorsal horn with degeneration of C fibre afferent terminals in lamina II of the substantia gelatinosa and sprouting of Aβ mechanoreceptor afferents (which normally terminate in laminae III and IV) into lamina II,[12] which may be the mechanism by which mechanical allodynia is generated.

There is now evidence in humans for considerable reorganization of primary somatosensory and motor cortices and in subcortical structures following amputation.[13] Cortical reorganization may be seen very soon after amputation.[14] The degree of cortical reorganization is strongly correlated with perceived pain intensity,[15] and it can be shown to reduce following effective treatment of pain.[16] Thalamic reorganization has also been demonstrated in humans.[17] Evidence for this can be readily demonstrated in the clinic, where detailed sensory examination will often reveal a somatotopic representation of the phantom limb (particularly the extremity) on the chest wall, in the stump or on the face.

## Treatment

About one third of the published literature on phantom limb pain concerns treatment of the condition. Most of this is in the form of descriptive studies, small case series and anecdotal reports. At the time of writing there are three randomized controlled trials in the literature: two relating to the use of transcutaneous electrical nerve stimulation (TENS) and one recommending the use of intravenous calcitonin. An evidence-based approach is, therefore, difficult. A pragmatic approach to management is, therefore, recommended with the use of simple, safe, reversible treatments first but with rapid progression through non-interventional options with frequent assessment of efficacy. The rational use of pharmacotherapy may be largely guided by the literature on other neuropathic pain states, with all drug doses being escalated to efficacy or maximum tolerated dose.

Table 24.1 shows a summary of treatments for phantom limb pain.

### TENS and acupuncture

Several case series and reports describe the efficacy of TENS, and its use is also supported by a double-blind controlled trial.[18] There is no consensus regarding optimum electrode placement in the amputee, but stimulation of the contralateral limb is usually used. Where the patient has a clear somatotopic representation of the amputated limb, for example, on the chest wall or flank, the author has had success placing the electrodes over this 'map' in a position corresponding to the most painful part of the phantom. In this way paraesthesiae can be elicited in the phantom limb.

Acupuncture is also a safe, simple, low morbidity intervention that has been successfully used in the treatment of phantom limb pain,[19] although there is little in the literature to support proof of efficacy.

### Mirror-box

Interesting observations have been made with the use of a device containing a vertically placed mirror so that the mirror reflection of the patient's intact limb is 'superimposed' on the perceived position of the phantom.[20] Patients can be given the sensation of movement in the phantom by movement of the intact limb. In four out of five patients with painful clenching of the phantom hand, short-term relief of symptoms was achieved when the mirror box allowed them to 'unclench' the phantom. Such descriptions provide a fascinating insight into the complex interaction between vision, touch and phantom sensations, although it is not clear what role such a simple device may play in the long-term management of phantom limb pain. Indeed the use of such a device has been reported as dramatically increasing phantom limb pain in one patient (personal communication).

### Pharmacotherapy

A number of drugs have been described as useful in the management of phantom limb pain, but the evidence for efficacy is poor as most are isolated case reports or, at best, case series.

**Table 24.1** Treatments for phantom limb pain

| Stump care/ prosthetics | Simple non-invasive therapies | Pharmacotherapy for phantom limb pain | Pharmacotherapy for neuropathic pain | Destructive lesions of CNS | Central stimulation techniques |
|---|---|---|---|---|---|
| Revisionary surgery | TENS | Ketamine | Tricyclic antidepressants | DREZ | Spinal cord stimulation |
| Use of prosthesis | Acupuncture | Gabapentin | SSRIs | Cordotomy | Motor cortex stimulation |
| | Hypnosis | Beta blockers | Anticonvulsants | | Deep brain stimulation |
| | Mirror-box | Fentanyl (it) | Ion channel blockers | | |
| | | Clobazam | GABA agonists | | |
| | | LSD | Ketamine | | |
| | | Chlorpromazine | Opioids | | |
| | | Capsaicin | Capsaicin | | |
| | | Narcotic/antidepressant combination | | | |
| | | Lamotrigine | | | |
| | | Fluoxetine | | | |
| | | Clonazepam | | | |
| | | Amitriptyline | | | |
| | | Calcitonin | | | |
| | | Tizanidine | | | |

CNS, central nervous system; DREZ, dorsal root entry zone ; GABA, $\gamma$-aminobutyric acid; LSD, lysergic acid diethylamide; SSRIs, selective serotonin (5-hydroxytryptamine) selective inhibitors; TENS, transcutaneous electrical nerve stimulation

Current practice does not reflect the evidence available. A small double-blind study of intravenous ketamine versus placebo showed that ketamine reduced the early incidence of stump and phantom limb pain.[21] The more prolonged use of this drug by the subcutaneous route has been described in a case series, but psychomimetic effects may limit its use.[22] More importantly, there are no large studies to suggest its efficacy in the long term. A small double-blind trial in which randomization was not described showed tizanidine in a dose of 12 mg per day to be superior to placebo.[23] The use of calcitonin is supported by a well-conducted (small) trial,[24] but this therapy is not commonly used. There are numerous other case reports describing success with a number of chemically diverse agents. There is more evidence to guide the prescriber in the general neuropathic pain literature, and systematic reviews are now available. It would seem sensible to start therapy with a tricyclic antidepressant, moving on to additional anticonvulsant therapy where necessary. It should be noted that strong opioid analgesia may be as effective as other classes of drug in managing this difficult and distressing condition. Treatments for neuropathic pain are described in Chapter 6.

## Central stimulation techniques

Stimulation of the central nervous system may be indicated for the management of phantom limb pain. As these techniques are invasive and expensive, it would seem sensible to use them when other simpler interventions have failed. Published case series of the use of spinal cord stimulation (over prolonged periods) for patients with a variety of conditions, some of whom had phantom limb pain, conclude that patients with phantom limb pain probably do less well than those with other neuropathic pain syndromes.[25] Because of the uncertainty about outcome, a period of trial stimulation is strongly recommended before insertion of an implantable pulse generator.

Stimulation of the motor cortex was first described for the treatment of central post stroke pain,[26] but it has more recently been described for the treatment of other neuropathic pain conditions including phantom limb pain. The literature includes a series of eight patients, two of whom had phantom limb pain,[27] and a well conducted, procedurally detailed trial from a multidisciplinary team, again including two patients with phantom limb pain in whom the technique was useful.[28] Stimulation of the motor cortex is usually an extradural procedure, and stimulation of the cortex responding to the upper limb is more technically feasible than stimulation of the leg.

The literature on deep brain stimulation for this indication is even more sparse, small numbers of patients with phantom limb pain being included in much larger series.[29] Deep brain stimulation is more invasive, carries a higher morbidity and is less available than other central stimulation techniques and should not routinely be recommended.

## Destructive lesions of the central nervous system

Dorsal root entry zone (DREZ) lesioning has been described in the treatment of phantom limb pain.[30] There is little in the literature to support the use of cervical anterolateral cordotomy. These procedures are invasive and irreversible, and the propensity for development of later additional neuropathic sequelae leave the place of such procedures in doubt.

## Stump care and prosthetics

Immediate fitting of stump prostheses appears to be helpful in the management of phantom limb pain. Generally, revisionary surgery to the amputation stump is not helpful for stump pain or phantom limb pain in the absence of demonstrable stump pathology. However, if local infection, presence of bone spurs or neuroma entrapment in the scar is present local stump surgery may be helpful.

# Prevention

The notion that phantom limb pain might be prevented was given impetus by the publication in 1988 of a small trial in which patients given preoperative epidural analgesia were reported as having a lower incidence of phantom limb pain than patients without this preoperative therapy.[31] These observations have been confirmed in other similar studies,[32] although studies were often small and lacked details of blinding and randomization. Other techniques, such as intraneural infusion of local anaesthetic pre- and postoperatively, might also reduce the incidence of phantom limb pain although results from this technique are contradictory.[33,34] More recently, a large, methodologically rigorous trial investigating the effects of preoperative epidural analgesia concluded that it is not possible to reduce phantom limb pain with such techniques.[35] The role of preventive techniques thus needs clarification.

Despite the disappointing results of recent studies of preemptive techniques, a number of simple measures are likely to help. Patients should be warned of the likelihood of postoperative phantom sensations and the possibility of phantom limb pain, and they should be assessed early in the postoperative period in this regard. Optimal management of postoperative pain is strongly recommended, and patients should be given appropriate information from a credible source at all stages of their care.

# Conclusion

Phantom limb pain is a distressing, disabling condition with profound implications for the well being of patients and carers. In many cases, the condition remains refractory to treatment and, despite the huge number of therapies described in the scientific literature, few if any are highly successful. Rapid advances in neuroscience have shed some light on this puzzling condition, but it remains a considerable challenge for both clinicians and scientists.

# References

1. Kooijman CM, Dijkstra PU, Geertzen JH, et al. Phantom pain and phantom sensations in upper limb amputees: an epidemiological study. *Pain* **87**: 33–41, 2000
2. Jensen TS, Krebs B, Nielsen J, Rasmussen P. Immediate and long term phantom limb pain in amputees: incidence, clinical characteristics and relationship to preamputation pain. *Pain* **21**: 267–278, 1985
3. Nikolajsen L, Jensen TS. Phantom limb Pain. *Br J Anaesth* **87**: 107–116, 2001
4. Angrilli A, Koster U. Psychophysiological stress responses in amputees with and without phantom limb pain. *Physiol Behaviour* **68**: 699–706, 2000
5. Hill A. The use of pain coping strategies by patients with phantom limb pain. *Pain* **55**: 347–353, 1993
6. Katz J, Melzack R. Pain 'memories' in phantom limbs; review and clinical observations. *Pain* **43**: 319–336, 1990
7. Sherman RA, Sherman CJ. Prevalence and characteristics of chronic phantom limb pain among American veterans. Results of a trial survey. *Am J Phys Med* **62**: 227–238, 1983
8. Kooijman CM, Dijkstra PU, Geertzen JHB, Elzinga A, Schans CP. Phantom pain and phantom sensations in upper limb amputees: an epidemiological study. *Pain* **87**: 33–34, 2000
9. Nikolajsen L, Ilkjaer S, Kroner Kchristensen JH, Jensen TS. The influence of preamputation pain on postamputation stump and phantom pain. *Pain* **72**: 393–405, 1997
10. Wall PD, Gutnick M. Ongoing activity in peripheral nerves: the physiology and pharmacology of impulses originating from a neuroma. *Exp Neurol* **43**: 580–593, 1974
11. Devor M, Seltzer Z. Pathophysiology of damaged nerves in relation to chronic pain. In: Wall PD, Melzack R, eds. *Textbook of Pain 4th edition*. London: Churchill Livingstone, 1999, pp. 129–164
12. Woolf CJ, Shortland P, Coggeshall RE. Peripheral nerve injury triggers central sprouting of myelinated afferents. *Nature* **355**: 75–78, 1992

13. Flor H, Elbert T, Muhlnickel W, Pantev C, Weinbruch C, Taub E. Cortical reorganisation and phantom phenomena in congenital and traumatic upper extremity amputees. *Exp Brain Res* **119**: 205–212, 1998
14. Grusser SM, Winter C, Schaefer M, et al. Perceptual phenomena after unilateral arm amputation: a pre and post-surgical comparison. *Neurosci letts* **302**: 13–16, 2001
15. Grusser SM, Winter C, Muhlnickel W, et al. The relationship of perceptual phenomena and cortical reorganisation in upper extremity amputees. *Neuroscience* **102**: 263–272, 2001
16. Huse E, Larbig W, Flor H, Birbaumer N. The effect of opioids on phantom limb pain and cortical reorganisation. *Pain* **90:** 47–55, 2001
17. Davis KD, Kiss ZHT, Luo L, et al. Phantom sensations generated by thalamic microstimulation. *Nature* **391**: 385–387, 1998
18. Katz J, Melzack R. Auricular transcutaneous electrical nerve stimulation (TENS) reduces phantom limb pain. *J Pain Symptom Manage* **6**: 73–83, 1991
19. Xing G. Acupuncture treatment of phantom limb pain – a report of nine cases. *J Trad Chinese Med* **18**: 199–201, 1998
20. Ramachandran VS, Rogers-Ramachandran D. Synaesthesia in phantom limbs induced with mirrors. *Proc Roy Soc London* – Series B Biological Sciences **263**: 377–386, 1996
21. Nikolajsen L, Hansen CL, Nielsen J, Keller J, Arendt-Nielsen L, Jensen TS. The effect of ketamine on phantom pain: a central neuropathic disorder maintained by peripheral input. *Pain* **67**: 69–77, 1996
22. Stannard CF, Porter GE. Ketamine hydrochloride in the treatment of phantom limb pain. *Pain* **54**: 227–230, 1993
23. Vorobecichick IM, Kukushkin ML, Reshetniak VK, et al. The treatment of phantom pain syndrome with Tizanidine. *Zhurnal Neuropatologii i Psikhiatri Imeni* **97**: 36–39, 1997
24. Jaeger H, Maier C. Calcitonin in phantom limb pain: a double-blind study. *Pain* **48**: 21–27, 1992
25. Kumar K, Toth C, Nath RK, Laing P. Epidural spinal cord stimulation for treatment of chronic pain – some predictors of success. A 15 year experience. *Surg Neurol* **50**: 110–120, 1998
26. Tsubokawa T, Katayama Y, Yamamoto T, et al. Chronic motor cortex stimulation in patients with thalamic pain. *J Neurosurg* **78**: 393–401, 1993
27. Saitch Y, Shibata M, Hirano S, et al. Motor cortex stimulation for central and peripheral deafferentation pain. Report of eight cases. *J Neurosurg* **92**: 150–155, 2000
28. Carrol D, Joint C, Maartens N, et al. Motor cortex stimulation for chronic neuropathic pain: a preliminary study of 10 cases. *Pain* **84**: 431–437, 2000
29. Kumar K, Toth C, Nath RK. Deep brain stimulation for intractable pain: a 15 year experience. *Neurosurgery* **40**: 736–746, 1997
30. Saris SC, Iacono RP, Nashold BS. Successful treatment of phantom pain with dorsal root entry zone coagulation. *Appl Neurophysiol* **51**: 188–197, 1988
31. Bach S, Noreng MF, Tjellden NU. Phantom limb pain in amputees during the first 12 months following limb amputation, after preoperative lumbar epidural blockade. *Pain* **33**: 297–301, 1988
32. Katsuli-Liapis I, Georgakis P, Tierry C. Preemptive extradural analgesia reduces the incidence of phantom pain in lower limb amputees. *Br J Anaesth* **76**: 125, 1996
33. Fisher A, Meller Y. Continuous post-operative analgesia by nerve sheath block for amputation surgery – a pilot study. *Anesth Analg* **72**: 300–303, 1991
34. Pinzur MS, Garla PGN, Pluth T, Vrbos L. Continuous postoperative infusion of a regional anaesthetic after an amputation of the lower extremity. *J Bone Joint Surg* **78**: 1501–1505, 1996
35. Nikolajsen L, Ilkjaer S, Kroner Kchristensen JH, Jensen TS. Randomised trial of epidural bupivacaine and morphine in prevention of stump and phantom pain in lower limb amputation. *Lancet* **350**: 1353–1357, 1997

# 25 Cardiac Pain

## Nicholas L Padfield

## Angina pectoris

Angina pectoris is a condition characterized by pain retrosternally with variable radiation to the left arm, the back, the neck, and the jaw through to the ear. It can arise as a result of myocardial ischaemia caused by an imbalance between oxygen supply and demand. It must be differentiated from chest pain arising in a similar distribution from:

- Oesophageal pain caused by acid reflux through an incompetent cardiac sphincter, spasm or over distension of a stenotic portion of the oesophagus by food or tumour
- Chest disease – pleuritis, pericarditis, mesothelioma
- Pulmonary disease – embolism, infarction, tumour
- Aortic disease – aneurysm, dissection
- Chest wall disease – Tietze's syndrome (discomfort in the costochondral and costosternal joints on palpation), myofasciitis of the thoracic muscles.

## Clinical features

Eliciting the precise symptoms will help the diagnosis. True angina pectoris will be provoked by exertion, and it will only last a few seconds once the exertion ceases. It is also responsive to nitrates. Myocardial infarction will last from minutes to hours and is not responsive to nitrates.

Oesophageal spasm can be provoked by ingestion of irritants, such as highly spiced food, alcohol and acids. It may not occur immediately after ingestion but hours later, thus making its diagnosis difficult.

Pulmonary embolism will cause sudden-onset severe chest pain with signs varying from cyanosis and sympathetic overactivity to profound cyanosis, cardiac decompensation and death.

Conditions such as pleurisy, pericarditis and mesothelioma will be constantly painful, and chest wall conditions will be localized and exacerbated by local palpation.

Dissection of the aorta may be an acute event, in which case the onset of symptoms will be sudden and, depending on the site, there may be differential pulses and signs of lower limb or buttock ischaemia in severe cases. Leaking abdominal aortic aneurysms may produce low retrosternal pain but may be accompanied by other signs of acute blood loss, and there may be a pulsatile mass palpable in the abdomen.

### Pain in myocardial infarction

The pain in myocardial infarction may arise without exertion and may indeed come on whilst digesting a particularly heavy meal. Occasionally, it is preceded by a feeling of chest discomfort or slight dyspnoea or unpleasant gastric sensations, often described as stomach fullness or indigestion.

The initial phase is characterized by a deep central and visceral pain, described as a tight band across the chest, which lasts for a few minutes. It is most commonly anterior, and least commonly posterior or inferior. It is often accompanied by intense nausea and vomiting and diffuse sweating. Patients often have a sense of impending death or extreme alarm.

The following phase comes on anything from 10 minutes to a few hours later, where the pain reaches parietal structures and changes in nature to a deep referred pain. This may be the first perceived pain, and it is defined as a squeezing or pressing sensation that tends to radiate. The spatial localization is now more precise. Muscular tenderness can develop in the pectorals and deep interscapular muscles and, less commonly, in the deltoids after a delay of a few hours to days. There can also be areas of cutaneous hyperalgesia in areas of referred pain.

## Pain in angina pectoris

The pain in angina pectoris can have the same site, quality and radiation as infarction pain, but it is less severe, and rarely accompanied by the feeling of impending catastrophe. If muscular tenderness accompanies these attacks, it remains in between attacks.

Angina has been reclassified into the following syndromes:

- Stable angina
- Unstable angina
- Variant angina.

There is also syndrome X – intermittent coronary artery spasm with normal coronary arteries.

Stable angina is usually angina with effort. A classic feature is the disappearance of pain after the use of nitroglycerine or the inhalation of amyl nitrite.

Unstable angina has the following features:

- Crescendo angina – i.e. more severe or frequent episodes of angina superimposed on a pre-existing pattern of relatively stable exertional angina
- Angina at rest as well as following minimal exertion.

Variant angina[1] occurs exclusively at rest in the absence of exertion or emotional stress, and it is associated with S–T segment elevations on the electrocardiogram (ECG). However, angiography demonstrating spasm has been associated with both S–T elevation as well as S–T depression, thus blurring the boundaries between Prinzmetal's and unstable angina.

## Syndrome X

In patients with syndrome X, there is a pattern of chronic stable angina but with normal coronary arteries on angiography. In some patients during exercise testing some S–T segment depression would occur, but in others there is no detectable ischaemia. It is thought that this condition represents an exaggerated response of small coronary artery vessels to vasoconstrictor stimuli.

## Valvular heart disease

- Aortic valve stenosis – angina can be present in up to two-thirds of symptomatic patients. It is typically angina of effort and is due to disease around the coronary ostia or myocardial hypertrophy where increased oxygen demand exceeds supply.
- Aortic incompetence – often arises as a result of atherosclerotic disease around the coronary ostia, combined with low diastolic perfusion pressure.

- Mitral valve stenosis – 15% of patients have a similar pain to that of angina pectoris.
- Mitral valve prolapse – pain is rarely reported but the concomitant finding of chest wall myofascial trigger points often is.
- Cor pulmonale – in many cases of acute cor pulmonale patients experience a true visceral pain that has the same qualities and radiation as myocardial infarction. However, during exacerbations brought on by exertion the patient becomes more cyanosed (angor caeruleus), whereas in infarction they tend to become paler (angor pallidus). It can last several hours – i.e. longer than angina – and can be exacerbated by deep inspiration.
- Aortic dissection – This pain is often unbearable and the patients will writhe around in agony seeking relief. Although the pain is like that of angina, patients will describe it as 'tearing, ripping or stabbing'. It also tends to move from the initial site to lower down the body as the dissection progresses. It is most commonly felt in the anterior chest with proximal dissection, and between the shoulder blades if the dissection is distal.
  Intractable nausea and vomiting, diffuse sweating and hiccup frequently accompany this pain.

## Mechanisms of cardiac pain

Controversy continues over the nature and cause of pain in myocardial disease. Since cardiac pain can occur in the absence of ischaemia and, conversely, periods of myocardial ischaemia can be painless, the link between ischaemia and pain is neither strong nor unequivocal.

There is consequently a shift in thinking from the ischaemia-centred practice and management of angina as greater understanding of the central, as well as peripheral, mechanisms are understood. Pain clinicians have embraced this new approach more readily than cardiologists, who still adhere to the traditional pain–ischaemia model.

The heart, like other visceral organs, does not possess a discrete peripheral nociceptive pathway and, therefore, the pathogenesis of angina involves interacting cardiac intrinsic nerves, the autonomic nervous system and the central nervous system (CNS).

Several clinical characteristics of angina pectoris are reflected in the nature of the cardiac nervous system. The extent of silent ischaemia, the slow onset of angina during the ischaemic cascade, the diffuse character of the visceral component of the pain and the referred pain. Of the putative myocardial pain messengers, so far only adenosine fulfills Lewis criteria for a cardiac pain messenger. Dependent on the pattern of ischaemic release, adenosine appears to stabilize or sensitize afferent cardiac nerves with silent or painful ischaemia as a result. Through spatiotemporal summation sensitization may result in an alarm whereby the myocardium signals centrally its precarious state. The activity of adenosine-sensitized afferent nerves may become enhanced by additional stimuli, such as potassium, protons, substance P and bradykinin. Primary and secondary afferents from the intrinsic and extrinsic intrathoracic cardiac nervous systems project towards the CNS via sympathetic and vagal elements. The majority of primary afferents have their cell bodies in extrinsic cardiac ganglia and only a minority in the dorsal root ganglia. No cardiotopical representation exists in the intrathoracic ganglia. The majority of neurones in intrinsic and extrinsic cardiac ganglia are interneurones integrating cardiac inotropic and vasomotor functions on a beat-to-beat basis. Multisynaptic transmission over secondary afferents may not only delay the anginal pain message; as somatic afferents also connect to the intrathoracic ganglia, these multisynaptic transmissions may also be a basis for referred pain or pain inhibition. Dorsal root afferents appear to convey only excitatory impulses. Probably due to interneurones, cardiac nodose ganglia activities can become either excitatory or inhibitory. Cardiocardiac reflexes occur from the axonal level up to the brain stem cerebral levels.

The brain defense system including the basal ganglia, the limbic system and the prefrontal, but not the sensory, cortex are activated during myocardial ischaemia indicating its traumatic nature. The reflexogenic nature of angina pectoris is evident as similar CNS activation occurs in silent ischaemia as occurs in angina pectoris, but with less intense prefrontal activation; while in Syndrome X more intense activation occurs. Therapeutic interference of the reflex mechanism by sympathectomy, electrical stimulation or pharmacological interventions can counteract angina pectoris and relax the reflexogenic stress and vasomotor drive on the heart.[2]

Activation of the spinal thalamic tracts is unlikely to be the sole mechanism of pain. It is known that angina can often be associated with skeletal muscle referred pain, thus suggestting the association with non-cardiac muscle hyperalgesia. There is indirect evidence for the role of the sympathetic system since denervation of the sympathetic supply to the heart arising from the upper four thoracic dermatomes has repeatedly proven beneficial. The exact nature of the sympathetic involvement is less clear.

It is likely that the pain arises from the release of pain-producing substances and these, in turn, can cause a hyperalgesia and an ischaemic neuropathy of the cardiac nerves. The corollary for this is the development of an ischaemic neuropathy in peripheral atherosclerotic vascular disease affecting the legs.

# Treatment of cardiac pain

Successful management of cardiac pain must address not only the somatic sensory and medical issues but also the psychological cognitive issues. When deciding upon a treatment strategy, the psychological distress of angina must not be overlooked – indeed this can account for a great deal of the apparent disability. Patients who have survived a myocardial infarct will recall vividly the sense of impending death or catastrophe and will have been frightened by it. Severe angina will have a similar cognitive impact on the sufferer. In every case, the experience of angina is individual to the particular patient, and there is no relationship between the unpleasantness of their experience and the severity of their cardiac disease. Success in management, therefore, lies in a multifaceted approach.

Treatment, therefore, follows these sequential phases:

- Attention to lifestyle – cessation of smoking, appropriate exercise regimen, weight reduction, diet, correcting or optimizing other medical related issues like hypertension, hyperlipidaemias, diabetes mellitus
- Cardiac medical treatment per se, such as anti-arrhythmics, beta blockade, calcium channel blockers, amiodarone, digitalis, optimizing serum potassium
- Nitrites and analgesics
- Coronary artery angioplasty/stenting
- Corrective surgery – coronary artery revascularization, valvular repair or replacement, resection/repair/stenting of thoracic aortic aneurysm
- Neuromodulation – transcutaneous electrical neurostimulation (TENS), spinal cord stimulation when corrective surgery is either not feasible or too risky
- Gene therapy, laser transmural endomyocardial revascularization and heart transplant.

However, as success is predicated by following the biopsychosocial model, this needs to start at the first doctor–patient contact. Cognitive behavioural therapy, teaching pacing activities, stress reduction, relaxation techniques and developing individualized effective coping strategies will all play an important part in relieving the distress and suffering.

## Pain intervention in cardiac pain

This will encompass:

- TENS
- Treatment of myofascial associated pain

- Upper thoracic/lower cervical sympathetic blockade, chemical or radiofrequency – see appendix for details of technique
- Spinal cord stimulation—see appendix for details of technique.

The use of low-dose antidepressants along with appropriate stretching exercises may help with the referred muscular pain in the chest or interscapular regions. Discrete trigger areas may respond to local acupuncture or injection with local anaesthetic and steroid – often overlooked in angina patients! Occasional short courses of non-steroidal anti-inflammatory drugs (NSAIDs) may be helpful, not only for their effect on cyclooxygenase but on cannabinoid receptors. It must be remembered that even intractable angina is episodic and that slow release morphine preparations are NOT appropriate – indeed, they usually result in constipation, sweating, dry mouth and weight gain and can pose a considerable challenge for detoxification.

### Transcutaneous electrical neurostimulation

Transcutaneous electrical neurostimulation can be very helpful where there is a lot of associated muscular pain. However, it should be used with caution when there is a cardiac pacemaker in situ[3,4] and, ideally, in consultation with a cardiologist.

### Sympathetic blockade

Thoracic sympathetic blocks have been performed for many years after a prognostic local anaesthetic block, chemically with either 6% aqueous phenol or 90% alcohol. Because of the lack of control of the spread of the injected neurolytic agent, techniques employing radiofrequency thermocoagulation have been gaining popularity. None of these techniques are without risk of pneumothorax, reported as 4% incidence even in experienced hands,[5] or causing neuropathic pain in adjacent sensory nerves.

This can be particularly vexing to the patients on top of their angina.

### Spinal cord stimulation

Spinal cord stimulation (SCS) has been successfully employed for many years in the management of so-called intractable angina. It is quoted as having a greater than 80% success rate in angina patients and greater then 70% success rate in patients with vasospastic conditions. It appears to work by antidromic activation of large afferent fibres and, possibly, by the activation of supraspinal loops via the brain stem projecting to the thalamocortical system, although less than 10% of the pain pathways involved are relayed this way.

In micropipette studies in rats, using a chronic sciatic constriction injury neuropathic pain model, the induced increase in glutamate and reduction of γ-aminobutyric acid (GABA) appear to be restored to normal by spinal cord stimulation. Opioids do not appear to be involved. It is likely that SCS has a vasodilatory effect in ischaemia mediated by calcitonin gene related peptide and nitric oxide released peripherally within the microvasculature of the heart. It also modulates autonomic function as ganglion blockade reduces the effect of SCS, as does selective nicotinic and alpha-adrenergic blockade. It also appears to evoke differential release of catecholamines in heart tissue. Atrial pacing studies have conclusively shown that it does not mask the onset of cardiac ischaemia.[6] In general, pacemakers, especially bipolar and multiprogrammable ones, do not pose a problem to SCS unless very high SCS voltages are used.[7]

**Evidence base**  There are no meta-analyses of randomized controlled trials. The majority of the published literature consists of prospective trials, some of which are randomized but rarely blinded because of methodological problems. One study, over a 10-year period, of 19 consecutively implanted patients whose disease was classified as New York Heart Association functional groups III/IV showed that annual admission rates and mean time in hospital per patient per year was significantly reduced by SCS.[4] The place of SCS is discussed amongst newer techniques, such as transmyocardial laser revascularization and long-term intermittent urokinase therapy.[3]

**Cardiac and vascular effects**   In cardiac patients, a positron emission tomographic study demonstrated an apparent homogenization of myocardial blood flow during SCS. In the same study, patients' exercise tolerance, dypiridamole stress tests and nitrate consumption over a 6 week period of SCS all significantly improved.[8]

Another study using Doppler flow studies in patients with coronary ischaemia failed to demonstrate any significant changes in flow velocity as when the SCS was then turned on no further increase in average flow velocity was observed.[9,10]

**Central nervous system effects**   The anti-anginal effects of SCS may have a CNS component involving known cerebral antinociceptive pathways. In a study of nine patients, the effects of SCS were studied in the CNS with photon emission photography (PET). Relative changes in regional cerebral blood flow (rCBF) related to stimulation compared with non-stimulation were assessed and analysed using the method of statistical parametric mapping. Increased regional cerebral blood flow was observed in the left ventrolateral peri-aqueductal grey matter, the medial prefrontal cortex, Brodman area (BA) 9/10, the dorsomedial thalamus bilaterally, the left medial temporal gyrus (BA 21), the left pulvinar of the thalamus, bilaterally in the caudate nucleus, and the posterior cingulated cortex (BA 30). Relative decreases in rCBF were noticed bilaterally in the insular cortex (BA 20/21 and BA 38), the right inferior temporal gyrus (BA 19/37), the right inferior frontal gyrus (BA 45), the left inferior parietal lobulus (BA 40), the medial temporal gyrus (BA 39) and the right anterior cingulated cortex (BA 24). It was concluded that SCS used as an additional treatment for angina applied at T1 modulates regional blood flow in brain areas known to be associated with nociception and in areas associated with cardiovascular control.[10]

**Sympathetic effects**   It had been postulated that the anti-ischaemic effect of SCS was mediated through a reduction in sympathetic tone. In a study where patients were paced to an atrial rate that produced moderate angina, cardiac and body noradrenaline levels were measured. The patients were then rested for 50 minutes and then paced to the same level that produced moderate angina but this time the SCS was turned on. With the SCS, body noradrenaline levels were significantly reduced, though the cardiac noradrenaline levels were not at comparable pacing rates. They concluded that the results of this study indicate that the previously postulated anti-ischaemic effect of SCS is not due to reduced cardiac sympathetic activity. However, SCS decreases overall sympathetic activity, which may benefit the heart, possibly by reducing oxygen demand.[11]

## Miscellaneous

Other cardiological/surgical options, such as percutaneous transmyocardial laser revascularization or even a heart transplant, may be considered, but such procedures carry a considerable mortality and should be a last resort. These treatments are clearly outside the scope of the pain clinician, but they need to be evaluated and compared with established pain treatments that carry a much lower morbidity and mortality while conferring in the majority of cases equal benefits to the patient. It should no longer be acceptable to entertain treatments that carry 10% mortality just because the patients are seriously incapacitated with a very restricted quality of life, if safer and alternative treatments, proven to be effective, are available.

# References

1. Prinzmetal M, Kennamer R, Merliss R, et al. A variant form of angina pectoris. *Am J Med* **27:** 375–388, 1959
2. Sylven C. Neurophysiological aspects of angina pectoris. *Zeitschrift fur Kardiologie* **86:** 95–105, 1997
3. Schoebel FC, Frazier OH, Jessurun GA, et al. Refractory angina pectoris in end-stage coronary artery disease evolving therapeutic concepts. *Am Heart J* **143:** 587, 1997
4. Murray S, Carson KG, Ewings, PD, Collins PD, James MA. Spinal cord stimulation significantly decreases the need for acute hospital admission for chest pain in patients with refractory angina pectoris. *Heart* **82:** 89–92, 1999
5. Mannheimer C, Carlsson C-A, Ericsson K, et al. Transcutaneous electrical nerve stimulation in severe angina pectgoris. *Eur Heart J* **3:** 297–302, 1982
6. Raj P, Rauck RL, Racz G. Autonomic blocks In: Raj P, ed. *Pain Medicine* . St Louis: Mosby, 1996, pp. 227–258
7. Mannheimer C, Eliasson T, Andersson B. Effects of spinal cord stimulation in angina pectoris induced by pacing and possible mechanisms of action. *Br Med J* **307:** 477–480, 1993
8. Romano M, Zucco F, Baldini MR, Allaria B. Technical and clinical problems in patients with simultaneous implantation of a cardiac pacemaker and a spinal cord stimulator. *PACE* **16:** 1639–1644, 1993
9. Hautvast RW, Blanksma PK, DeJongste MJ, et al. Effect of spinal cord stimulation on myocardial blood flow assessed by positron emission tomography in patients with refractory angina pectoris. *Am J Cardiol* **77:** 462–467, 1996
10. Norsell H, Eliasson T, Albertsson P, et al. Effects of spinal cord stimulation on coronary blood flow velocity. *Coronary Artery Dis* **9:** 273–278, 1998
11. Hautvast RW, Ter Horst GJ, DeJong BM, et al. Relative changes in regional cerebral blood flow during spinal cord stimulation in patients with refractory angina pectoris. *Eur J Neurosci* **9:** 1178–1183, 1997
12. Norsell H, EliassonT, Mannheimer C, et al. Effects of pacing-induced myocardial stress and spinal cord stimulation on whole body and cardiac norepinephrine spillover. *Eur Heart J* **18:** 1890–1896, 1997

# Further Reading

Andersen C, Hole P, Oxhoj H. Does pain relief with spinal cord stimulation for angina conceal myocardial infarction. *Br Heart J* **71:** 419–442, 1994

Braunwald E, ed. *Heart disease*, 5th edn. Philadelphia: WB Saunders, (Chronic coronary artery disease. pp. 1289–1365; Diseases of the Aorta. pp. 1546–1581; Valvular heart disease. pp. 1007–1076), 1997

Chandler MJ, Brennan TJ, Garrison DW, Kim KS, Schwartz PJ, Foreman RDA. Mechanism of cardiac pain suppression by spinal cord stimulation: implication for patients with angina pectoris. *Eur Heart J* **14:** 96–105, 1993

Collins P, Fox KM. Pathophysiology of angina. *Lancet* **335:** 94–96, 1990

De Jongste MJL, Haaksma J, Hautvast RWM, et al. Effects of spinal cord stimulation on myocardial ischaemia during daily life in patients with severe coronary artery disease. A prospective ambulatory electrocardiographic study. *Br Heart J* **71:** 413–418, 1994

De Jongste MJL, Nagelkerke D, Hooyschuur CM, et al. Stimulation characteristics, complications and efficacy of spinal cord stimulation systems in patients with refractory angina; a prospective feasibility study. *PACE* **17:** 1751–1760, 1994

Eliasson T, Jern S, Augustinsson LE, Mannheimer C. Spinal cord stimulation in severe angina pectoris. *Coronary Artery Dis* **5:** 845–850, 1996

Eliasson T, Augustinsson LE, Mannheimer C. Spinal cord stimulation in severe angina pectoris-presentation of current studies, indications and clinical experience. *Pain* **41:** 255–265, 1996

Eliasson T, Albertsson P, Hardhammar P, et al. Spinal cord stimulation in angina pectoris with normal coronary arteriograms. *Coronary Artery Dis* **4:** 819–827, 1993

Kujacic V, Eliasson T, Mannheimer C, et al. Assessment of the influence of spinal cord stimulation on left ventricular function in patients with severe angina pectoris; an echocardiographic study. *Eur Heart J* **14:** 1238–1244, 1993

Mannheimer C, Carlsson CA, Eriksson K, et al. Transcutaneous electrical stimulation in severe angina pectoris. *Eur Heart J* **3**: 297–302, 1988

Mannheimer C, Eliasson T, Andersen B. Effects of spinal cord stimulation in angina pectoris induced by pacing and possible mechanisms of action. *Br Med J* **307**: 477, 1993

Mannheimer C, Eliasson T, Augustinsson LE, et al. Electrical stimulation versus coronary artery bypass surgery in severe angina pectoris. The ESBY study: *Circulation* **97**: 1157–1163, 1998

Mobilia G, Zuin G, Zanco P, et al. [Effects of spinal cord stimulation on regional blood flow in patients with refractory angina. A positron emission tomography study.] Effetti della stimolazione spinale epidurale sul flusso miocardiaco regionale in pazienti con angina pectoris refrattaria. Uno studio con tomografia ad emissione di positroni. *Giornale Italiano di Cardiologia* **28**: 1113–1139, 1998

Muray S, Carson KGS, Ewing's PD, James MA. Spinal cord stimulation significantly decreases the need for acute hospital admission for chest pain in patients with refractory angina pectoris. *Heart* **82**: 89–92, 1999

Sanderson JE, Ibrahim B, Waterhouse D, Palmer RBG. Spinal electrical stimulation for intractable angina-long-term clinical outcome and safety. *Eur Heart J* **15**: 810–814, 1994

# 26 Post-stroke Pain

## Robin S Howard and Anthony G Rudd

It is very common for pain to occur following a stroke causing significant disability. This is usually related to a variety of causes, including musculoskeletal pain (especially involving the shoulder), spasticity, headache, deep vein thrombosis, pressure sores, fractures and instrumentation.[1-4] A number of recent reviews have emphasized the clinical features, aetiology and mechanisms of post-stroke pain.[5-11] In this chapter we will review the mechanisms and treatment of central post-stroke pain (CPSP) and discuss other causes of post-stroke pain.

## Central post-stroke pain

Central post-stroke pain (CPSP) may be considered as a form of central pain, which follows a vascular event affecting the ascending pathways and/or their brainstem or cortical relays. It is usually associated with abnormal sensibility to temperature and to noxious stimulation.[12] The term 'thalamic pain' is often used to signify CPSP arising from any sort of vascular event regardless of its aetiology or site.

Dejerine and Roussy[13] described six patients who, following stroke, developed central pain, which was severe and paroxysmal. The pain was associated with hemianaesthesia, impaired deep sensation, and astereognosis as well as mild hemiplegia without contractures, choreoathetosis and hemiataxia on the paralysed side. In three patients, post-mortem studies showed that the lesions extended to include the posterior limb of the internal capsule, involving thalamocortical projections from the posterior thalamus.

### Anatomy of lesions causing CPSP

Antemortem localisation of lesions responsible for CPSP was previously difficult, and most lesions have been defined from autopsy studies. However, the development of newer imaging techniques, in particular magnetic resonance imaging (MRI), has enabled accurate localization of parenchymal involvement. Most imaging studies have shown CPSP is associated with lesions which include the ventroposterior thalamic region (Figure 26.1).[14,15] This region of the thalamus receives particularly rich spinothalamic projections.[16] Leijon et al.[15] showed 9 of 27 patients with CPSP had lesions in the thalamus, although these were usually not restricted to the thalamic nuclei. Other authors have suggested that between 25%[17] and 60%[18] of patients with CPSP have lesions in the thalamic region. In most studies, the lesions have occupied the ventroposterior portion of the thalamus but are rarely localized and generally extend laterally and superiorly.[7,14,15,17,19,20,21]

Lesions involving cortical and brainstem regions may also give rise to CPSP. Edinger first noted that the epileptic aura may be associated with pain, suggesting cortical involvement, and this has been suggested by others.[14,15,19,22-24] Lesions in other cortical regions can occasionally be associated with CPSP, these included the cortical and subcortical region of the

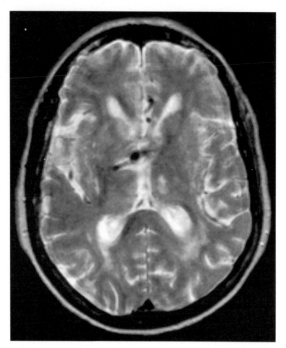

**Figure 26.1**   Left sided thalamic infarct in a patient with central post-stroke pain.

first somatosensory area (SI) and the insular region – secondary somatosensory area (SII),[22,24,25] however, localization to cortical regions remains imprecise, as there is likely to be considerable involvement of subcortical white matter, particularly in the insular region.[24,26] Central post-stroke pain may also be associated with medullary lesions and with pontine and midbrain stroke, particularly infarction in the territory of the posterior inferior cerebellar artery.[7,14,27]

## Aetiology of strokes causing CPSP

All forms of cerebrovascular disease have been reported to cause CPSP. However, the most common aetiology is infarction in the territory of the thalamostriate artery, which involves the ventroposterior part of the thalamus, and the posterior inferior cerebellar artery (PICA), which supplies the lower brainstem.[15,28,29] Central post-stroke pain may follow intracerebral haemorrhage (ICH)[26] and, occasionally, after subarachnoid haemorrhage (SAH) with intracerebral extension or infarction secondary to severe vasospasm.[30] Aneurysms[31] and arteriovenous malformation may also cause CPSP, secondary to mass effect or secondary haemorrhage.[32,33] However, the localization rather than the size of the lesion seems to be the most critical factor in predicting the development of CPSP.

## Incidence

The incidence of CPSP is extremely difficult to elucidate. There are many causes of pain following stroke and the onset of the pain may be delayed. In a prospective study of 191 patients, 8.4% developed central pain but 18% of those with somatosensory developed CPSP.[17] In a retrospective study, McGowan[34] described CPSP in 25% of patients with brainstem stroke.

## Pathophysiology

The lesions that cause central pain vary widely, but it is accepted that the thalamus plays an important role in the aetiology of CPSP. In particular, the ventroposterior region and the medial-intralaminar region are involved, as is the reticular nucleus. Large parts of the ventroposterior nucleus receive nociceptive inputs, as well as receiving inputs via the lemniscal pathways. However, most patients with CPSP have abnormal pain and temperature sensation but normal threshold to touch, vibration and joint position sense; therefore the lesion appears to involve the spinothalamic pathways including the indirect spinoreticulothalamic and spinomesencephalic projections, but it does not have to involve the dorsal column–medial lemniscal pathway. It has been suggested that the crucial lesion causing CPSP may involve the reticulothalamic projections, which leaves the more medially and inferiorly terminating projections anatomically intact.[11,18]

Because of the variety of lesions affecting somatosensory projections that may give rise to CPSP, it is difficult to establish a unifying explanation for the origin of the pain. Most theories have suggested that CPSP is either due to the excitation in damaged sensory pathways or the effects of impaired inhibitory pathways. It has been considered to be due to abnormal excitation from an 'irritable cortical focus'.[13] Certainly, epilepsy may be associated with pain and, following stroke, epileptic aura may be characterized by pain.[17,22] Also ictal changes have been recorded from midbrain and thalamus in patients with CPSP.[35–37] Lesions of the dorsal column–medial lemniscus may lead to a disinhibition of spinothalamic pathways leading to CPSP, but more recently it has been proposed that a lesion 'disconnecting' thalamocortical pathways may also be important, and deafferentation phenomena may explain the abnormal spontaneous and evoked burst activity in the thalamus following stroke.[22] However, it remains unresolved whether neurogenic pain is necessarily associated with excitation in spinothalamic pathways at the thalamic or cortical level, but post-stroke pain has been reported in patients whose entire thalamus on one side has been infracted.[38]

The role of sympathetic mechanisms remains uncertain, but they have long been thought to be important because of the presence of signs of abnormal sympathetic activity in association with CPSP including oedema, decreased sweating, and reduced skin temperature. Some of these patients respond to sympathetic blockade, but it is uncertain whether this is a primary or secondary phenomenon.[39]

## Clinical Features

Central post-stroke pain is highly variable in character, severity and distribution. In particular, the history may be vague and 'non-anatomical' leading to a diagnosis of psychogenic pain. It is necessary to exclude underlying causes of post-stroke pain related to immobility: these may include shoulder and skin pain. The onset of CPSP may be highly variable, with approximately 50% developing pain within a few days or during the first month while, in the remainder, the onset of pain may be delayed by up to 6 months, with the longest reported delay being 34 months,[15,17,34] and it may develop as sensory impairment is improving.[7] The nature of CPSP is highly variable, whilst the classical description of severe, intolerable, burning pain is common, a significant number of patients experience a stinging or aching pain of less severity even with thalamic lesions.[15] Others describe the pain as tearing, pricking or lancinating. Although the pain may not be excruciating, it is frequently irritating and constant. Hyperaesthetic sensation is commonly associated with CPSP. The abnormal sensory disturbances include spontaneous or evoked abnormal sensations, radiation of sensation from the stimulus site, prolonged response latency, after discharges and temporal summation. There may be increased sensation to a painful stimulus or allodynia if pain results from a stimulus that does not normally evoke pain. In CPSP, 85% of patients have spontaneous dysasthesiae, 41% evoked dysasthesiae and 41% paraesthesiae.[40,41]

**237**

The pain is often extensive and diffuse, frequently having a hemisensory distribution which affects the face in a minority of cases.[15] However, in some patients, the pain may be highly localized to the face, an arm or even a hand. Brainstem lesions often lead to CPSP involving the ipsilateral face (especially periorbital regions) and contralateral body.[7,14,15,19] This pattern is caused by injury to the ipsilateral spinal trigeminal nucleus and the crossed spinothalamic tract. Large lesions of the ventroposterior thalamus or the posterior limb of the internal capsule may cause bilateral pain.[23] Most spontaneous central pain is present constantly with no pain free intervals.[40] Central post-stroke pain is commonly permanent, but it may remit spontaneously and completely. A few cases have been described in which a new supratentorial stroke abolishes the pain.[42]

A variety of stimuli may influence the severity of the pain. It may be worsened by cutaneous stimuli, body or limb movements, cold or strong emotion. Allodynia (pain evoked by a stimulus that is not usually painful) is common in CPSP. Psychological factors including depression are common in patients with CPSP, but it not clear whether these worsen the pain or are simply secondary to the chronic pain.

On examination, virtually all patients with CPSP have somatosensory symptoms and signs. There is considerable variation in the range of somatosensory abnormalities associated with CPSP, ranging from subtle alterations in sensory threshold to hemianaesthesia in the painful region. The most common sensory abnormality is abnormal temperature and pain sensibility in the territory of the pain, even with normal threshold to touch and vibration sensation. However, 85% of patients will also have coexisting hyperaesthesiae and dysaesthesiae. This finding suggests that all patients with central pain have lesions affecting spinothalamic afferent pathways but only some have lesions that also affect the dorsal column–medial lemniscus pathways.[14,18,29,40] Patients may show clinical signs of autonomic involvement of the affected side, and the painful area may have changes in sweating and appear cool and vasoconstricted. The pattern of sensory involvement will depend on the site of the lesion. Following ventroposterior thalamic lesions, there is often a general loss of all modalities, whilst, after a low brainstem infarct causing lateral medullary syndrome (Figure 26.2), there is a crossed dissociated sensory loss. Brainstem strokes usually have more profound spinothalamic deficits compared with thalamic and subthalamic strokes.

Approximately half have motor abnormalities, including hemiataxia or involuntary movements.[15] Other neurological abnormalities, including agnosia, apraxia, visual and speech disturbances, may be present in a few patients depending on the site of the lesion.[27,40] Central post-stroke pain following thalamic stroke has been reported more often in association with right sided lesions.[43]

## Investigations

Abnormalities of somatosensory evoked potentials, which test the function of dorsal column–medial lemniscus pathways, correlate with abnormalities of touch and vibration.[20] However, laser-evoked cerebral potentials are usually abnormal when elicited from the affected side of patients with CPSP, confirming typical spinothalamic dysfunction and small fibre mediated involvement. Peripheral stimulation of spinothalamic afferents in CPSP shows abnormalities of long latency cortical-evoked potentials, which correlate with abnormalities in temperature and pain sensation but not to touch and vibration.[44-46]

## Management

Central post-stroke pain can be extremely difficult to treat and responds poorly to a variety of physical, pharmacological and interventional procedures. All treatments carry potential side-effects and, therefore, patients must be fully counselled and they should realize that treatments

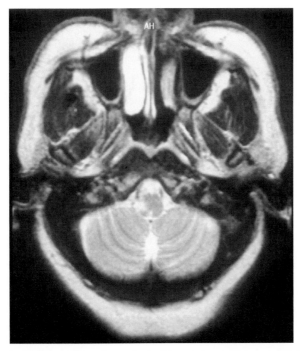

**Figure 26.2** Lateral medullary syndrome in a patient with central post-stroke pain. High signal is shown laterally in the right side of the medulla.

are often empirical and have not been subjected to rigorous, controlled clinical trials. Furthermore, they must recognize that treatment is often aimed at symptomatic relief rather than curing the pain.

The first line of management is the treatment of any nociceptive component such as infection, skin changes and abnormal posture as these enhance CPSP. A large variety of drugs have been used to treat CPSP, and some patients do gain benefit in an unpredictable fashion, but there is no consistent pattern of response in controlled trials. The relevant studies have been discussed in a number of recent reviews.[47,48]

## Medical

- Tricyclic antidepressants are the most valuable drugs available for the treatments of CPSP and 50–90% of patients derive benefit: the non-selective drugs seem to be most helpful. In a single controlled trial, 66% of patients responded to amitriptyline regardless of whether the CPSP had a thalamic or non-thalamic aetiology,[49,50] but other studies of tricyclics have failed to support these results. The benefits of amitriptyline are probably independent of any depression in most patients, but they are dose-dependent. A favourable response in CPSP has been shown using doxepin.[49] The mechanisms of action of antidepressants in CPSP is uncertain, but it is likely to relate both to their effects on reuptake of 5-hydroxytryptamine (5-HT, serotonin), including selective 5-HT blockers like desimipramine, maprotiline and mianserin, and possibly also the adrenergic system.
- Antiepileptic drugs are frequently used to treat CPSP.[51] Carbamazepine is the best studied – there is a small but significant effect in reducing central pain in a small group of patients with CPSP.[50] Other open studies and anecdotal reports have suggested an important role for gabapentin, phenytoin and valproate if carbamazepine is ineffective or

not tolerated. Other drugs which have been used to treat CPSP include vigabatrin, topiramate, clonazepam and barbiturates.

- Local anaesthetics and antiarrythmic drugs were used because of the putative hyperexcitability of the damaged CNS. There are occasional reports of systemic lignocaine and oral mexilitine being effective in treating CPSP.[52]
- Analgesics may be beneficial to a minority of patients and opioids are used in some with varying benefit. Clonidine (an α2-agonist) has been used in CPSP, as has the β2-agonist propranolol, which may enhance the actions of doxepin. One small study suggested a possible benefit of physostigmine and pyridostigmine. The beneficial role of intrathecal baclofen, enhancing inhibitory γ-aminobutyric acid (GABA) mediated processes, has been described.[53]

### Neurosurgical ablative procedures

Many different lesioning procedures have been undertaken but no reliable technique has been found.[8,54,55] The results are not favourable because of unacceptably high complication rates or return to postoperative pain levels after some time. Previously, open medullary and mesencephalic tractotomies and other procedures were undertaken, but these have been replaced by stereotactic techniques with lower morbidity and mortality, greater accuracy and less risk of postoperative dysasthaesiae.[27] Stereotactic mesencephalic tractotomy is well tolerated but less effective and usually combined with additional medial thalamotomy to produce consistent long term relief of CPSP.[27] When the central pain is confined to the face, trigeminal tract stimulation may obviate the need for stereotaxis.

### Stimulation

Whilst enthusiasm for ablative procedures has waned, there has been increasing use of stimulation procedures. Transcutaneous electrical nerve stimulation (TENS) is simple and easy to administer, however, it can only be effective if the dorsal column–medial lemniscal pathways are still functionally intact and the patient has not lost touch and vibration sensation to the painful region.[56]

- Deep brain stimulation involves a neurosurgical procedure but is well tolerated.[57] Areas that have been stimulated include ventrobasal thalamus (including ventroposterior lateral and medial nuclei) the periventricular and periaqueductal grey matter and adjacent nuclei.[58] Others have suggested capsular stimulation may be more effective.[23] However, these techniques have not been subjected to adequate trials, and there remains uncertainty about the site, frequency and level of stimulation.[59,60]
- Motor cortex stimulation depends on extradural stimulation of premotor cortex leading to stimulation of descending non-nociceptive sensory pathways present in the motor cortex. However, the mechanism may be more complex involving inhibitory processes in the ipsilateral thalamus and brainstem as well as the cingulated gyrus and orbitofrontal cortex.[61]
- Sympathetic blockade, either general or through regional intravenous sympathetic blockade, has been suggested as a treatment for CPSP, particularly if there is coexisting hyperpathia. Loh[39] described three patients with CPSP who experienced remarkable relief of their pain, and disappearance or improvement in their hyperpathia following sympathetic blockade, although the effect was short-lasting.

### Behavioural and psychological

The role of cognitive behavioural therapy and psychiatric support is considerable.[62]

# OTHER CAUSES OF POST-STROKE PAIN

A variety of systemic complications may lead to pain following stroke.

## Musculoskeletal pain

Musculoskeletal pain as a late complication of stroke has been reported in 31% of hospitalized stroke patients,[63] shoulder hand syndrome in 27–41%[64,65] and painful shoulder 4%.[3] In an observational study following 108 patients for 6 months post-stroke,[66] over 63% of patients developed hemiplegic shoulder pain. The wide range of reported incidence probably reflects the lack of accepted definitions, differences in the populations of patients studied and differences in study methodology. The underlying reasons for the development of post-stroke shoulder pain has not been studied. It does not appear to be related to shoulder subluxation, although in one study the incidence of problems was reduced from 27% to 8% by increased awareness amongst staff of the risks of shoulder trauma.[64] Frequency increases with increasing disability, and it is consequently more commonly found in patients in rehabilitation settings than in community studies. Even though the evidence is absent, it makes sense to take measures to reduce the risk of trauma to the paralysed shoulder, by avoiding the use of overhead arm slings[67] and supporting the paralysed arm, especially during the period of reduced muscle tone. Strapping of the shoulder is, however, ineffective.[68] Shoulder pain can be extremely disabling for patients. Even if motor recovery is good, an immobile shoulder can render the arm virtually useless.

Treatment of established pain should start using simple analgesics or non-steroidal anti-inflammatory drugs (NSAIDs). High intensity transcutaneous electrical nerve stimulation (TENS) has been shown, in one randomized controlled trial of 60 patients, to be effective for some patients.[69] Early studies with small numbers of patients supported the use of intra-articular steroid injections,[70] however, this has not been supported in a more recent trial.[71] Bobath physiotherapy was compared with cryotherapy in a randomized trial showing no significant differences in recovery rates between the two groups.[72]

## Headache

Few studies have examined the frequency and causes of headache associated with stroke. Vestergaard et al.[73] questioned 280 consecutively admitted acute stroke patients about headache and prior headache. Twenty seven percent experienced headache from 3 days before to 3 days after stroke, with 50% of those with intracerebral haemorrhage, 26% of those with cortical infarction and 15% with lacunar infarction. Headache was more common in posterior circulation strokes and literalized in 33% of cases. No association was found between size of cortical infarct and the likelihood of headache.

## Deep venous thrombosis

Other causes of pain include deep venous thrombosis (DVT), which occurs in up to 50% of unselected hospitalized stroke patients when actively sought using sensitive imaging, such as MRI or venography, and it is almost invariably in the hemiparetic limb or bilateral. Pain however is relatively uncommon.

## Pressure sores

In the largest available study of post-stroke medical complications,[3] 18% of the 607 hospitalized patients had skin breaks or pressure sores. While some pressure sores may be inevitable, occurring before presentation of stroke, many can be avoided by good nursing care and the appropriate use of pressure relieving mattresses and cushions. Once present they can be the cause of severe pain, significantly delaying recovery from stroke.

## Depression

Depression may affect as many as half of all stroke patients with rates ranging from 5–50%.[3,74] Pain can be a presenting symptom of depression, and it can certainly make pre-existing pain worse. Randomized controlled trials of antidepressant medication for post-stroke depression have been few, of small size and often with methodological flaws. There is no convincing evidence that either tricyclic antidepressants or the selective serotonin (5-hydroxytryptamine) reuptake inhibitors are any more effective than placebo, but most clinicians still use them, in the absence of any alternatives.

# References

1. Warlow CP, Dennis MS, van Gijn J. *Stroke – A Practical Guide to Management.* Oxford: Blackwell, 1996, pp. 508–509
2. Andrews K, Greenwood RJ. Physical consequences of neurological disablement In: Greenwood R, Barnes MP, McMillan TM, Ward CD, eds. *Neurological Rehabilitation.* Edinburgh: Churchill Livingstone, 1993, pp. 199–219
3. Davenport RJ, Dennis MS, Wellwood I, Warlow CP. Complications after acute stroke. *Stroke* **27:** 415–420, 1996
4. Kalra L, Yu G, Wilson K, Roots P. Medical complications during stroke rehabilitation. *Stroke* **26:** 990–999, 1995
5. Boivie J. Central pain. In: *Textbook of pain. 4th edition.* Wall PD, Melzac R, eds. Edinburgh: Churchill Livingstone, 1989, 879–914
6. Schott GD. From thalamic syndrome to central post stroke pain. *J Neurol Neurosurg Psychiatrist* **61:** 560–565, 1996
7. Riddoch G. The clinical features of central pain. *Lancet* 234: **I:** 1093–1098, 1150–1156, 1205–1209, 1938
8. Tasker RR, de Carvalho G, Dostrovsky JO. The history of central pain syndromes with observations concerning pathophysiology and treatment. In: Casey KL, ed. *Pain and Central Nervous System Disease – The Central Pain Syndromes.* New York: Raven, 1991, pp. 31–58
9. Bonica JJ. Introduction: semantic, epidemiologic, and educational issues. In: Casey KL, ed. *Pain and Central Nervous System Disease: The Central Pain Syndromes.* New York: Raven, 1991, pp. 13–29
10. Casey KL, ed. *Pain and Central Nervous System Disease: The Central Pain Syndromes.* New York: Raven Press, 1991
11. Bowsher D. Central pain. *Pain Rev* **2:** 175–186, 1995
12. Merskey H, Bogduk N, eds. *Classification of chronic pain. Description of chronic pain syndromes and definitions of pain terms. 2nd ed.* Seattle: IASP Press, 1994, pp. 43–48.
13. Dejerine J, Roussy G. Le syndrome thalainique. *Rev Neurol (Paris)* **14:** 521–532, 1906: English translation in: Ronenberg DA, Hochberg FH, eds. *Neurological classics in modern translation.* New York: Hafner Press, 1977, 189–200. Extract in: Wilkins RH, Brody LA. The thalamic syndrome. *Arch Neurol* 20: 559–562, 1969
14. Bowsher D, Leijon G, Thuomas K-A. Central post-stroke pain: correlation of magnetic resonance imaging with clinical pain characteristics and sensory abnormalities. *Neurology* **51:** 1351–1352, 1998
15. Leijon G, Boivie J, Johansson I. Central post-stroke pain – neurological symptoms and pain characteristics. *Pain* **36:** 13–25, 1989
16. Boivie J. An anatomical reinvestigation of the termination of the spinothalamic tract in the monkey. *J Comp Neurol* **168:** 343–370, 1979
17. Andersen G, Vestergaard K, Ingeman-Nielsen M, Jensen TS. Incidence of central post-stroke pain. *Pain* **61:** 187–193, 1995
18. Bowsher D. Central pain: clinical and physiological characteristics. *J Neurol Neurosurg Psychiat* **61:** 62–69, 1996
19. Garcin R. Thalamic syndrome and pain central origin. In: Soulairac A, Cahn J, Charpentier J, eds, *Pain.* London: Academic, 1968, pp. 521–541
20. Schott B, Laurent B, Mauguiere F. Les douleurs thalamiques: etude critique de 43 cas. *Rev Neurolog (Paris)* **142:** 308–315, 1986

21. Bogousslavsky J, Regli F, Uske A. Thalamic infarcts: clinical syndromes, etiology, and prognosis. *Neurology* **38**: 837–848, 1988
22. Schmahmann JD, Leifer D. Parietal pseudothalamic pain syndrome. Clinical features and anatomic correlates. *Arch Neurol* **49**: 1032–1037, 1992
23. Fields HL, Adams JE. Pain after cortical injury relieved electrical stimulation of the internal capsule. *Brain* **97**: 169–178, 1974
24. Michel D, Laurent B, Convers P, et al. Douleurs corticales. Etude clinique, electrophysiologique et topographique de 12 cas. *Rev Neurol (Paris)* **146**: 405–414, 1990
25. McNamara PJ, Tanaka Y, Miyazaki M, Albert ML. Pain associated with cerebral lesions. *Pain* **44**(Suppl 5): S434–436, 1991
26. Sandyk R. Spontaneous pain, hyperpathia and wastings of the hand due to parietal lobe haemorrhage. *Eur Neurol* **24**: 1–3, 1985
27. Tasker RR. Management of nociceptive deafferentation and central pain by surgical intervention. In: HL Fields, ed. *Pain Symptoms in Neurology*. London: Butterworth, 1990, pp. 143–190
28. Lewis-Jones H, Smith T, Bowsher D, Leijon G. Magnetic resonance imaging in 36 cases of central post-stroke pain (CPSP). *Pain* **42**(Suppl 5): S278, 1990
29. Vestergaard K, Nielsen J, Andersen G, Ingeman-Nielsen M, Arena Nielsen L, Jensen TS. Sensory abnormalities in consecutive unselected patients with central post-stroke pain. *Pain* **61**: 177–186, 1995
30. Bowsher D, Foy PM, Shaw MDM. Central pain complicating infarction following subarachnoid haemorrhage. *Br J Neurosurg* **3**: 435–442, 1989
31. Stoodley MA, Warren ID, Oatey PE. Thalamic syndrome caused by unruptured cerebral aneurysm. *J Neurosurg* **82**: 291–293, 1995
32. Breuer AC, Cuervo H, Selkoe DJ. Hyperpathia and sensory level due to parietal lobe arteriovenous malformation. *Arch Neurol* **38**: 722–724, 1981
33. Silver ML. 'Central pain' from cerebral arteriovenous aneurysm. *J Neurosurg* **14**: 92–97, 1957
34. MacGowan DJL, Janal MN, Clark WC. Central post-stroke pain and Wallenberg's lateral medullary infarction: frequency, character, and determinants in 63 patients. *Neurology* **49**: 120–125, 1997
35. Young BG, Blume WT. Painful epileptic seizures. *Brain* **106**: 537–554, 1983
36. Young GB, Barr HWK, Blume WT. Painful epileptic seizure involving the second sensory area. *Neurology* **19**: 412–418, 1988
37. Wilson WP, Nashold BS. Epileptic discharges occurring in the mesencephalon and thalamus. *Epilepsia* **9**: 265–273, 1968
38. Parrent AG, Lozano AM, Dostrovsky JO, Tasker RR. Central pain in the absence of functional sensory thalamus. *Stereotact Funct Neurosurg* **59**: 9–14, 1992
39. Loh L, Nathan PW, Schott GD. Pain due to lesions of central nervous system removed by sympathetic block. *Br Med J* **282**: 1026–1028, 1981
40. Boivie J, Leijon G. Clinical findings in patients with central post-stroke pain. In: Casey KL, ed. *Pain and central nervous system disease: the central pain syndromes*. New York: Raven, pp. 65–75
41. Boivie J, Leijon G, Johansson I. Central post-stroke pain – a study of the mechanisms rough analyses of the sensory abnormalities. *Pain* **37**: 173–185, 1989
42. Soria ED, Fine EJ. Disappearance of thalamic pain after parietal subcortical stroke. *Pain* **44**: 285–288, 1991
43. Nasreddine ZS, Saver JL. Pain after thalamic stroke: right diencephalic predominance and clinical features in 180 patients. *Neurology* **48**: 1196–1199, 1997
44. Casey KL, Beydoun A, Boivie J, et al. Laser-evoked cerebral potentials and sensory function in patients with central pain. *Pain* **64**: 485–491, 1996
45. Holmgren H, Leijon G, Boivie J, Johansson I, Ilievska L. Central post-stroke pain-somatosensory evoked potentials in relation to location of the lesion and sensory signs. *Pain* **40**: 43–52, 1990
46. Mauguiere F, Desmedt JE. Thalamic pain syndrome of Dejerine-Roussy. Differentiation of four subtypes assisted by somatosensory evoked potentials data. *Arch Neurol* **45**: 1312–1320, 1988
47. Leijon G, Boivie J. Pharmacological treatment of central pain. In: Casey KL, ed. *Pain and central nervous system disease: the central pain syndromes*. New York: Raven, 1991; pp. 257–266
48. Bowsher D, Nurmikko T. Central post-stroke pain. Drug Treatment Options. *CNS Drugs* **5**: 160–165, 1996
49. Leijon G, Boivie J. Treatment of neurogenic pain with antidepressants. *Nordisk Psykiatrisk Tidsskrift* **43**: 83–87, 1989

50. Leijon G, Boivie J. Central post-stroke pain – a controlled trial of amitriptyline and carbamazepine. *Pain* **36**: 27–36, 1989
51. Swerdlow M. Anticonvulsants in the therapy of neuralgic pain. *Pain Clin* **1**: 9–19, 1986
52. Awerbuch GI. Treatment of thalamic pain syndrome with Mexiletone. *Ann Neurol* **28**: 233–235, 1990
53. Taira T, Tanikawa T, Kawamura H, Iseki H, Takamura K. Spinal intrathecal baclofen suppresses central pain after stroke. *J Neurol Neurosurg Psychiat* **57**: 381–382, 1994
54. Sjolund BH. Role of transcutaneous electrical nerve stimulation, central nervous system stimulation, and ablative procedures in central pain syndromes. In: Casey KL, ed. *Pain and central nervous disease: the central pain syndromes.* New York: Raven, 1991, pp. 267–274
55. Tasker RR. Pain resulting from central nervous system pathology (central pain). In: Bonika JJ, ed. *The Management of Pain.* Philadelphhia: Lea & Febiger, 1990, pp. 264–280.
56. Leijon G, Boivie J. Central post-stroke pain – the effect of high and low frequency TENS. *Pain* **38**: 187–191, 1989
57. Duncan GH, Bushnell MC, Marchand S. Deep brain stimulation: a review of basic research and clinical studies. *Pain* **45**: 49–59, 1991
58. Richardson DE, Akil H. Long term results of periventricular gray self-stimulation. *Neurosurgery* **1**: 200–202, 1977
59. Meyerson BA, Undblom U, Underoth B, Und G, Herregodts P. Motor cortex stimulation as treatment of trigeminal neuropathic pain. *Acta NeurochirSuppl (Wien)* **58**: 150–153, 1993
60. Levy RM, Lamb S, Adams JE. Treatment of chronic pain by deep brain stimulation: long term follow-up and review of the literature. *Neurosurgery* **21**: 885–893, 1987
61. Tsubokawa T, Katayma Y, Yamamoto T, Hirayama T, Koyama S. Chronic motor cortex stimulation in patients with thalamic pain. *J Neurosurg* **78**: 393–401, 1993
62. Pither CE. Nicholas MK. Psychological approaches in chronic pain management. *Br Med Bull* **47**: 743–761, 1991
63. Dromerick A, Reding M. Medical and neurological complications during inpatient stroke rehabilitation. *Stroke* **25**: 358–361, 1994
64. Braus DF, Krauss LK, Strobel J. The shoulder-hand syndrome after stroke: a prospective clinical trial. *Ann Neurol* **36**: 728–733, 1994
65. Chalsen CG, Fitzpatrick KA, Navia RA, Bean SA, Reding MJ. Prevalence of the shoulder-hand pain syndrome in an inpatient stroke rehabilitation population: a quantitative cross-sectional study. *J Neurol Rehab* **1**: 137–141, 1987
66. Wanklyn P, Forster A, Young J. Hemiplegic shoulder pain (HSP): natural history and investigation of associated features. *Dis Rehab* **18**: 497–501, 1996
67. Kumar R, Metter EJ, Mehta AJ, Chew T. Shoulder pain in hemiplegia: the role of exercise. *Am J Phys Exercise Rehab* **69**: 205–208, 1990
68. Hanger HS, Whitewood P, Brown, et al. A randomised controlled trial of strapping to prevent post-stroke shoulder pain. *Clin Rehab* **14**: 370–380, 2000
69. Leandri M, Parodi CI, Corrieri N, Rigard S. Comparison of TENS treatments in hemiplegic patients. *Arch Phys Med Rehab* **57**: 588–591, 1976
70. Dekker JHM, Wagenaar RC, Lankhorst GJ, de Jong BA. The painful hemiplegic shoulder: effects of intra-articular triamcinolone acetonide. *Am J Phys Med Rehab* **76**: 43–48, 1997
71. Snels IAK, Beckerman H, Twisk JWR, et al. Effect of triamcinolone injections on hemiplegic shoulder pain. A randomised controlled trial. *Stroke* **31**: 2396–2401, 2000
72. Partridge CJ, Edwards SM, Mee R, Langenberghe HVK. Hemiplegic shoulder pain: a study of two methods of physiotherapy treatment. *Clin Rehab* **4**: 43–49, 1990
73. Vestergaard K, Anderson G, Nielsen MI, Jensen TS. Headache in stroke. *Stroke* **24**: 1621–1624, 1993
74. Eastwood MR, Rifat SL, Nobbs H, Ruderman J. Mood disorder following cerebrovascular accident. *Br J Psychiat* **154**: 195–200, 1989

# 27 Scar Pain

*Stephan Weber*

Most scar tissue forms within the 10 days to 6 weeks after surgery. Scar pain is defined as persistent pain in a healed postoperative scar of more than 3 months' duration with *allodynia* and *hyperalgesia* adjacent to the scar with no sensory loss other than over the scar itself.

As will be outlined later, scar pain is multidimensional, i.e. it involves neurophysiological systems and causes emotional and behavioural reactions. Therefore, the clinical manifestations are as diverse as the conditions causing scar pain.

## Pathophysiology

The precise mechanisms are still debated, but it is likely that changes occur throughout the nervous system, from the peripheral nociceptor to the brain. It is speculated that afferent C fibre burst initiates long-lasting events that result in changes in spinal processing. This will then alter the response to successive inputs:

- Following a peripheral tissue injury, experiments[1] demonstrated an increase in $Na^+$ channel expression predominantly in unmyelinated small-diameter primary afferent neurones, leading to spontaneous activity originating from that terminal. There is also an increased sensitivity to allogenic agents, such as histamines, 5-hydroxytryptamine (5-HT, serotonin), kinins, lipidic acids, cytokines – tumour necrosis factor (TNF-a) and interleukins – and various peptides such as substance P (SP) and calcitonin gene-related peptide (CGRP). However, neuronal sensitization by cytokines occurs centrally as well as in the periphery, and includes mechanisms such as upregulation of SP receptors in the dorsal horn.
- Neuroma formation might also occur due to disorganized nerve regeneration, mainly of unmyelinated nerve fibres, leading to ephaptic transmission. Neuroma embedded in scar tissue have impaired blood supply, and an hypoxic/bradytrophic environment may be one of many possible triggers of noxious impulses.
- Prolonged C fibre activation also alters the pattern of gene transcription in dorsal root ganglion (DRG) cells and dorsal horn neurones. This results in an increased expression of the capsaicin or vanilloid receptor-1 (VR1) in these regions.[2] Capsaicin stimulates the VR1 receptor to a similar degree to that caused by noxious heat. In addition, the terminal also develops an increased sensitivity to a variety of other products, such as bradykinin, prostaglandin and adrenaline.
- Myelinated Aβ fibres, which transmit the sensation of touch and pressure, sprout from their site of termination in lamina III to lamina II and, thereby, gain access to dorsal horn neurones involved in processing nociceptive input. This could be demonstrated in animal studies[3] and is an explanation for *allodynia* following normally innocuous Aβ fibre stimulation.
- The normal DRG possesses hardly any sympathetic innervation. Sprouting from sympathetic neurones into the DRG occurs after peripheral injury, functionally coupling these

efferent neurones with afferent sensory input terminals. This results in increased activity in the DRG cells.

- In the dorsal horn the input of various sensory qualities from primary afferents are controlled and modulated by interneurones. They are presynaptic to large central afferent neurones. An important class of these neurones contain the *inhibitory amino acids* γ-aminobutyric acid (GABA) and glycine. It appears that the excitatory effects of Aβ fibres are under their modulatory control. Peripheral injury can lead to cell death of GABA- and glycine-containing neurones in the dorsal horn area and, consequently, to loss of the intrinsic modulatory systems that alter afferent evoked excitation. Thus, a stimulus such as touch leads to a facilitated response of wide dynamic range (WDR) neurones, causing pain behaviour (allodynia) in the affected individual.
- A different group of interneurones in the dorsal horn release the *excitatory amino acids* glutamate and aspartate when excited by C fibres. They stimulate and increase the sensitivity of WDR cells via $N$-methyl-D-aspartate (NMDA) receptors by triggering the release of intracellular calcium ions. Calcium ($Ca^{2+}$) ions acting as secondary messengers initiate protein kinase C activation and phospholipase C and nitric oxide synthetase production. The result is an alteration of membrane ion channel function, lowering the membrane threshold and so increasing the responsiveness of the nociceptive system.

## Aetiology and prevalence

Scar pain may develop at any site of the body where skin is breached beyond the stratum corneum and formation of granulation tissue occurs. A surgical procedure is the most likely reason, but scar formation can equally be caused by trauma. It is debatable if neuroma formation due to a cut nerve or continuous C fibre stimulation, or both, is the pacemaker. But other form of injuries such as burns or deep abrasion secondary to falls can cause persistent scar pain.

There are only few studies investigating scar pain, and the majority look at the prevalence of scar pain after specific surgical interventions. However, procedures likely to give rise to scar pain include:

- Abdominal wall surgery (e.g. hernia repair)
- Pfannenstiel incisions (e.g. Caesarean section, hysterectomy)
- Mastectomy
- Sternotomy/thoracotomy (e.g. coronary artery bypass grafting/lung resection).

### Abdominal wall & thoracic surgery

Following surgery involving the abdominal wall, such as inguinal hernia repair, the reported prevalence of late or persistent pain varies from 0–37%. A recent study[4] found that pain in the groin area persisted 1 year after surgery in 28.7%, and 11.0% reported that pain was interfering with work or leisure activity.

Equally high is the reported prevalence of protracted pain following cardiac bypass surgery. In a Swedish study questioning patients 1 year following surgery, 28% reported chest discomfort different from that which they experienced prior to surgery.[5] Most patients experienced modest pain intensity, but some (1%) reported severe pain. Eisenberg et al.[6] reported that 56% of patients suffered chronic anterior chest wall pain and described a subcategory of patients who suffered exclusively from midline scar pain. Another study[7] reported a prevalence of chronic post-thoracotomy pain of 80% at 3 month, 75% at 6 months and 61% after 1 year. Severe pain was reported by 3.5% of patients.

## Pfannenstiel incisions

Pfannenstiel incisions for various gynaecological and obstetric interventions can cause prolonged pain. The majority of studies looked at scar endometriosis, which presents as a periodic recurrence of pain and occasional swelling in the scar just prior to menstruation. This finding is pathognomonic. The prevalence for scar endometriosis following Caesarean section ranges from 0.03–1.7%.[8] Surgical excision is the treatment of choice, providing both diagnostic and therapeutic intervention.

## Mastectomy

Mastectomy causes protracted pain and the prevalence of post-mastectomy varies between 20%[9] and 46%.[10] A recent study reported the prevalence of hyperaesthesia (as opposed to hyperalgesia) in the scar as 3% after one year.[11] The difficulty in assessing scar pain following mastectomy is that the symptoms troubling patients are varied, ranging from numbness to paraesthesia and pain.

# Assessment

Good clinical practice demands an accurate diagnosis by taking a targeted history from the patient followed by physical examination. This approach should minimize unsuccessful treatment strategies and subsequent patient (and clinician!) dissatisfaction. Obtaining original operation notes might be helpful. It is prudent to exclude any progressive illness (e.g. malignancy), the presence of an organic lesion or a surgically rectifiable cause (e.g. foreign material, herniation, scar endometriosis).

The patient has most likely undergone surgery at least 3 months previously and is now complaining of pain adjacent to the scar, which can be *continuous, spontaneous* or *paroxysmal*. The latter can be perceived as an electric shock-like sensation. Generally the patient will describe the skin sensations as burning, stabbing or pricking. Also:

- Light touch or clothes rubbing against the scar can cause pain (allodynia).
- A noxious stimulus might evoke a disproportionate response (hyperalgesia).

It is established that a painful neuroma can be localized to a discreet spot. On palpation of this spot, pain radiates in the normal distribution of the involved peripheral nerve.[12]

# Management

At present, there is no conclusive data available comparing pharmacological and interventional strategies for treating scar pain. Parallels might exist with other chronic pain syndromes, such as neuropathic pain, leading to the assumptions that they – despite a different aetiology – might share the same pathophysiology. For that reason, clinicians may employ a treatment strategy for scar pain that has been successfully used in other conditions.

The following treatment modalities are by no means mutually exclusive, but they should be used as a treatment continuum – i.e. increasing levels of intervention and complexity.

## Pharmacological

If not already tried and exhausted, simple oral analgesia should be the first therapeutic step, since injections or other invasive techniques will unavoidably cause the patient temporarily additional discomfort or pain. This puts the practitioner under the pressure to 'deliver' and, if not immediately successful, may cause the patient to lose confidence in further interventions.

## Topical

- Capsaicin cream in concentrations of 0.025% or 0.075% has been used in a variety of pain conditions ranging from osteoarthritis, to trigeminal neuralgia and scar pain. It is readily absorbed and selectively binds to the VR1 receptor. The signal gets transmitted to the dorsal horn ganglia, evoking the release of SP and CGRP. Repeated stimulation of the VR1 receptor causes depletion of SP as neurotransmitter and so cessation of transduction of noxious stimuli in the dorsal horn. The patient should be instructed to apply the cream wearing gloves and to avoid contact with open wounds and eyes. The size of a lentil is then massaged into the scar and surrounding tissue until no cream remains. It is prudent to inform the patient to expect a burning sensation for the first hour or so after application. This sensation will be worsened if the patient is taking a hot bath or shower just before or after application. However, the burning will disappear after a few days of regular use. The patient may then increase the amount of cream, or use the 0.075% instead of the 0.025% concentration. Compliance can be difficult; the cream must be applied three to four times daily, and it will worsen the patient's pain at least initially. Application of EMLA cream or lignocaine gel might increase the compliance. After 2 weeks, cessation of the scar pain can occur and the dosage interval can be reduced to twice daily. Discontinuation of therapy can be attempted after 3 months.
- Lignocaine in the form of self-adhesive patches (Lidoderm 5%) is a relatively new way of applying this local anaesthetic for longer period of time to painful skin and overcoming the impractical use in the form of a gel. Lignocaine blocks $Na^+$-channels selectively, leading to a diminution of ectopic activity by altering the generator that leads to the facilitated state. The patch contains 700 mg of lignocaine (50 mg per g of adhesive). The dimension of the patch is approximately $20 \times 15$ cm, and it can be cut to an appropriate size covering the painful area. It should be worn for 12 hours and then taken off for 12 hours. This should be continued for approximately 2 months.

## Systemic

- Tricyclic antidepressants (TCA) – these have been used for some time in treating continuous burning dysaesthetic pain. The mechanism of action focuses on reuptake inhibition of noradrenaline and 5-HT in the central nervous system (CNS), causing inhibition of afferent nociceptive neurones in the dorsal horn via efferent pathways. The common muscarinic side-effects, such as dry mouth, constipation, sedation, blurred vision, hypotension and urinary retention, are often a reason for poor patient compliance. However, comparatively low doses are required to treat pain compared with those for depression, so patients are less likely to experience common side-effects. Furthermore, the sedative properties may be desirable, as insomnia due to pain is a frequent problem in this group of patients, adding to their suffering. It is equally important to explain to the patient that the drug is not being used to treat depression, although elevation of mood may occur as pain improves. In the author's opinion, there is little to choose between the various drugs of this group. However, there seems to be some predilection amongst pain clinicians for one drug or another. The most frequently prescribed drug is amitriptyline: 25 mg per day commenced at night is the starting dose, 10 mg per day being a more appropriate dose in the frail and elderly. This is increased by 10–25 mg per day at 7–14 day intervals to a maximum dose of 150 mg per day, depending on therapeutic success and careful monitoring for side-effects. Should side-effects occur at any incremental dose, the patient is advised to reduce the amount to the previous dose. Dothiepin can be used instead and may be better tolerated.

The initial dosage is 25 mg per day and is increased up to 75 mg per day in weekly intervals, again, depending on effectiveness and absence of side-effects. Once an effect is established the patient can attempt to discontinue the drug after several months.

- Anticonvulsants – this group of drugs is useful in scar pain where the patient is complaining of shooting sensations or lancinating pain. The mode of action is thought to be by blocking $Na^+$ channels and suppression of spontaneous activity in C and Ad fibres (carbamazepine). Two other possible mechanisms are action via NMDA receptor sites and GABA inhibition (sodium valproate, clonazepam). Carbamazepine is an established treatment for pain conditions with a burning sensation,[13] most evident in trigeminal neuralgia and postherpetic neuralgia. The treatment is started with 100 mg twice daily and increased gradually to response. The maximum dose of 1.6 g in three divided doses should not be exceeded. Monitoring of hepatic function, haematology and looking out for skin reaction is mandatory. Failure to respond or the appearance of side-effects might warrant the use of sodium valproate, which may be better tolerated. However, there is no evidence in the literature for its efficacy.[14] Gabapentin has gained increasing popularity over recent years in the treatment of neuropathic pain. Treatment is started with 300 mg per day and increased daily by 300 mg until cessation of the symptoms is achieved or the maximum dose of 2.4 g is reached. Clinical trials demonstrate effectiveness in postherpetic neuralgia and mixed neuropathic pain states, but there are no direct trials comparing it with carbamazepine. A recent Cochrane review could not find any evidence that gabapentin has a higher efficacy than carbamazepine,[15] the latter being a cheaper drug.
- Local anaesthetics – lignocaine at 5 mg/kg bodyweight infused over 30–60 minutes is worthwhile trying in patients where there has been very little progress in treating allodynia. Interestingly, the dose needed is smaller than those that block conduction in a normal nerve. If successful, pain relief can last weeks and the patient can be started on oral mexiletine.
- Non-steroidal anti-inflammatory drugs (NSAIDs) – as spinal prostaglandin synthesis is an important pacemaker in the maintenance of hypersensitivity states, their use might be beneficial, either by topical application as a gel[16] or orally, absence of contraindications permitting. However, the effectiveness of NSAIDs and even selective cyclooxygenase 2 inhibitors in treating pain caused by nerve injury and their long-term effects is still controversial.
- There is no evidence to support the use of opioids for scar pain, although tramadol and oxycodone have been shown to be useful in some neuropathic pain states.
- Oxpentifylline – this has been successfully used in the treatment of pain caused by hypertrophic scar formation even though the evidence is anecdotal.[17] This substance is used to treat claudication and Raynaud's disease. The transforming growth factor (TGF) family of growth factors is believed to be primarily responsible for excessive scar formation. Oxpentifylline is thought to reduce local TNF-$\alpha$ production in the keloid. The recommended dose varies from 400 mg twice to three times daily. Reduction of scar pain was observed within 7–14 days.

## Local infiltration techniques

- Steroids – these have been found to suppress ectopic discharges from experimental neuromas and to have a short-lasting suppressive effect on transmission in normal C fibres.[18] Injection into painful scars is usually performed in combination with a local anaesthetic, most frequently bupivacaine. This approach should be the next step in line after oral medication has failed. Even though pain relief might be short lived, it can be repeated 2–3 times at weekly intervals in the attempt to 'stun' the ectopic centre. If this approach fails to alleviate the pain, it still provides useful diagnostic information.
- Aminoglycosides – painful scars display increased CGRP and SP innervation at the base of the epidermis. Aminoglycoside antibiotics interact with voltage-operated $Ca^{2+}$ chan-

nels, suppressing ectopic or spontaneous activity primary afferent nociceptive pathways. It has been used in combination with lignocaine for treatment of trigeminal neuralgia.[19,20] Injecting scars with 1 g streptomycin dissolved in 5–10 ml 1% lignocaine at weekly intervals for 5 weeks is a practical approach. At these doses, ototoxicity is unlikely to occur.

## Neuromodulation

- Acupuncture is a technique worthwhile considering in scar pain. Intradermal needling has been used successfully for intractable abdominal scar pain.[21]
- Transcutaneous nerve stimulation (TENS) is devoid of side-effects. Location of the scar itself can also be a limiting factor because certain anatomical regions are impractical for the placement of electrodes.
- Spinal cord stimulation falls also into the category of neuromodulation, but is the most invasive and possibly most expensive procedure in pain management. It is certainly only to be considered after all other interventions have failed to produce a result, and the insertion, maintenance and follow-up should be left for special units.

## Interventional procedures

The least destructive interventional procedure should be employed first and, depending on the outcome, gradually progress to more destructive techniques if indicated.

- Sympathetic nerve blocks – these can be considered if there is sympathetically-maintained pain in the scar. Diagnostic blocks with local anaesthetics such as bupivacaine are the first step and, if successful, might warrant the injection of neurolytic drugs such as 6% phenol. For example, a stellate ganglion block for persistent scar pain following mastectomy is an option. However, caution is indicated, since there is the possibility for post-denervation neuralgia. Radiofrequency lesioning of the ganglion is an option. The risk of inadvertent adjacent nerve injuries is reduced with this technique.
- Cryotherapy – this has been used to treat scar pain following thoracotomy, hernia repair and neuroma formation in other scars. For the above named procedure it is advised to take care to identify the appropriate nerve. Cryoablation and radiofrequency lesions can be repeated if analgesia lasts more than 3–6 months. A problem with all neurolytic procedure is the regrowth of axons at a rate of 1–3 mm/day. This gives rise to the potential growth of (new) painful neuromas, thus limiting the duration of pain relief. Despite this, prolonged analgesia has been observed, possibly by affecting the plasticity of the nervous system.

## Psychological

Scars can be mutilating, and there appear to be powerful psychoemotional factors that play a role in the development of scar pain. The prevalence and severity of scar pain following surgical procedures often reduces with time. However, for patients who continue to suffer with severe pain, this may be of little comfort. In these circumstances, or when other forms of intervention have failed to produce results, pain management programmes should be considered.

## Conclusion

In general, prevention is better than cure. With evidence of neuronal plasticity, particularly after surgery and trauma, early intervention or even prevention may be the way forward. This includes minimally invasive surgery, preemptive analgesia and improved wound care. In spite of the range of treatments available, successful management of scar pain can remain a challenge for patient and pain clinician.

# References

1. Cummins TR, Dib-Hajj SD, Black JA, Akopian AN, Wood JN, Waxman SG. A novel persistent tetrodotoxin-resistant sodium current in SNS-null and wild-type small primary sensory neurons. *J Neurosci* **19**: RC43, 1999
2. Caterina MJ, Schumacher MA, Tominaga M, Rosen TA, Levine JD, Julius D. The capsaicin receptor: a heat-activated ion channel in the pain pathway. *Nature* **389**: 816–824, 1997
3. Woolf CJ, Shortland P, Coggeshall RE. Peripheral nerve injury triggers central sprouting of myelinated afferents. *Nature* **355**: 75–78, 1992
4. Bay-Nielsen M, Perkins FM, Kehlet H. Pain and functional impairment 1 year after inguinalherniorrhaphy: a nationwide questionnaire study *Ann Surg* **233**: 1–7, 2001
5. Meyerson J, Thelin S, Gordh T, Karlsten R. The incidence of chronic post-sternotomy pain after cardiac surgery - a prospective study. *Acta Anaesthesiol Scand* **45**: 940–944, 2001
6. Eisenberg E, Pultorak Y, Pud D, Bar-El Y. Prevalence and characteristics of post coronary artery bypass graft surgery pain (PCP). *Pain* **92**: 11–17, 2001
7. Perttunen K. Chronic pain after thoracic surgery: a follow-up study. *Acta Anaesthesiol Scand* **43**: 563–567
8. Wolf GC, Singh KB: Cesarian scar endometriosis: A review. *Obstet Gynecol Survey* **44**: 89–94, 1989
9. Stevens PE, Dibbie SL. Prevalence, characteristics, and impact of mastectomy pain syndromes: an investigation of women's experiences. *Pain* **61**: 61–68, 1995
10. Smith WCS, Bourne D, Squair J, Phillips DO, Chambers A. A retrospective cohort study of post mastectomy pain syndrome. *Pain* **83**: 91–95, 1999
11. Tasmuth T, von Smitten K, Kalso E. Pain and other symptoms during the first year after radical and conservative surgery for breast cancer. *Br J Cancer* **74**: 2024–2031, 1996
12. Novak CB, van Vliet D, Mackinnon SE. Subjective outcome following surgical management of lower extremity neuromas. *J Reconstr Microsurg* **11**: 175–177, 1995
13. Killian JM, Fromm GH. Carbamazepine in the treatment of neuralgia. Use of side effects. *Arch Neurol* **19**: 129–136, 1968
14. Drewes AM. Andreasen A. Poulsen LH. Valproate for treatment of chronic central pain after spinal cord injury. A double-blind cross-over study. *Paraplegia* **32**: 565–569, 1994
15. Wiffen P, Collins S, McQuay H, Carroll D, Jadad A, Moore A. Anticonvulsant drugs for acute and chronic pain (Cochrane Review). *Cochrane Library* Issue 2, 2002. Oxford: Update
16. Irving AD. Morrison SL. Effectiveness of topical non-steroidal anti-inflammatory drugs in the management of breast pain. *J Roy Coll Surg Edin* **43**: 158–159, 1998
17. Wong TW, Lee JY, Sheu HM, Chao SC. Relief of pain and itch associated with keloids on treatment with oxpentifylline. *Br J Dermatol* **137**: 151–152, 1997
18. Johansson A, Bennett GJ. Effect of local methylprednisolone on pain in a nerve injury model. A pilot study. *Region Anesthes* **22**: 59–65, 1997
19. Kreiner M. Use of streptomycin-lidocaine injections in the treatment of the cluster-tic syndrome. Clinical perspectives and a case report. *J Cranio-maxillo-facial Surg* **24**: 289–292, 1996
20. Bittar GT, Graf-Radford SB. The effects of streptomycin/lidocaine block on trigeminal neuralgia: a double blind crossover placebo controlled study. *Headache* **33**: 155–160, 1993
21. Kotani N, Kushikata T, Suzuki A, Hashimoto H, Muraoka M, Matsuki A. Insertion of intradermal needles into painful points provides analgesia for intractable abdominal scar pain. *Regional Anaesth Pain Med* **26**: 532–538, 2001

# 28 Pain of Unknown Origin

## Nicholas L Padfield

Occasionally the pain physician will be presented with patients who complain of pain for which, up to that moment, no physical cause has been found. These patients come from varied sources. They may come from:

- Exasperated colleagues who have thoroughly investigated the cause without success
- As self referrals seeking another opinion
- From primary care physicians who are themselves convinced that there is no physical cause for the pain.

The patients themselves also present with a wide range of psychological 'baggage'. This may have arisen because of the numerous medical opinions that have been sought and/or proffered as to cause, treatment and prognosis. The patient may enjoy the aura of mystery that gives importance and meaning to their pain. Such patients are likely to have many cognitive, emotional and behavioural issues that will cloud the history and confound the physical signs and, indeed, the attention received may perpetuate the pain and reinforce illness behaviour.

The nature of the pain in terms of site, duration, periodicity, quality and intensity has often been long forgotten. This is a perplexing state for the patient as well as the pain physician. It is against this background that the pain physician must return to basic scientific principles in the evaluation of physical signs and symptoms. Ideally, these should be reliable, reproducible, consistent and valid – regrettably too often a counsel of perfection.

It can be a battle of wills to prise the information out of the patient, as often the patient will mulishly persist in describing symptoms in affective rather than descriptive terms. As such interviews are time consuming and frustrating for the physician, it is all too easy to attribute the cause as psychogenic. However, true psychogenic pain – i.e. that which arises without any organic stimulus/trigger – is rare. It must also not be forgotten that the intensity of the physical stimulus of pain does not correlate with disability. Because illness behaviour is likely to be prevalent in this difficult population of patients, the pain physician must impart a sense of reality to the patient's hopes, expectations, fears and beliefs from the outset. Indeed the whole tenor of the first consultation will determine the course of the entire professional relationship and the course of the consultant episode. Never promise anything that cannot be delivered and always admit the limits of your knowledge.

## History

Wherever possible, the physician must be satisfied as to the pathophysiology of the pain. Thus is it:

- Nociceptive by activation of physiologically normal nociceptive nerve fibres (i.e. sharp, well localized, etc)?
- Somatic?
- Visceral?

- Neuropathic by injury to the nervous system (i.e. burning, poorly localized, etc)?
- Sympathetically maintained (i.e. with vascular and trophic changes)?
- Vascular i.e. ischaemic, migrainous?
- A combination of mechanisms?

Since patients in this category often have symptoms that at first do not follow anatomical distribution, it worth spending time on defining the quality of the pain. It will certainly test consistency of symptoms as reported in the initial and subsequent consultations. This can often prove to be the most important source of information for the pain clinician.

The medical history must detail the following where possible:

- Precipitating cause or event – if any (e.g. trauma, surgery, infection, alcohol, bereavement)
- Onset
  - gradual i.e. degenerative
  - sudden i.e. as a result of some physical change that should be exhaustively investigated, such as metastatic erosion causing nerve compression or ischaemia, both central and peripheral, due to emboli, lymphatic infiltration, parasites
- Qualifying descriptors – periodicity, duration, diurnal variation
- Associated factors
- Provoking and relieving factors
- Employment history
  - type of job and the inherent physical demands
  - days off sick
  - job satisfaction/ promotion prospects/ stress
  - exposure to toxic chemicals
- Social and family
- Hobbies and sports
- Pleasurable activities
- Interpersonal relationships/skills (social isolation?)
- Manipulation within immediate social group and secondary gain from pain reporting and behaviour
- Education
- Information available and accessible (i.e. internet, published articles, newspapers and magazines, television and radio, relatives and friends)
- Fears and beliefs – comprehension and evaluation of available information
- Systematic enquiries
  - general health, energy, sleep, appetite, weight
  - medications, alternative medicines, recreational drug use
  - allergies, medications, foods, chemicals
  - previous hospitalization for significant medical disease (e.g. diabetes mellitus)
  - tuberculosis, encephalitis, multiple sclerosis, HIV, autoimmune diseases, psychological disease
  - any previous pain experiences or patient or family member or friends
- Significant life events
  - divorce
  - death of significant other
  - unemployment/ redundancy
  - moving house
  - birth of children or sibling.

There may be other suspicious factors in the history that may make the pain clinician sceptical about taking all the reported symptoms at face value. The demeanour of the patient, and also who is brought in or left outside the consultation, may indicate dysfunctional family or social dynamics. One must not overlook the possibility of schizophrenia or borderline personality disorder, and frank clinical depression is not uncommon in this category of patients. The patients thought content, delusions or suicidal ideation may be apparent for the first time with a sympathetic and responsive audience.

Patients may present increasingly often with bruised and battered psyches as a result of unsatisfactory consultations with rushed, unsympathetic colleagues and huge delays in obtaining differing medical opinions in our failing NHS. Their experience of the medical profession may result in fear, scepticism or downright contempt, and it is against this background that the pain clinician has to salvage the trust and confidence of the patient.

The history may indicate a musculoskeletal cause but, because the sclerotomal/myotomal pain representation may mimic a number of other clinical disease entities, it is these which will have been exhaustively investigated without result. An example of this would be psoas myofasciitis mimicking renal pain or gallbladder pain. It is immensely satisfying when baffled surgical or medical colleagues refer such patients as an act of desperation and the pain is alleviated by an appropriate local anaesthetic and steroid injection. Sadly, though, such a diagnostic triumph is the exception rather than the rule, and, if all screening tests fail to produce a satisfactory diagnosis, the pain clinician is left with having to manage the patient along empirical lines.

## Common categories

Examples of commonly presenting pain of unknown origin (when history and examination along with diagnostic tests do not produce a diagnosis/obvious cause) include:

- Some types of headache
- Some types of facial pain, e.g. glossodynia
- Abdominal pain
- Whole-limb pain
- Pelvic pain
- Total body pain.

In such cases, diagnosis is further hampered by other confusing features, for example, inconsistencies between symptom reporting and physical signs. While every effort must be made to discover the cause, it must be remembered that such exhaustive attention in terms of the clinician's time and the extent and nature investigation will only reinforce the patient's conviction of serious illness.

This is particularly so in hysterical conversion. In this situation, there are changes in sensory perception that do not correspond to organic nerve distribution and may be influenced by suggestion. The reporting of any anaesthesia or change in sensation that stops abruptly at the midline or does not fit a segmental nerve supply (e.g. has a glove and stocking distribution) may indicate hysteria. This impression may be reinforced by subsequent physical examination revealing a different area of anaesthesia or change in sensation. Nerve conduction studies should be performed in any event to confirm or rule out the diagnosis of peripheral neuropathy.

If the patient still has intact stereognosis in an area of alleged anaesthesia and can perform delicate tasks that require an intact sensorium, hysteria is a likely cause.

# Management

The first thing patients with pain whose origin is unknown want is reassurance that:

- They have not got cancer
- They have not got a progressive debilitating illness
- They will not experience a deterioration of their pain and functioning.

This, in turn, means that they must be engaged in their pain management. They must have explanations of treatment strategies in terms that mean something to them. Medical technical terminology never impresses anxious patients, and this is not an appropriate time to show how clever you are!

The treatment strategies will depend on the impression the pain clinician will have made of the contribution of nociceptive, neuropathic and psychological components of the patients distress and/or disability.

These then translate into the employment of:

- Interventional techniques to seek to map the area of pain with anaesthetic coverage by a targeted block to try and find the site of pain generation
- Pharmacological therapies targeted to particular mechanisms of neurogenic pain genesis, e.g. channel specific blockers, anticonvulsants, $N$-methyl-D-aspartate antagonists, opiate receptors, cholecystokinin antagonists
- Psychological therapies, such as cognitive behavioural programmes, behavioural modification and relaxation techniques.

# 29 Pain Control in Advanced Cancer

## Brendan Amesbury

Pain is a common phenomenon in advanced cancer, occurring in approximately 70% of patients. It is important to note that 80% of patients with pain will have more than one pain, although as many as 30% of patients will not experience pain. It should be possible to achieve satisfactory pain relief in 95% or more of cases, but often the figure is lower than this. In some cases, the cause of the pain will not be directly due to the cancer but will be due to other disease processes. The pain of malignant disease may have physical, psychological, social and spiritual dimensions, and this must be taken into consideration when planning treatments.

## Management of cancer pain

- Accurate diagnosis of the cause of pain is essential and is obtained by taking a good history and performing an appropriate examination and investigations.
- Give the correct treatment – it may not always be an analgesic.
- Give treatment regularly, before pain returns.
- Treatment should be by mouth, if possible, not injection.
- Frequent review and dose adjustments are necessary.

### History, examination, investigations and diagnosis

The history should include full assessment of each pain including site, character, severity, precipitating and relieving factors, radiation and response to current and previous treatments. It should be determined if one or more pains are present and the same process conducted for each pain. Body or pain charts and visual analogue scales may be useful to identify painful areas and severity of pains. Consideration should be given to the medical history, particularly the current cancer history, for example, recently diagnosed metastatic disease. Previous problems should also be considered, such as peptic ulcer disease, arthritis and heart disease. Attention should be paid to psychological problems (such as depression, insomnia, fear or tiredness), to social factors (such as family support or loneliness) and to spiritual matters, for example, anger with God or unresolved issues from the patient's past. The examination should be a full general examination, including all the painful areas and relevant systems. Explanation of the cause of symptoms, reassurance about treatment and frequent follow-up all help to alleviate pain.

Plain X-rays and other radiological investigations are sometimes indicated. Biochemical, haematological and microbiological tests may also be helpful.

It is important to make a diagnosis for the cause of each pain.

### Total pain

The concept of 'total pain' encompasses psychological, social and spiritual factors, as well as the physical aspects of pain. Patients experience overwhelming pain from all directions and the support of the whole team is necessary to help them cope with their immense distress.

**257**

# Causes of cancer pain

Most cancer pains are caused by stimulation of nociceptive nerve endings. A burning or shooting pain may indicate a neuropathic pain, caused by compression or invasion of a nerve by the tumour.

- **Bone metastases** – there is constant, occasionally intermittent, aching pain, often in multiple sites. The pain is worse on movement, and it may improve with rest. There may be tenderness over the bone. Treat with both a non-steroidal anti-inflammatory drug (NSAID) and an analgesic according to the WHO analgesic ladder ranging from paracetamol, to weak opioid, to strong opioid.[1] Radiotherapy is also very effective in controlling bone pain.
- **Invasion of hollow organ by tumour** – there is a constant or irregular ache or spasm over the site of pain, which may be worse with eating and improve with vomiting and rest. The patient may have a distended abdomen with a tender mass on examination. Treat with analgesics.
- **Bowel colic or spasm** – there is intermittent colicky pain with possible radiation. The pain may be worse after eating. Bowel function may be disturbed and pain may be due to constipation. Treat with analgesics and consider antispasmodics, for example, hyoscine butylbromide.
- **Liver metastases** – there is a constant ache or sharp pain, localized to the right upper quadrant. Hepatomegaly and tenderness may be present. Treat with analgesics and dexamethasone to reduce oedema and liver capsule distension.
- **Invasion of coeliac plexus by tumour** – there is a boring epigastric ache, which may radiate to the back. The patient may have local tenderness or mass. Treat with analgesics and consider a coeliac plexus block.
- **Bladder spasm** – there is intermittent colicky suprapubic pain with possible suprapubic tenderness. Treat the cause if possible, for example, infection or blood clots. Treat spasm with hyoscine butylbromide or oxybutynin.
- **Ureteric colic** – there is intermittent colicky pain in the loin, which may radiate to the groin. Loin tenderness is possible. Treat with hyoscine butylbromide and NSAIDs.
- **Chest wall or rib pain** – there is a constant aching pain. The patient may have local tenderness, which may be worse or stabbing in nature on breathing. Treat with NSAIDs and analgesic. Consider intercostal nerve block, interpleural local anaesthetic or transcutaneous electrical nerve stimulation (TENS).
- **Diffuse abdominal pain due to peritoneal metastases** – there is a constant aching pain, and possibly sharp exacerbations. Pain may be worse on movement, and there may be local tenderness or a mass palpable. Treat with analgesics.
- **Soft-tissue invasion** – often there is an aching pain at the site of tumour, and swelling if the site is superficial. Treat with analgesics, NSAIDs and possibly steroids.
- **Neuropathic pain** – this is a constant or intermittent stabbing or burning pain, often in a dermatomal distribution associated with altered sensation, which is usually caused by nerve compression or infiltration. Treat with analgesics and antidepressants, anticonvulsants or antiarrhythmics for their pain-modifying action and consider steroids if nerve compression may be involved.
- **Headache of raised intracranial pressure** – headache may be localized or general. Reduce oedema with dexamethasone or possibly radiotherapy. Analgesia may require paracetamol or opioid.
- **Epidural spinal cord compression from metastatic disease** – pain is localized to the vertebral body with possible radicular pain in a dermatome and sensory changes and progressive weakness in the limbs. Bladder and bowel sphincter symptoms occur late. Treat with dexamethasone and radiotherapy and consider spinal decompression.

- **Painful muscle spasm** – painful spasm and muscle contractures can occur in a limb following a hemiplegia, or in the presence of a painful metastasis in a long bone. Treat with diazepam or baclofen.
- **Infection of a fungating tumour** – bacterial superficial soft-tissue infection can be very painful, often when the tumour itself has not been painful. Treat with appropriate antibiotics following microbiological swab for culture and sensitivity.
- **Pain related to treatment** – for example, postsurgical incisional pain, postradiation mucositis or proctitis and painful peripheral neuropathy following chemotherapy. Treatment depends on the nature of the problem.

## Common causes of non-cancer-related pain

- Osteoarthritis
- Simple tension headache
- Constipation
- Oral or oesophageal thrush
- Pleurisy
- Infected pressure sore
- Distended bladder
- Iatrogenic causes
- Adverse drug reactions.

# Analgesics

## The World Health Organization analgesic ladder

The use of different classes of analgesic drugs has been promoted by the World Health Organization (WHO) for some years by the use of the WHO analgesic ladder.[1] This involves the progression from a

- Non-opioid analgesic (for example, paracetamol) to a
- Weak opioid (for example, co-proxamol) to a
- Strong opioid (for example, morphine).

At every stage in the analgesic ladder the use of co-analgesics such as NSAIDs, antidepressants, anticonvulsants and benzodiazepines is important to optimize analgesia.

Note: The term *opioid* refers to all drugs, both naturally occurring and synthetic, that have morphine-like activity and are antagonized by naloxone. *Opiate* refers to naturally occurring drugs obtained from the poppy, such as morphine and codeine. Thus, morphine is both an opioid and an opiate, while a synthetic drug such as diamorphine is only an opioid.

## Non-opioid analgesics

For mild pain initial treatment with paracetamol is appropriate. The dose is normally 1 g 4-hourly to a maximum of 4 g/day, although a dose frequency of five times a day is commonly used in palliative medicine.[2]

## Weak opioids

If pain is not controlled by paracetamol, use of a weak opioid is required, this being the next step up the WHO analgesic ladder. Various weak opioids are available, for example, co-proxamol (dextropropoxyphene 32.5 mg and paracetamol 325 mg), dihydrocodeine and combinations

**259**

of dihydrocodeine and paracetamol. Co-proxamol is commonly used in palliative care settings with a dose of two tablets five times a day being used regularly.[2] If analgesia is not obtained with one weak opioid, there is no benefit to be obtained by changing to another drug of the same class, and so a strong opioid should be used.

## Strong opioids

### Morphine
Morphine is the strong opioid of choice.

- **Preparations** – there are several different preparations available in the UK. There is an immediate-release elixir administered every 4 hours made in two different strengths, and an immediate-release tablet administered every 4 hours with three tablet sizes. Slow-release tablets and capsules acting over 12 hours and a slow-release suspension acting over 12 hours are also available. Slow-release 24-hour capsules are used less commonly. The slow-release preparations are produced in several different strengths.
- **Morphine pharmacology and metabolism** – morphine acts in the brain and spinal cord and is a mu opioid receptor agonist. Morphine is well absorbed from the gastrointestinal tract, mainly in the proximal small bowel. There is extensive first-pass metabolism, which leads to a reduced bioavailability of oral morphine when compared with parenteral use. Morphine is metabolized to morphine-3-glucuronide and then to the active analgesic metabolite, morphine-6-glucuronide (M6G). M6G is excreted by the kidney and accumulates in patients with renal failure when a reduction in dose and increase in dose interval may be required.
- **Administration of morphine** – if possible, morphine is given by mouth at regular 4-hourly intervals, five times a day, and the aim of the treatment is to keep the patient pain-free all the time. The patient's response to treatment should be monitored frequently, and the dose altered according to response. There is a direct relationship between dose and response and, with an opioid-responsive pain, no ceiling dose. The dose can range from 2.5 mg 4-hourly to 500 mg or more 4-hourly, although very few patients will need such high doses. Most patients will need less than 200 mg in 24 hours.
- **Starting dose of morphine** – this is 10 mg 4-hourly but the starting dose should be reduced to 5 mg in the elderly or those with known renal failure. Morphine elixir or immediate-release tablets are normally used initially because of the speed of onset and ease of manipulation. Morphine should be given regularly, 4-hourly, *five times a day*, and increases of 33–50% be made when increasing the dose, e.g. 10 mg to 15 mg; to 20 mg; to 30 mg; to 40 mg; to 60 mg. The patient should be reviewed frequently, particularly when treatment is initiated. Patients may well need increases of the regular 4-hourly dose and top-up doses for breakthrough pain of the same size as the regular dose before analgesia is achieved. Dose increases are normally made every 1–2 days and should take account of the breakthrough doses needed. The majority of patients do not need a dose in the middle of the night. Regular assessment of pain and titration of the dose are continued until pain control is achieved. If pain continues, it is important to increase the dose and not the frequency. The use of 4-hourly dosing meaning five times a day is very important.
- **Long-term treatment** – once satisfactory analgesia is achieved, many patients will be able to change to slow-release tablets or capsules given twice a day, although some patients will prefer to continue the 4-hourly elixir or tablets. Conversion to slow-release medication is done by totalling the 24-hour dose of morphine, dividing by two and giving this dose as a slow-release preparation twice a day. Once stable, some patients will continue on the same morphine dose, but many will need gradual increases of the dose as their disease progresses. Top-up doses of immediate release morphine may still be needed occasionally for breakthrough pain.

## Alternatives to oral morphine

The various alternatives to morphine can be useful when the side-effects of morphine are difficult to control, such as nausea and vomiting, or when confusion and drowsiness are major problems. Pain control may improve swapping from one opioid to another, a process known as opioid switch.[3]

- Fentanyl is primarily a μ-opioid receptor agonist and is available as a transdermal patch in which the duration of action of the patches is 3 days. It is available in four patch strengths releasing 25, 50, 75 and 100 μg per hour and is particularly useful in patients who find swallowing difficult. (For conversion ratios see the British National Formulary.[4]) There may be a lower incidence of constipation, nausea and vomiting, drowsiness and confusion when compared with morphine.[5] Fentanyl is also produced as a lozenge for absorption through the buccal mucosa – oral transmucosal fentanyl citrate (OTFC). It is useful for breakthrough pain when a patient is on transdermal fentanyl or other opioids.[6] The dose of OTFC appears to be unrelated to the regular opioid dose. The lozenges come in strengths ranging from 200 to 1600 μg. Fentanyl may be useful in patients with renal failure.
- Oxycodone is a κ-opioid receptor agonist and may help some pains which have responded poorly to the μ-agonist action of morphine.[7] Oxycodone is available as an immediate release liquid or tablet and also as a slow release preparation. 5 mg oxycodone is equivalent to 10 mg morphine.
- Methadone is a μ- and δ-opioid receptor agonist and is available as 5 mg tablets or a liquid preparation and is given 8–12 hourly, or possibly less frequently. It may be useful in patients with pain poorly responsive to morphine. It has variable metabolism and can accumulate and cause problems with side-effects, and is therefore best used only by doctors with experience of its use. Methadone may be useful in patients with renal failure.
- Hydromorphone is a μ-receptor agonist available as immediate- and slow-release capsules and is an alternative to morphine, which may have a different side-effect profile within individual patients. It is about seven times more potent than morphine.
- Dextromoramide has short durations of action, which may be useful for painful procedures.

## Side-effects of strong opioids

- Nausea or vomiting occurs in many patients taking opioids and often lasts for 3 or 4 days. It can be controlled with haloperidol 1.5 mg daily or metoclopramide 10 mg tds, which may later be stopped. If nausea persists it may be due to causes other than the opioid.
- Drowsiness occurs commonly at the start of treatment with opioids but usually only lasts for a few days, although it can recur with increased doses of morphine.
- Hallucinations and confusion may occur, particularly in elderly patients. If these problems continue to be troublesome, a switch to an alternative strong opioid may be necessary.[3] Dehydration may also contribute to the toxicity of opioids and subcutaneous fluids are sometimes used for rehydration.
- Constipation occurs in virtually every patient on an opioid and prophylactic treatment with laxatives is almost mandatory. Co-danthramer or co-danthrusate or a combination of lactulose and senna are most commonly used. Rectal measures such as suppositories or enemas may also be needed.
- Occasional problems occur with a dry mouth (also consider oral *Candida*), sweating, itch and myoclonic jerks (reduce opioid dose or switch to another, and consider midazolam).
- Addiction to opioids is an occasional concern for the prescribing doctor or for the patient. It is not a significant practical problem, provided the treatment is given appropri-

ately. Psychological addiction, i.e. active drug-seeking behaviour, is almost never seen in practice and an increased demand for morphine usually reflects an increased need for analgesia.
- Respiratory depression is seen very rarely if opioid doses are increased with care and in response to the clinical situation. If respiratory depression does occur, the dose should be reduced and biochemical evidence of renal failure sought.
The use of naloxone to reverse the effects of opioids may result in an alert patient, but one in considerable pain. It may be simpler to discontinue the opioid and observe the patient.

### Subcutaneous administration of opioids using the syringe driver

The oral route is preferred for the administration of opioids but subcutaneous administration using a portable syringe driver will become necessary for many patients.[8] This will be required in cases of:

- Uncontrolled nausea and vomiting
- Dysphagia
- Progressive weakness leading to an inability to swallow medication.

The syringe driver is a small and unobtrusive device, which does not interfere with the patient's contact with his or her family in the same way that, for example, an intravenous infusion does. The dose of opioid required for 24 hours is placed in the syringe and the syringe driver delivers the drugs continuously over 24 hours via a butterfly needle.

- Diamorphine is normally used as the opioid of choice subcutaneously because of its greater solubility compared with morphine. There is debate about the relative potency of oral morphine and subcutaneous diamorphine. Some centres use a 3:1 conversion ratio, with 15 mg oral morphine being equivalent to 5 mg subcutaneous diamorphine. Other centres use a 2:1 ratio. In clinical practice, the patient's response to changing treatment is most important, and doses often require increasing as disease progresses.
- Nausea and vomiting may be treated by adding antiemetics, such as haloperidol (5–10 mg over 24 hours), cyclizine (100–150 mg over 24 hours), metoclopramide (10–40 mg over 24 hours) or levomepromazine (6.25–50 mg over 24 hours) to the syringe driver.
- Gastrointestinal obstruction occurs in some patients with intra-abdominal malignancy – intermittent or complete obstruction with vomiting and colicky abdominal pain may occur. Vomiting can normally be controlled using the antiemetics as described above, administered subcutaneously via a syringe driver. The bowel stimulant action of metoclopramide may make vomiting worse in cases of high bowel obstruction and is, therefore, not commonly used in such situations. Colicky pain can be controlled using hyoscine hydrobromide (20–40 mg over 24 hours). An opioid analgesic will frequently also be required.
- Anxiety and distress that are not due to treatable causes, for example, pain or distended bladder or rectum, may be controlled using midazolam (20–100 mg in 24 hours) in the syringe driver.

# Co-analgesics

Co-analgesics are drugs used with, or instead of, analgesics to enhance pain control. The drugs may or may not have intrinsic analgesic activity.

## Non-steroidal anti-inflammatory drugs

Non-steroidal anti-inflammatory drugs are frequently used for controlling pain for metastatic bone disease. Optimum doses should be used and change to an alternative NSAID considered if one is not successful. Radiotherapy may also be helpful in bone pain. Diclofenac may be used subcutaneously. There is a risk of gastric and duodenal ulceration, particularly if NSAIDs are used at the same time as steroids. Appropriate gastro-protection with an $H_2$-antagonist, proton pump inhibitor or prostaglandin analogue should be considered. NSAIDs will often be part of the treatment for advanced cancer pain as most pains have an inflammatory element and will respond, to some degree, to NSAIDs.

## Steroids

Steroids have a place in pain control in several settings in advanced cancer. The predominant effect is due to a decrease in oedema surrounding a tumour mass, which reduces the pressure caused by the tumour mass and improves pain control. Dexamethasone is usually used because of its greater (7-fold) potency compared with prednisolone. For liver metastases, dexamethasone in a dose of 4–8 mg/day should be used in conjunction with an analgesic. Nerve compression pain may respond to opioid and non-opioid analgesics and the addition of steroids (dexamethasone may be used at 4–12 mg/day) may improve pain control. Headache caused by raised intracranial pressure secondary to peritumour oedema, whether due to primary or secondary disease, responds well to dexamethasone in often quite high doses, for example, up to 24 mg/day. The lowest possible maintenance dose should be used once symptoms are controlled. Analgesics may also be necessary to control the headache. Steroids should be given early in the day as patients may experience insomnia due to their stimulant effect. The response to treatment should be closely monitored and doses reduced if possible. If no benefit is noted, the steroids should be discontinued. Side-effects, particularly the moonface of Cushing's syndrome, and the development of or disturbance of control of diabetes may cause some problems with continued usage of steroids.

## Antidepressants and anticonvulsants

Antidepressants and anticonvulsants can be used for neuropathic pain. Neuropathic pain is often difficult to control satisfactorily. The pain may be described as a burning or stabbing pain in a dermatomal distribution associated with altered sensation. Neuropathic pain may be due to invasion or compression of nerves by tumour, or may be indirectly related to the cancer as a paraneoplastic syndrome, or may be treatment-related, for example, chemotherapy induced neuropathy.

Neuropathic pain commonly has one of three basic characters:

- Continuous burning pain
- Intermittent stabbing or shooting pain
- Allodynia – light touch, for example, clothing-causing pain.

Analgesics, often opioids, may have some effect on the pain and may be used initially, but other drugs that have a pain-modifying action will often be needed.[10] An antidepressant (for example, amitriptyline 10–75 mg at night) may be used for constant burning pain. An anticonvulsant may be appropriate for intermittent pain. The three most commonly used anti-convulsants are carbamazepine (200–800 mg/day), gabapentin (300 mg increasing to 1800 mg/day) and sodium valproate (400–1200 mg/day). The benefits are often limited by side-effects. Steroids may also improve the control of neuropathic pain, e.g. dexamethasone 4–12 mg/day.

## Muscle relaxants

Muscle relaxants (diazepam/baclofen) may be necessary to control the uncomfortable muscle spasm which may follow a painful bone metastasis or hemiplegia secondary to a brain tumour.

## Bisphosphonates

There is good evidence to support the use of bisphosphonates to improve the pain of metastatic bone disease.[11] Intravenous infusions of pamidronate (60–90 mg) clodronate (1500 mg) or zolendronic acid (4 mg) are given every 3–4 weeks.

## Other medication for neuropathic pain

Other medication for neuropathic pain – ketamine,[12] clonidine, mexiletine, oxycodone and methadone may all help patients with neuropathic pain. Specialist advice should be sought before using these drugs.

# Psychological Support

## Depression

Depression is common in people with advanced cancer, but poorly diagnosed and under-treated. A depressed patient will have pain that is harder to control, and the use of antidepressants should be made early in a person's illness.

Anxieties and fears about the illness, its complications and prognosis can be addressed by honest and effective communication between patient and doctor.[13,14] Some patients need support and guidance in developing coping strategies. The palliative care team social workers have a major role to play in this area.

Support from family and friends is vital, and it is much easier in an atmosphere of full knowledge and understanding of the problem presented. Collusion (the hiding of knowledge) between patient and family can be very destructive, and addressing it often improves the pain control as well as family relationships.

Chaplains and other ministers may be very helpful as patients may have great spiritual and existential difficulties. Some patients become angry with God, or have other anxieties about their faith.

For some patients the problems of changes in body image and sexuality, and the financial concerns brought about by terminal illness have a significant impact on levels of pain.

## Effective communication with patients

Patients need their health carers to have high quality communication skills, to enable accurate and clear information to be given to patients and also to elicit the concerns patients have about the diagnosis, treatment and prognosis. Good quality communication will reduce the level of pain experienced and increase the patient's quality of life.[13,14] The communication skills of health care professionals can be improved by training courses.

# Other therapies

## Complementary therapies

Some patients may benefit from massage or aromatherapy massage as part of their pain control and relaxation management.[15]

## Transcutaneous electrical nerve stimulation

Transcutaneous electrical nerve stimulation may help to control the pain of advanced malignancy. TENS stimulates peripheral nerves via the intact skin using two small electrodes connected to a portable stimulator. It may help the pain of bone metastases, visceral pain or neuropathic pain. Similar benefit may also be obtained from acupuncture.

## The team approach

For some patients pain control is achieved by the work of other members of the team, for example, chaplain, physiotherapist, occupational therapist, art therapist and other members of staff.

## Spinal opioids and local anaesthetics and nerve blocks

Spinal opioids and/or local anaesthetics (either intrathecal or epidural) can be used on occasions. Opioid side-effects are less than with oral administration as doses are lower, and better pain control has been reported in some cases. Improved analgesia may occur with the addition of local anaesthetic. Peripheral nerve blocks, such as interpleural and intercostal blocks, may also help the pain of advanced malignant disease. Advice should be sought from specialist anaesthetists experienced in pain control (see also Chapter 33).

## Active treatments

It is important to consider active anticancer treatments as possible pain control measures, including:

- Radiotherapy for the pain of bone metastases, headache from brain tumours, nerve compression pain and soft-tissue infiltration
- Chemotherapy for control of small-cell lung cancer and locally advanced breast cancer
- Hormone manipulation for carcinoma of breast or prostate
- Prophylactic orthopaedic pinning of a metastasis in a long bone to prevent a fracture
- Surgery for the formation of a stoma or a bypass procedure to relieve bowel obstruction.

Advice from colleagues in oncology and surgery should be requested if appropriate.

## Professional support

A network of support services for patients with advanced cancer is available throughout the UK. Most acute trusts have hospital-based palliative care teams of nurse specialists, consultant physicians and other professionals. Referral of hospital patients to these teams is often helpful to both patient and medical and nursing staff. Most cities and towns have local hospice services offering inpatient and home care facilities. The community clinical nurse specialists and physicians visit patients and families at home and provide advice on pain and symptom control to the primary care team. Psychosocial support is offered to the patient and family.

Many organizations exist to provide support and information to patients. In addition to the nationwide charity *Cancer BACUP* many local support and self-help groups are in existence.

# References

1. World Health Organisation. National Cancer Control Programmes. Policies and managerial guidelines. Geneva: World Health Organisation, 2002.

2. Hanks GW, Justins DM. Cancer pain: management. *Lancet* **339**: 1031–1036, 1992

3. Zeppetella G, Bates C. Expert clinical opinion for the utility of opioid switching. In: Hillier R, Finlay I, Miles A, eds. *The Effective Management of Cancer Pain, 2nd edition*. London: Aesculapius Medical Press, 2002

4. British Medical Association and the Royal Pharmaceutical Society of Great Britain. *British National Formulary, 45th edition*. London: British Medical Association, 2003

5. Ahmedzai S, Brooks D. Transdermal fentanyl versus sustained-release oral morphine in cancer pain: preference, efficacy and quality of life. *J Pain Symptom Manage* **13**: 254–261, 1997

6. Coluzzi PH, Schwartzberg L, Conroy JD, et al. Breakthrough cancer pain: a randomised trial comparing oral transmucosal fentanyl citrate (OTFC) and morphine sulfate immediate release (MSIR). *Pain* **91**: 123–130, 2001

7. Watson CPN, Babul N. Efficacy of oxycodone in neuropathic pain. *Neurology* **50**: 1837–1841, 1998

8. Dickman A, Littlewood C, Varga J. *The Syringe Driver. Continuous Subcutaneous Infusion in Palliative Care*. Oxford: Oxford University Press, 2002

9. Amesbury B. Converting from oral morphine to subcutaneous diamorphine. *Palliat Med* **14**: 165–166, 2000

10. Makin M, Smith J. Scientific evidence and expert clinical opinion for the use of co-analgesics. In: Hillier R, Finlay I, Miles A, eds. *The Effective Management of Cancer Pain, 2nd edition*. London: Aesculapius Medical Press, 2002

11. Mannix K, Ahmedzai SH, Anderson H, et al. Using bisphosphonates to control the pain of bone metastases: evidence-based guidelines for palliative care. *Palliat Med* **14**: 455–461, 2000

12. Finlay I. Ketamine and its role in cancer pain. *Pain Reviews* **6**: 303–313, 1999

13. Faulkner A, Maguire P. *Talking to Cancer Patients and Their Families*. Oxford: Oxford Medical Publications, 1994

14. Walker G, Bradburn J, Maher J. *Breaking Bad News*. London: King's Fund Publishing, 1996

15. Buckley J. Massage and aromatherapy massage: nursing art and science. *Int J Palliat Nursing* **8**: 276–280, 2002

# Further Reading

Doyle D, Hanks GW, MacDonald N, eds. *Oxford Textbook of Palliative Medicine, 2nd edn*. Oxford: Oxford University Press, 1999

Regnard CFB, Tempest S. *A Guide to Symptom Relief in Advanced Disease, 4th edn*. Manchester: Haigh & Hochland, 1998

Twycross RG, Wilcox A. *Symptom Management in Advanced Cancer, 3rd edn*. Oxford: Radcliffe Medical Press Ltd, 2001

Twycross RG, Wilcox A, Charlesworth S, Dickman A. *Palliative Care Formulary, 2nd edition*. Oxford: Radcliffe Medical Press, 2002

# 30 Palliative Care: Interventional Approach

## Karen H Simpson

## Cancer pain

Worldwide, there are more than 9 million patients with cancer related pain. The prevalence of pain in cancer varies with the nature of the cancer, the stage of the disease and the assessment methods used. More than 50% of patients with cancer in hospitals and hospices have pain; advanced disease is painful in more than 75% of cases.[1] Most patients with cancer have more than one site of pain, therefore, it is unlikely that simple interventions can provide a total or permanent solution. Breakthrough pain (flares of pain that interrupt controlled background pain) and incident pain (pain on movement) are common, and often difficult to manage; these are more likely to need interventional treatments. Rapidly escalating pain is an emergency that requires prompt assessment and intervention. Different issues are involved in the assessment and treatment of pain at the end of life, when complex interventional techniques may become inappropriate.

Children with cancer pain need special consideration, for example age-appropriate assessment tools, staff training and availability of therapies for procedure-related pain. Interventional methods of pain control are often technically challenging in small children. The elderly and those with learning difficulties who have cancer pain may have several problems, such as cognitive impairment, effects of co-morbidity on drug handling and use of polypharmacy. Non-drug pain management therapies may be appropriate in these groups.

Adequate pain relief can be achieved by at least 75% of cancer patients who receive optimal analgesic management using simple techniques, such as those suggested by the World Health Organization analgesic ladder (see Chapter 29). An important barrier to good pain management is lack of knowledge about basic analgesic drugs, rather than failure to use interventional therapies. Pain management services can play an important role in the education of health care professionals.

## Palliative care

Palliative care is defined as the active, total care of the patient with active progressive life-threatening disease.[2,3] It involves a variety of health care professionals who work as a multi-professional team. Palliative care provides a model for continuing management, including control of pain and symptoms, maintenance of function, psychosocial and spiritual support for the patient and family, and comprehensive care at the end of life. Specialist pain management should form part of good palliative care. It is vital that pain specialists are integrated into the total care of the patient, and that they liaise with primary care, oncology and palliative care services. If interventional pain management techniques are to be used, it is important that appropriate education and facilities exist in palliative care units and the community for the ongoing management of the patient. It is not acceptable to use such techniques until appropriate ongoing care is organized.

# Assessment of cancer pain

Definition of the extent of disease and the nature of the underlying aetiology of the pain is important.[4–6] An accurate history, a full physical examination, a review of laboratory and radiographic tests, and appropriate further investigations are mandatory before planning pain management. Patients with malignant disease may have altered anatomy and physiology, due to weight loss or tumour progression, which is important when considering interventions. An increase in pain intensity following a stable period necessitates new evaluation of the underlying aetiology. Some emergencies in cancer patients may present with pain (e.g. back pain due to spinal cord compression, pathological fractures); these need prompt evaluation and treatment. Specific methods of investigating cancer pain – e.g. ultrasound, radioisotope, single photon emission computerized tomography (SPECT), computed tomography (CT), positron emission tomography (PET) and magnetic resonance imaging (MRI) with biopsy – should be used if necessary. These may be particularly relevant if interventional techniques are planned. Comprehensive assessment must consider other medical problems, physical function and psychosocial and spiritual issues. It is important to be aware of cultural differences in the presentation, reaction to life-threatening illness and acceptance of and response to therapies.

Syndrome recognition is an essential part of pain assessment, as this may provide information relevant to treatment and prognosis. Common pain syndromes can be due to direct effects of tumour (e.g. bone metastases), anticancer therapies (e.g. surgery, drugs), general debility (e.g. pressure sores) and from factors unrelated to the disease or its treatment (e.g. osteoarthritis). The contribution of chemical and mechanical factors with skeletal, neural and soft tissue pathology should be assessed. Factors other than pain are important, including physical symptoms (e.g. fatigue, nausea, anorexia and constipation), coexistent psychological symptoms and psychiatric disorders (e.g. anxiety and depression), functional status, family dynamics, spirituality, social support systems, medical support systems and financial resources.[13] Pain predominantly sustained by psychological factors appears to be rare in the cancer population. However, psychological factors are important in determining the impact of the pain on the patient's life and their response to pain. Patients with long-standing chronic pain from a benign condition, who then develop pain from cancer, can be difficult to manage; these patients may be referred to the pain management specialist. In this situation, behavioural issues should be addressed in parallel with any interventional technique.

# Management of cancer pain[7–11]

It is important to use and develop evidence-based practice in the management of cancer pain, however, much of the evidence is incomplete. Clinicians often need to make treatment decisions based on less robust evidence, particularly when considering interventional methods. The use of any strategy for analgesia requires careful evaluation of the appropriateness, feasibility, benefits, burdens and risks.[12] Adequate explanation and consent is an important part of pain management. Interventional pain therapies must be integrated into the oncological management of the patient, this may include both primary anticancer therapy and palliative care. Therapies aimed at the underlying pathology may also be useful in the management of cancer pain, including radiotherapy, pharmacotherapy (e.g. chemotherapy, hormonal, biological and antibiotic therapy), and surgery. Other medical problems (e.g. anaemia, infection and hypercalcaemia) may require treatment.

## Drug treatment[3,7,11]

Most patients with cancer pain can be effectively managed with an optimal oral opioid regimen and co-analgesics. Some patients who are unable to achieve a favorable balance between opioid analgesia and side-effects require an alternative approach. Other patients may be unable to swallow or absorb drugs enterally, thus limiting prescribing. Patients with end-stage disease, cachexia or hepatorenal compromise may have altered analgesic drug handling. Coincident use of steroids, chemotherapy or biological therapies may narrow analgesic options, for example, non-steroidal anti-inflammatory drugs (NSAIDs) may be contraindicated. Patients often achieve better pain control if drug therapy is integrated with other analgesic modalities (multimodal therapy).

## Specialist pain management techniques

Nerve blocks or spinal drugs may be used when pain is localized to specific dermatomes or involves the sympathetic nervous system. The patient must be well enough to tolerate the procedure and benefit from its effects. When a nerve block is performed, it may then be necessary to reduce the patient's analgesic drugs to prevent side-effects. Sepsis or uncorrectable coagulopathy contraindicates most interventional treatments. Spinal cord compression is an important risk that must be considered in all patients undergoing spinal injection.

### Nerve and plexus blocks[9,12]

Simple nerve blocks using local anaesthetic, with or without depot steroid, can be useful in the management of cancer pain (e.g. infiltration of localized painful primary or metastatic tumour). Many common painful conditions can be treated in this way, such as trigger points or shoulder, hip, and sacroiliac joint injection. Local anaesthetic blocks may aid diagnosis and localization of the cause of pain, but systemic effects from absorbed local anaesthetic may confound their prognostic value.[13] Incident or breakthrough pain, for example, from a pathological fracture or an acutely ischaemic limb, may be relieved using local or regional techniques. A brachial plexus, lumbar plexus, intrapleural, epidural or spinal injection, or temporary catheter may give relief and allow time for alternative treatment to be instituted.

### Spinal drug delivery

Patients with pain responsive to oral opioids, but with intolerable side-effects, may be candidates for spinal drugs.[14] Epidural or intrathecal drugs can be delivered long term by percutaneous or fully implanted infusion systems; these can be highly effective for cancer pain. There is some very preliminary evidence of increased survival in those with implantable pumps.[15] Before embarking on such treatment, it is imperative that there is a system for caring for catheters and infusion devices for prolonged periods in a hospice or palliative care setting, or in the community. This requires investment in education, equipment and reliably produced, stable and sterile drug supplies.

A variety of opioids have been used spinally, such as morphine, diamorphine, hydromorphone, and fentanyl. Time to onset, duration of action, uptake, distribution and side-effects depend on the opioid pharmacokinetics and receptor affinity. Recommendations have been made about the choice of drugs, generally favouring a trial of opioids first.[16] Conversion of oral to spinal doses of opioid can be difficult, and each patient must be individually treated. The usual rule is oral: epidural: intrathecal 100:10:1. It is best to estimate the dose in the lower range and then titrate up. Usually, the oral opioid dose is immediately reduced by 50%, and then reduced further as the spinal dose increases. Whist cancer pain is often an urgent issue, it is rarely an emergency, and so dosage titration should not be rushed. If one opioid is not effective, or the patient becomes tolerant to it, then switching to another opioid may be worthwhile. The side-effects of opioids include nausea, vomiting, urinary retention, pruritus, constipation, sedation, confusion, myoclonus, polyarthralgia, endocrine dysfunction, and peripheral oedema. Some opioids have adverse effects on immune function; the significance of this in cancer pain is unknown. Care is needed in those who do not have opioid-responsive pain (e.g. brachial or lumbar plexopathies). If there is no response to spinal opioid alone, then addition of other drugs may be useful. Spinal clonidine provides potent analgesia whether used alone or in combination with opioids. The main side-effects are hypotension, dry mouth, drowsiness, dizziness, and constipation. Sudden withdrawal of clonidine can precipitate agitation and hypertension. Intrathecal bupivacaine is useful and neurological side-effects do not usually occur with less than 25 mg per 24 hours.[17] The use of ropivacaine or levobupivacaine would be expected to reduce side-effects, but there is no evidence for this.[18] If large volume infusions are anticipated, then external pumps may be preferable as internal systems usually have small chambers.

There is controversy about the relative merits of intrathecal and epidural drug administration. Large-volume epidural injections or infusions may precipitate spinal cord compression. Epidural invasion by tumour is common and can compromise epidural drug delivery.[19] Changes in the amount of epidural fat in those with cancer can influence drug handling. Catheters placed in the epidural space are more likely to become blocked by fibrosis than intrathecal catheters; this may lead to loss of analgesia. Epidural catheters have a high rate of infection and technical complications. In a study of 91 patients with 137 epidural catheters over a period of 4326 catheter days, 43% had technical complications and 12 patients had deep infections.[20] Intrathecal drugs do not have to pass the physical barrier of the dura to get to their site of action and so can be used in lower doses. This is an important advantage when considering the frequency of syringe driver changes necessary to maintain analgesia with an external system. It is the only method of drug delivery possible when using fully implanted systems. The intrathecal route produces more problems in the first 20 days, but, thereafter, the complication rate for epidural rises to 55% and intrathecal falls to 5%. Cerebrospinal fluid (CSF) leak is the main intrathecal complication within the first 20 days, and epidurals frequently obstruct or dislodge after the first 20 days.[21] The intrathecal route does not pose a greater infection risk than epidural drug delivery. There is no evidence that externalized, tunnelled intrathecal catheters have a higher infection risk than epidural catheters. In a study of 200 adults with external intrathecal catheters treated for 1–575 days, where there were defined protocols for catheter care, 93% had perfect function of the system.[22] However, occult infection may be more common than is realized: about 20% cultures from cassettes, syringes and filters may be colonized without clinical evidence of infection. Pathogens are usually skin flora. The only factor significantly associated with infection is prolonged catheter placement time. The catheter hub is the most common site for entry of infection with external systems; to reduce this, filter changes should be done monthly, as a minimum. Overall, intrathecal drug delivery provides better pain control and fewer complications than epidural drug administration.[23] It has lower incidence of catheter occlusion, lower malfunction rate, lower dose requirement, fewer side-effects and better pain control.

Silicone-rubber intrathecal catheters have been used as a cost-effective method for spinal drug delivery for patients with a limited prognosis (less than 1 month). Implantation can be performed under local anaesthesia and sedation. Catheters should be tunnelled to reduce the risk of dislodgement. Drug delivery is possible by bolus injections, continuous infusion or patient-controlled administration. Disadvantages include catheter migration, kinking, dislodgement, or other mechanical problems. There is a risk of infection, especially in those with stomas or immune compromise. A single dose of antibiotic should be given at catheter insertion. Local guidelines on catheter care can limit complications.

Fully implantable intrathecal infusion pumps should probably be used for patients who are likely to survive for longer. It takes some time to recover from the procedure, and so is inappropriate in those with only a few weeks to live. In the future, infusion devices may have the facility for patients to self-administer bolus doses, which could be helpful in managing breakthrough pain. Health economic data suggests that a prognosis of 3–4 months is reasonable.[24] The normal battery life of a programmable pump depends on the flow rate, and is about 5–7 years. It is important to test the patient's response to spinal opioids before implanting a system. There are many different approaches to efficacy trials. Some practitioners only use the epidural approach and others, only the intrathecal approach. Some use daily sequential bolus dosing, increasing the dose daily until the appropriate dose is attained, while others use continuous infusions. Some believe that the trial should include a single-blinded placebo control, either given as a bolus or as a continuous infusion. Whatever the method for trial that is chosen, the trial must be adequate for the practitioner and patient to make a rational decision regarding the efficacy of the impending implantation. Refilling of the pump is performed through the central fill port. It is important not to avoid inadvertent subcutaneous injection of the highly concentrated drug mixture, as this would produce disastrous side-effects. Reprogramming errors can be reduced by careful protocols for checking. Overfilling, battery failure, pump failure and flipping of a freely movable pump can occur. Cerebrospinal fluid leaks can occur around the intrathecal catheter and may cause headache or cerebrospinal fluid hygromas. Most of these are self limiting, and draining of the fluid is unnecessary and may lead to contamination of the fluid. Pump pocket seromas are usually self limiting, and should not be drained unless they are causing problems. Mechanical catheter complications include breaking, dislodgement, kinking, disconnection and obstruction at the tip. After careful aspiration of the catheter, simple injection of non-ionic contrast into the pump side port may help in the diagnosis. As the patient approaches the end of life, the pain may change in character or distribution. The small pump reservoir may mean that, at this stage, an alternative method of analgesia must be used. It is important not to try to rely on the pump to solve a pain problem that it was never intended to manage, but to be ready to use other methods as an adjunct or even an alternative.

Although serious complications are extremely rare when a system for safe practice of spinal analgesia has been implemented, spinal infection and bleeding can occur, with potentially disastrous consequences. Long-term catheter placement close to the spinal cord may lead to the growth of expanding sterile granulomas around the catheter tip, which may cause cord compression and myelopathy. It is mandatory to have a system for monitoring for early signs of these complications, which can include leukocytosis, back pain, increasing leg weakness or bladder problems, and a system for rapid action should such symptoms occur. Early recognition, contrast enhanced MRI, and early surgery are important in treating bleeding or infection. Infections can be disastrous; therefore, strict asepsis, preoperative antibiotics and vigilance are mandatory. If infection involves the implant, failure to remove it can lead to persistence and spread of the infection.

## Neurolytic blocks

Nerve destruction is a simple, single, often effective intervention that is usually cheap. However, serious complications, including severe neurological deficits, are possible. Duration of analgesia after a neurolytic block is limited to about 3–6 months; but some blocks can be successfully repeated. Gasserian ganglion block using glycerol under fluoroscopy may be useful, but corneal anesthesia can occur, and inadvertent intrathecal injection may cause serious complications and death. Most neurolytic blocks of peripheral nerves should be reserved for patients with life expectancy of 1 year or less, as neuropathic pain may develop. An example would be phenol block of the intercostal nerves for a single anteriorly placed rib metastasis. Sympathetic blocks, and possibly subarachnoid neurolysis, less commonly cause lasting deafferentation pain, and may be considered in those with longer life expectancy.

Coeliac plexus block is effective for visceral cancer pain in the upper abdomen, where opioid therapy is often ineffective and usually complicated by emesis.[25] It should be considered early whilst the patient is fit enough to tolerate the technique. Coeliac plexus block alone will not relieve pain due to tumour infiltration of the posterior abdominal wall that involves somatic afferent nerves. Fluoroscopic guidance should be used for the percutaneous technique, but some clinicians use CT or ultrasound guidance as alternatives to fluoroscopy. Injection of 50 ml 50% alcohol is performed bilaterally anterior to the L1 vertebra. In 73–92%

of cases, at least partial relief is maintained until death.[26–28] Reports of poor or short-lasting pain relief may be due to an insufficient injected volume of alcohol.[25,27] Intraoperative coeliac plexus block improves pain, reduces opioid analgesic consumption, improves function and increases duration of survival.[29] Transient adverse effects include local pain (96%), diarrhoea (44%) and postural hypotension (38%). If diarrhoea is troublesome, it can be treated with octreotide. Impotence may result. Neurological complications, such as paraplegia and incontinence, can occur but are rare.[30] Patients must be warned of these rare but devastating problems.

Phenol blocks of the superior hypogastric plexus[31,32] or bilateral lumbar sympathetic block may relieve pain from pelvic organs. Local tumour extension may cause somatic nociceptive pain and may limit the effectiveness sympathetic blocks. Neurolytic lumbar sympathectomy can also be useful for ischaemic leg pain in those who are unfit for surgery. Bilateral block has also been used to treat tenesmus from perineal tumour. These techniques are simple, but they must be performed under fluoroscopy. Adverse effects include postural hypotension, lateral thigh pain due to genitofemoral neuritis, impotence, and renal or ureteric trauma. Block of the ganglion of Impair may be useful for pain from pelvic malignancy.

Intrathecal neurolytic block can be performed by subarachnoid injection close to the affected nerve roots with 0.3–0.6 ml hypobaric ethanol (96%) with the patient's painful side up, or hyperbaric phenol (5% in glycerol) with the painful side down. This technique is now used much less often because better pharmacological methods are available that have less risk of severe complications. Saddle block with 0.6 ml phenol in those with a colostomy and permanent bladder catheter is still a simple and useful technique.

## Spinal cord stimulation

The application of spinal cord stimulation (SCS) to cancer pain is very limited.[33] Success is not likely with nociceptive pain especially incident pain. The more widespread the malignancy and the more rapid its progression, the less likely SCS is to be of value. Wide areas of pain or changing pain may mean that many electrodes would be needed with increasingly complex programme. Clearly defined, localized pain or vascular pains are the best indications. Before exploring the use of expensive, invasive procedures, all other techniques should have been tried without success. The patient's life expectancy must be long enough to allow them to benefit from SCS; generally, cost-benefit can be achieved after 3–6 months of treatment. The patient and carers must be well informed about the burdens and benefits of SCS. There must be appropriate follow-up and maintenance organized to allow the use of SCS to be optimized.

## Surgery and interventional radiology[9]

Surgery for those with cancer can provide analgesia, for example, repair of bowel obstruction, stabilization of pathological fracture and vertebrectomy for metastatic disease. Neurosurgical procedures (e.g. thalmotomy, rhizototomy) can be useful for managing cancer pain. Intraventricular infusion of opioid has been used successfully for head and neck cancer pain management.[34] Percutaneous cervical cordotomy can be used in selected patients. Destruction of the anterolateral quadrant of the cervical spinal cord is performed using radiofrequency lesioning with fluoroscopic or CT guidance. Analgesia does not last, and the treatment should be restricted to patients not expected to survive for more than 1 year. It is only suitable for patients with pain below the C5 dermatome. It is very useful for difficult neuropathic pain.[35] Ventilatory depression is a significant complication; reduced ventilatory reserve on the side of the pain is a relative contraindication. Postoperative weakness of the ipsilateral leg occurs in more than 50% of patients, but, at 1 month, weakness is present in less than 2%. Other infrequent complications include ataxia, hemiparesis, headache and hypotension.

## Physical therapies[11,12,36]

Physical therapy can be useful in cancer pain management, for example, prevention of secondary painful myofascial or joint complications in those with weakened limbs. Physical modalities, such as the use of heat or cold, can be used. Non-invasive or minimally invasive stimulatory approaches, including counterirritation, transcutaneous electrical nerve stimulation (TENS) and acupuncture, are used empirically for some patients with cancer pain. These interventions are not supported by a strong evidence base at present.

## Conclusions

- Consider the needs of the patient and coexisting pathology in their social context.
- Assess and record pain regularly and accurately using appropriate tools.
- Allow the patient as much choice and control as possible.
- Consider the benefits and risks in each case.
- Choose evidence-based analgesia when possible.
- Choose methods that fit local needs (e.g. staff skill mix and availability, equipment).
- Choose safe and simple techniques; multimodal analgesia is often the best.
- Monitor and treat adverse effects.
- Educate health care professionals, patients and their carers.

Analgesia for those with cancer pain can be enhanced using techniques other than drugs. Good nursing care and psychological and spiritual support should never be forgotten in the context of total pain control. This approach requires a team of committed professionals working in a complementary way to the patients primary and secondary care teams, providing support and education when required.

## References

1. Hearn J, Higginson IJ. *Epidemiology of pain: pain associated with cancer. Task Force on Epidemiology.* Seattle: IASP Press, 1999
2. Twycross RG. *Symptom Management in Advanced Cancer.* Oxford: Radcliffe Medical Press, 1997
3. Hillier R, Finlay I, Miles A, eds. *Effective Management of Cancer Pain. 2nd edn.* London: Aesculapius Medical Press, 2002
4. Chemy NI, Portenoy RK. *Cancer pain: principles of assessment and pain syndromes.* In: Wall PD, Melzack R, eds, *Textbook of Pain, 4th edn.* Edinburgh: Churchill Livingstone, 1999, pp. 1017–1065
5. Higginson IJ. *Innovations in assessment: epidemiology and assessment of pain in advanced cancer.* Seattle: IASP Press, 1997
6. Ferrante FM, Bedder M, Caplan RA, et al. Practice guidelines for cancer pain management. A report by the American Society of Anesthesiologists Task Force on Pain Management, Cancer Pain Section. *Anesthesiology* 94: 1243–1257, 1996
7. Chemy NI, Portenoy RK. Practical issues in the management of cancer pain. In: Wall PD, Melzack R, eds. *Textbook of Pain, 4th edn.* Edinburgh: Churchill Livingstone, 1999, pp. 1479–1523
8. Hanks G, Portenoy RK, MacDonald N, Forbes K. Difficult pain problems. In: Doyle D, Hanks G, MacDonald N, eds. *Oxford Textbook of Palliative Medicine.* Oxford: Oxford University Press, 1998
9. Simpson KH, Budd K. *Cancer pain management. A comprehensive approach.* Oxford: Oxford University Press, 2000
10. Ashby M, Stoffell D. Therapeutic ratio and defined phase. A framework for ethical decision making in palliative care. *Br Med J* 302: 1322–1324, 1991
11. Doyle D, Hanks GWC, MacDonald N, eds. *Oxford Textbook of Palliative Medicine.* Oxford: Oxford University Press, 1998.
12. Wall PD and Melzack R, eds. *Textbook of Pain, 4th edn.* Edinburgh: Churchill Livingstone, 1999

13. Hogan QH, Abrams SE. Neural blockade for diagnosis and prognosis: A review. *Anesthesiology* **86:** 216–241, 1997

14. Mercadante S. Problems of long-term spinal opioid treatment in advanced cancer patients. *Pain* **1:** 1–13, 1999

15. Staals PS, Smith TJ, Deer TR, et al. Prediction of improved survival in a randomised clinical trial of therapy for refractory cancer pain with an implanted drug delivery system to comprehensive medical management. In: *Abstracts of 10th World Congress on Pain.* Seattle: IASP Press, 2002 pp. 192

16. Bennett C, Burchiel K, Buscher E, et al. Clinical guidelines for intraspinal infusion: report of an expert panel. Poly-Analgesia Consensus Conference. *J Pain Symptom Manage* **20:** S37–43, 2000

17. Van Dongen RTM, Crul BJP, de Bock M. Long term intrathecal infusion of morphine and morphine/bupivacaine mixtures in the treatment of cancer pain: a retrospective analysis of 51 cases. *Pain* **55:** 107–111, 1993

18. Dham P, Lundberg C, Jansen M, et al. Comparison of 0.5% intrathecal bupivacaine with 0.5% intrathecal ropivacaine in the treatment of refractory cancer pain. *Reg Anesth Pain Med* **25:** 480–487, 2000

19. Applegren L, Nordborg C, Sloberg M, et al. Spinal epidural metastasis: implications for spinal analgesia to treat "refractory" cancer pain. *J Pain Symptom Manage* **13:** 25–42, 1997

20. Smitt PS, Tsafka A, Teng-van de Zande F, et al. Outcome and complications of epidural analgesia in patients with chronic cancer pain. *Cancer* **83:** 2015–2022, 1998

21. Crul BJ, Delhaas EM. Technical complications during long-term subarachnoid or epidural administration of morphine in terminally ill cancer patients: a review of 140 cases. *Reg Anesth* **16:** 209–213, 1991

22. Nitescu P, Sjoberg M, Applegren L, et al. Complications of intrathecal opioids and bupivacaine in the treatment of "refractory" cancer pain. *Clin J Pain* **11:** 45–62, 1995

23. Dahm P, Nitescu P, Appelgren L, et al. Efficacy and technical complications of long-term continuous intraspinal infusions of opioid and/or bupivacaine in refractory nonmalignant pain: a comparison between the epidural and the intrathecal approach with externalized or implanted catheters and infusion pumps. *Clin J Pain* **14:** 4–16, 1998

24. Mueller-Schwefe G, Hassenbusch SJ, Reig E. Cost effectiveness of intrathecal therapy for pain. *Neuromodulation* **2:** 77–84, 1999

25. Sharfman WH, Walsh TD. Has the efficacy of celiac plexus block been demonstrated in pancreatic cancer pain? *Pain* **41:** 267–271, 1990

26. Eisenberg E, Carr DB, Chalmers TC. Neurolytic celiac plexus block for treatment of cancer pain: a meta-analysis. *Anesth Analg* **80:** 290–295, 1995

27. Mercadante S, Nicosia F. Celiac block: a reappraisal. *Reg Anesth Pain Med* **23:** 37–48, 1998

28. Coeliac plexus block. *www.jr2.ox.ac.uk/bandolier/booth/painpage/index.html*

29. Lillemo KD, Cameron JL, Kaufman HS, et al. Chemical splanchnicectomy in patients with unresectable pancreatic cancer. *Ann Surg* **217:** 447–457, 1993

30. Davis DD. Incidence of major complications of neurolytic coeliac plexus block. *J Roy Soc Med* **86:** 264–266, 1993

31. de Leon-Casasola OA, Kent E, Lema MJ, et al. Neurolytic superior hypogastric plexus block for chronic pelvic pain associated with cancer. *Pain* **54:** 145–151, 1993

32. Plancarte R, Amescua C, Patt RB, et al. Superior hypogastric plexus block for pelvic cancer pain. *Anesthesiology* **73:** 236–239, 1990

33. Simpson B. Spinal cord and deep brain stimulation. In: Wall PD, Melzack R, eds. *Textbook of Pain,* 4th edn. Edinburgh: Churchill Livingstone, 1999, pp. 1353–1383.

34. Ballentyne JC, Carr DB, Berkey CS, et al. Comparison of the efficacy of epidural, subarachnoid and intracerebroventricular opioid in patients with pain due to cancer. *Reg Anesth* **21:** S42–56, 1996

35. Lahuerta J, Lipton S, Wells JCD. Percutaneous cervical cordotomy: results and complications in a recent series of 100 patients. *Ann Roy Coll Surg Engl* **67:** 41–44, 1985

36. O'Gorman B, Elfred A. Physiotherapy. In: Simpson KH, Budd K, eds. *Cancer pain management. A comprehensive approach.* Oxford University Press: Oxford, 2000, pp. 63–74

# 31 Pain in Human Immunodeficiency Virus

## Caroline Bradbeer

Human immunodeficiency virus (HIV) is a blood borne retrovirus, which is lymphotropic and neurotropic; it damages the immune system, laying the body open to opportunistic infections and malignancies and also directly affects the brain and peripheral nervous system. Pain in HIV disease is caused by a constellation of conditions. Many of these are relatively acute, pain being just one symptom of the highly complex opportunistic conditions that are the province of the HIV specialist. Such conditions are unlikely to present to a pain clinic and are only touched on here. Other conditions, such as shingles, may be more common in HIV infection, but they are not specific to HIV nor are they altered clinically by the presence of HIV; many of these are covered elsewhere in this manual. The incidence of opportunistic conditions and neuropathic pain in those with HIV infection increases with a reduction in immunity, as measured by the decline in CD4 lymphocyte count.[1] When HIV infection is allowed to progress untreated, the terminal stages are characterized by some or all of the following: cachexia and weakness, severe diarrhoea, dementia, blindness and paralysis. Not surprisingly, pain is common, and the symptoms in late disease are no different from those in patients with cancer.[2] However, with the advent of effective anti-HIV therapy in the form of antiretrovirals (ARVs), it is possible in almost all cases to reverse this decline in immunity and, with it, the risk of developing many of the painful conditions hitherto associated with HIV.[2] Pain in HIV disease consequently presents a different spectrum now from that observed before 1996,[3] with pain due to the side-effects of the ARVs themselves becoming a more prominent feature. A study on ambulatory HIV-infected men before the era of combined ARVs showed the most common four pain symptoms to be due to: HIV-related headaches, herpes simplex, painful peripheral neuropathy and back pain.[4]

## General considerations

### Interrelations with pain symptoms

HIV infection is a potentially fatal, chronic infection that invariably carries a degree of stigma; obsession with the diagnosis, with concerns about health and with death is common. People with HIV infection often have psychiatric conditions and/or a drug and alcohol problem.[5] These problems may have antedated their acquisition of HIV (and even facilitated that acquisition) or have developed as a result of the traumatic effect of finding themselves to be infected. Therefore, their pain may be exaggerated by anxiety about the possible import of trivial symptoms, by underlying depression, by fear of disclosure of their HIV status or by effects related to substance misuse. Conversely, pain has an adverse effect on quality of life measurements even when other variables are controlled for, and a study on children shows it to be also associated with higher mortality.[6,7]

## Measuring pain

The prevalence of pain has been measured by many authors in HIV disease and been shown to be between 20 and 97%, this proportion varying with the degree of immunosuppression.[2,8] However, without a control group, it is difficult to quantify the impact of pain in those with HIV infection. Nevertheless, many studies have shown that pain in these patients is poorly managed, especially in those who are current or past drug users.[8,9]

## Factitious HIV infection

Patients falsely claiming to have HIV are surprisingly common; some appear to do this for monetary gain and others as part of a Munchausen syndrome. It is good practice to ensure evidence of infection and if in doubt to repeat the HIV test.[10]

## Causes of pain in HIV disease

The causes can be divided into four categories: pain due to direct affects of HIV; pain due to opportunistic diseases; pain secondary to ARV therapy; and pain from causes not directly related to HIV (Table 31.1). The first two categories are strongly related to the degree of immunosuppression, being unlikely if the CD4 count is above $200–300 \times 10^6$/litre. Pain secondary to therapy is usually related to the duration of therapy and/or the total dose. The degree of immunosuppression is an invaluable discriminator in assessing the likelihood of the cause of pain; serious, life-threatening, HIV-related conditions being rare in those with a CD4 count above $300 \times 10^6$/litre and being increasingly common as the levels decline below $200 \times 10^6$/litre.[4]

# Causes of pain symptoms in HIV infection

## Headache

Most headaches in HIV-infected patients are not serious, so one danger is that relatively trivial causes will go unrecognized and the patient will be subjected to unnecessary imaging and lumbar puncture.

- Sinusitis is a common and frequently overlooked cause of pain in HIV disease, especially in those with mild or moderate immunosuppression. It may present acutely or as a chronic headache with a post-nasal drip as the main localizing feature.
- Tension headaches, related to understandable anxiety, are also common as are other non-HIV related causes, such as migraine or viral meningitis.
- Headaches associated with fevers of a non-cranial aetiology are a common cause of concern in HIV patients. Since fevers of whatever cause naturally fluctuate, the diagnosis depends on observing that the headache is only present when the body temperature is raised, and in identifying the cause of the fever.
- Drug-related headache is commonly experienced on initiation of zidovudine and, less frequently, efavirenz therapy. It is almost always self-limiting, resolving within 3 weeks of the start of therapy but may occasionally persist and require a change of ARV regimen.
- Cryptococcal meningitis presents with headache in 80–90% of cases[11] and sufferers usually describe it as by far the worst headache they have ever experienced.
- Cranial space-occupying lesions are less likely to engender headaches and the common causes – toxoplasmosis and B-cell lymphoma – are difficult to distinguish clinically or on imaging, although toxoplasmosis is more likely to cause a fever.

| Table 31.1    Examples of painful conditions in HIV disease |
|---|
| **Direct effects of HIV infection** |
| • Meningoencephalitis – at seroconversion<br>• HIV neuropathy<br>• HIV headache<br>• Arthropathy<br>• Myopathy<br>• Painful diarrhoea of unknown cause<br>• Wasting, e.g. causing pressure sores |
| **Opportunistic conditions** |
| Often associated with mild immunosuppression (CD4 > 200 × $10^6$/litre)<br>• Oral candidosis<br>• Sinusitis<br>• Herpes zoster (shingles)<br>• Herpes simplex (genital and oral)<br>Associated with more profound immunosuppression (CD4 < 200 × $10^6$/litre)<br>• Cryptococcal meningitis<br>• Tuberculous meningitis<br>• Hydrocephalus secondary to the above<br>• Cerebral toxoplasmosis<br>• Cerebral lymphoma<br>• Oesophageal candidosis<br>• Bacterial gut infections<br>• Cytomegalovirus colitis |
| **Side-effects of antiretroviral therapies (ARVs)** |
| • Headache<br>• Peripheral neuropathy<br>• Pancreatitis<br>• Lipodystrophy, e.g. causing buttock-fat loss and discomfort in sitting |
| **Conditions only indirectly related to HIV** |
| • Tension headaches<br>• Alcoholic neuropathy<br>• Liver pain secondary to alcohol or hepatitis<br>• Infected injection sites, e.g. in drug users<br>• Opiate withdrawal<br>• Sexually transmitted infections, e.g. secondary syphilis<br>• Factitious HIV |

- HIV itself may cause meningoencephalitis and headache in 30%[12,13] at seroconversion, which is thought to be cytokine mediated. At this time the HIV antibody test will be negative but specific tests to identify the antigen should confirm the diagnosis. If a patient is diagnosed as having a seroconversion illness, he or she should be offered immediate ARV therapy, as this has been shown to improve prognosis.

- The so-called HIV headache[14] is also thought to be a direct effect of the virus and usually occurs in late-stage disease. It may be acute or chronic and has variable meningitic components. The CSF shows a mononuclear pleocytosis.

Managing severe opportunistic conditions is complex and should always involve an experienced physician. If such a cause of headache is suspected, essential basic tests include serum cryptococcal antigen and toxoplasmosis antibody levels, brain imaging and, having ensured no raised intracranial pressure, a lumbar puncture. The laboratory needs to be involved from the outset to advise on the correct samples of cerebrospinal fluid (CSF) to send.

## Gastrointestinal pain

- Oral pain and odynophagia are common and frequently found together. *Candida*, oral and oesophageal, and non-specific ulceration are the most common causes. A now little-used ARV drug, zalcitabine, can cause recurrent oral ulcers. *Candida* responds well to antifungals, but ulceration may be very difficult to manage. Oral ulcers can be treated with local steroid preparations but large areas of ulceration, especially in the oesophagus, may require thalidomide to heal. Oral pain is also commonly due to gingivitis, and this generally responds to metronidazole.
- Abdominal pain is frequently associated with diarrhoea and an infective cause. Diarrhoea is also a common side-effect of many of the ARV drugs, especially the protease inhibitors. Symptoms of intestinal obstruction occasionally occur and may indicate Kaposi's sarcoma or an intestinal lymphoma. More commonly, such pain will be due to constipation as a result of opiate use or abuse.
- Pancreatitis is an uncommon but life-threatening condition occurring predominately as a side-effect of therapy with the ARV drug, didanosine, especially when predisposing factors, such as high alcohol intake or some other drugs (e.g. systemic pentamidine) are present.
- Lactic acidosis is a serious, potentially fatal, side-effect of ARVs. It presents acutely with generalized gastrointestinal symptoms, pain, nausea, diarrhoea, and malaise. Liver function is abnormal and serum lactate raised. Once the diagnosis is suspected, in conjunction with an HIV specialist, therapy with ARVs should be stopped.
- Anorectal pain may be a consequence of chronic diarrhoea, but rectal herpes simplex infections are frequent in gay men, and there is also an increased incidence of anal carcinoma in HIV disease.

## Peripheral neuropathy

Although peripheral neuropathy is a common condition in untreated HIV disease, when it is thought to be a direct effect of the virus, it is now seen far more frequently as a complication of ARV therapy. The pathology in both cases appears to be a distal sensorimotor polyneuropathy (DSP). The mechanism for drug-induced DSP may be inhibition of nerve growth factor.[5] Electromyocardiograms (EMGs) show axonal neuropathy affecting large and small fibres.[13] The incidence of DSP, whatever the cause, increases as immunosuppression develops, beginning in the longest nerves and causing symptoms first in the soles of the feet. However, it may go unnoticed until the neuropathy has reached above the ankles, since it can be painless – some patients merely complaining of numbness.

When DSP is drug induced the main culprits among the ARVs are stavudine, didanosine and zalcitabine. Their effect is cumulative, related to the total dose, but with great individual variation in susceptibility. Examples of other drugs used in HIV disease that also cause neuropathies are dapsone, thalidomide and vincristine. Pain develops, or becomes more severe, during recovery following cessation of the culprit drug and may last for several weeks. The two mainstays of treatment are to ensure recovery of immunity and to stop, or reduce the dose of, any offending therapy. It is generally possible to find an alternative ARV, except in those patients with highly resistant virus, and this should be the aim. Symptomatic treatment may be necessary over the recovery period and in some patients, especially those with HIV-related DSP whose immunity needs time to respond to ARVs, this may be prolonged. In a tiny minority of others, there may currently be no alternative to their existing ARV regimen, and they may have to continue with their regimen despite the neuropathy. Treatments that have been tried include simple analgesics, carbamazepine, amitriptyline and more recently good results have been reported with gabapentin, levacecamine (acetyl-L-carnitine) and recombinant nerve growth factor.[15]

## Conclusion

HIV disease is multifactorial, but there are no specific painful conditions that require different management from any other group of patients. It remains important to exclude life-threatening disease, best done through close liaison with an HIV specialist, and then to tackle pain as with any other chronic disease.

## References

1. Kelleher T, Cross A, Dunkle L. Relation of peripheral neuropathy to HIV treatment in four randomised clinical trials including didanosine. *Clin Ther* **21**: 1182–1192, 1999
2. O'Neill WM, Sherrard JS. Pain in human immunodeficiency virus: a review. *Pain* **54**: 3–14, 1993
3. Glare PA. Pain in patients with HIV infection: issues for the new millennium. *Eur J Pain* **5**(Suppl A): 43–48, 2001
4. Singer EJ, Zorilla C, Fahy-Chandon B, et al. Painful symptoms reported by ambulatory HIV-infected men in a longitudinal study. *Pain* **54**: 15–19, 1993
5. Treisman GJ, Kaplina AI. Neurologic and psychiatric complications of antiretroviral agents. *AIDS* **16**: 1201–1215, 2002
6. Rosenfeld B, Breitbart W, McDonald MV, et al. Pain in ambulatory AIDS patients. II: Impact of pain on psychological functioning and quality of life. *Pain* **68**: 323–328, 1996
7. Gaughan DM, Hughes MD, Seage GA 3rd. The prevalence of pain in pediatric human immunodeficiency virus/acquired immune deficiency syndrome as reported by participants in the Pediatric Outcomes Study PACTG 219. *Pediatrics* **109**: 1144–1152, 2002
8. Frich LM, Borgbjerg FM. Pain and pain treatment in AIDS patients: a longitudinal study. *J Pain Symptom Manage* **19**: 339–347, 2000
9. Swica Y, Breitbart W. Treating pain in patients with AIDS and a history of substance use. *West J Med* **176**: 33–39, 2002
10. Mileno MD, Barnowski C, Fiore T, et al. Factitious HIV syndrome in young women. *AIDS Read* **11**: 269–277, 2001
11. Dismukes WE. Cryptococcal meningitis in patients with AIDS. *J Infect Dis* **157**: 624–627, 1988
12. Mirsattari SM, Power C, Nath A. Primary headache with HIV infection. *Headache* **39**: 3–10, 1999
13. Weisberg LA. Neuroligic abnormalities in human immunodeficiency virus infection. *South Med J* **94**: 266–275, 2001
14. Price RW. Neurological complications of HIV infection. *Lancet* **348**: 445–452, 1996
15. Moyle GJ, Sadler M. Peripheral neuropathy with nucleoside antiretrovirals: risk factors, incidence and management. *Drug Saf* **19**: 481–494, 1998

# 32 Psychological Interventions for Medical Patients in Pain

## Jay R Skidmore

Efforts at pain management, without attention to psychological factors, may be doomed to fail, or at least fall short of optimal outcomes. Even with acute pain, there are major differences in how various individuals respond to pain and to the treatments prescribed for pain.[1] But the longer that any type of pain persists, the greater role for psychological factors as mediated through the central nervous system.[2,3,4] Therefore, the purpose of this chapter is to assist physicians and surgeons by providing information about psychological interventions that have proven useful for medical patients who suffer with chronic pain.

The details of psychologic or psychobiological mechanisms in chronic pain are beyond the scope and purpose of this chapter. Instead, the emphasis will be on practical methods for psychological assessment and treatment with chronic pain patients.

In some cases, the physician may be able to utilize these psychological interventions directly with the patient. More often, the physician may simply want to refer the patient to a qualified clinical psychologist for collaborative care. Either way, it is likely that doctors will be more successful in pain management, and their patients better served, when the following guidelines for psychological interventions are considered.

## When will patients with chronic pain most need psychological interventions?

While some medical and surgical patients may benefit from psychological interventions for coping with acute pain, the focus of this chapter will be upon chronic pain. One of the pioneers in pain research, JJ Bonica[2] has defined chronic pain as:

> "...pain that persists a month beyond the usual course of an acute disease or a reasonable time for an injury to heal or that is associated with a chronic pathological process that causes continuous pain or the pain recurs at intervals for months or years. Some clinicians use the arbitrary figure of 6 months to designate pain as chronic, but this is not appropriate..."

Whether we should use 1, 3 or 6 months to specify chronic pain, there are indeed many patients who suffer persistent pain long after their injuries have healed. Other patients have chronic pain after a disease has resolved. This may be true even with patients who obtained the best medical and surgical treatments; although it is sometimes compounded by iatrogenic medical treatments. Lastly, and perhaps most sad, are those patients who suffer chronic pain due to an on-going malignant disease or pathological process that may be unlikely to ever resolve in this life. It has been my experience that pain chronicity – the longer a patient has to struggle with pain – increases the likelihood that a patient may require psychological services to assist with emotional distress and relationship problems, and/or readjustment to work and life goals.

Various researchers have suggested that people process and interpret pain in stages. According to one model of pain processing,[5,6] people pass through four stages:

- Sensory discrimination
- Affective and emotional arousal associated with pain perception
- Suffering
- Behavioral effects on activities of daily living.

Again, this suggests an order-in-time across which psychological symptoms may be expected, from fairly acute anxiety in the early stages, to depression, and then to disabilities in work and home life. Yet, it is important to consider how often these stages get recycled; for example, when some people avoid early problems with depression but later, after a loss of employment or frustration with persistent physical impairment, they become (understandably) very depressed and in need of psychological assistance.

Consequently, the question of when to refer for psychological care should probably be revisited over the course of the illness, the course of the rehabilitation process and the course of the patient's recovery. Sadly, in the vast majority of cases in both the USA and the UK, the referral for psychological care is likely to come very late – typically after patients have already suffered for several years with chronic pain.

# Which pain patients will benefit from psychological interventions?

Many people have persistent pain for months, years or indefinitely, following injury or illness, even after appropriate medical treatment. Common painful conditions include chronic back, hip or neck pain, other joint pains associated with arthritis, abdominal or chest pain (from specific pathologies or, more often, benign), various neuropathies and frequently recurring headaches. Less common conditions include post-burn pain and phantom limb pain. And, of course, many individuals have disease-related pain symptoms (e.g. from cancer) and/or endure recurrent painful medical procedures. While analgesic medicines can reduce pain in many cases, significantly, seldom do drugs take away the pain completely. Many people cope surprisingly well with some degree of chronic pain, and they resume active and meaningful lives. But others remain distressed, become less physically active and make the rounds of doctors and therapists looking for a cure. Occasionally, these patients find a cure, perhaps because their condition was wrongly diagnosed or mistreated. More often, they suffer from medical conditions for which an actual cure remains elusive or may be unrealistic, and the most reasonable option may be for them to learn better ways to manage their symptoms while getting back to life.

Patients who demonstrate the following types of symptoms or behaviours are among those most in need of psychological interventions.

## Anxious and somatizing patients

Some degree of anxiety is to be expected with anyone in response to pain, but individuals who appear more anxious than others, and especially those who remain overly-focused on the pain or other bodily symptoms, are clearly in need of psychological attention. At the least, this signals a need for further explanation or discussion about the medical condition, pain symptoms, or treatments. Questions of prognosis, or whether hurt = harm, may need to be addressed with a patient. When such reassurance is not enough, then the physician, therapist or nurse might use any number of stress reduction or relaxation techniques with the patient. Beyond this, patients who remain anxious and/or overly-focused on pain symptoms may require more specialized psychological treatment. Also, when the anxiety is associated with substantial physical injury and impairment, or other dire consequences, then it makes even more sense to provide specialized psychological care for helping patients rebuild their lives.

## Depressed and lonely patients

There has been considerable discussion about whether previously depressed individuals are more prone to develop chronic pain problems and, conversely, to what degree persistent pain may lead to depressive symptoms. Readers may wish to refer to the review by Fishbain[7] for details. But there remains little doubt that a significant number of chronic pain patients are likely to be clinically depressed. For example, a review of the research found 32–82% of patients seeking treatment from pain clinics due to back pain also had depressive symptoms.[8] In addition to various psychobiological factors, social isolation will increase the risks for depression. Any of the widely used scales can be utilized as screening tools, including the Beck, Zung or Hamilton measures. All patients treated in pain clinics should be screened; some may 'look fine' yet be emotionally distressed.

## Drug-dependent patients

Doctors differ greatly in their views about drug treatments for chronic pain, and also about how to define drug dependence. Yet, many physicians and their patients have found the following guidelines to be helpful:

- Keep current with drug research and guidelines related to chronic pain.
- Maintain drugs that (a) reduce pain, and (b) allow increased functioning.
- Decrease or discontinue drugs if functional activity levels are declining.
- Re-assess the usefulness of drugs every 6 weeks, or at least 6 monthly.
- For chronic pain, take the drugs on time-contingent (not prn) basis.
- Help patients to wean-off drugs that 'barely' provide pain relief.

Sometimes patients are drug dependent, and yet claim analgesic effects in order to get prescriptions renewed. But, more often, emotionally distressed patients will fail to obtain sufficient pain relief with typical drug doses, or they find 'nothing helps' yet want their drug treatment to continue. These patients do better after their psychological problems are addressed. In either case, it is often helpful to turn attention away from pain relief, solely, and toward the improvement of functional life activities as the major outcome. Obviously this will be a delicate balance, and one that may require gentle negotiation between the physician and the patient. When psychologists are involved, they should participate in discussions about drug or dosage changes, and be prepared to develop behavioural management plans. Moreover, the psychologist should be able to help the patient refocus on self-control methods for dealing with recurrent pain flare-ups. Admittedly, drug dependence and addiction problems are far more complex than this brief discussion implies, but, again, the purpose herein is to offer practical guidelines for pain clinic physicians to consider.

# Which types of psychological interventions will be most useful?

There are perhaps five major treatment arenas for psychological interventions with pain patients:

- Reduction of pain itself, in some cases
- Resolution of emotional distress, to some degree

- Improvement in coping skills for the self-management of chronic pain
- Improvement in health habits and overall well-being
- Assistance in rebuilding social and occupational activities and/or other meaningful life goals.

These may be best accomplished by a combination of the therapeutic relationship between patient and doctor (or psychologist, therapist or nurse) and the appropriate use of specific psychotherapeutic procedures. The following are the psychological interventions that are most widely used for treatment of patients with chronic pain.

## Stress reduction and relaxation training

Any method capable of reducing arousal of the sympathetic nervous system will be likely to reduce pain levels as well as emotional distress. Yet, unfortunately, one still hears clinicians say, 'There's nothing else to reduce your pain, so just try to relax.' On the contrary, doctors and nurses should gently encourage patients with this fact: if they can learn to relax, such that their mental states are eased, breathing slows and their muscle tension declines, then by definition the pain itself will almost certainly go down a bit. Behavioral methods of relaxation training include:

- Calm or diaphragmatic breathing
- Progressive muscle tension and release exercises
- Pleasant mental imagery
- Passive mental states (e.g., mindfulness meditation).

Some of these are quite simple (such as calm breathing, or muscle tension and release) and can be learned with common sense and practice, and then used by almost any health professional to help their patients learn to relax. This can be especially helpful for giving patients a practical technique to use with painful flare-ups or recurrent exacerbation of symptoms.

## Advanced psychophysiological therapies

Procedures like clinical hypnosis, biofeedback and more complex forms of relaxation training are best mastered with specialized training and supervized experience, as well as reference to the research literature, and integration with psychotherapeutic processes. While there is considerable overlap in these relaxation and psychophysiological procedures, there are also numerous complexities and specific applications that clinicians should understand prior to using such techniques with patients.[9,10] Hypnosis, in particular, has been subject to widespread use by amateurs on the one hand, and under-utilization by medical professionals on the other.[11] Decades of research at Stanford University School of Medicine as well as many other universities and hospitals[12] have clarified the variables associated with hypnosis for pain relief, and clinical guidelines have been published[13] that specify what approach works best, for whom, and with which medical conditions. However, the use of hypnosis for pain relief may have some of the same disadvantages as the anesthetics procedures – in particular, patients may get some pain relief but continue in rather dysfunctional living and, therefore, never really obtain 'enough relief' to be satisfied. Nonetheless, hypnosis along with analgesic medication can offer many patients a significant reduction in pain levels, which may be at least one legitimate portion of a broad approach to pain management.

## Cognitive and behavioural psychotherapies

Cognitive behavioural therapy (CBT) has become almost reified as an evidence-based approach to psychotherapy,[14] but it is more accurate to view CBT as a collection of empirical treatment procedures. Some authors refer separately to cognitive and behavioural treatment procedures, which may be useful.[15] One can think of cognitive therapies as including such techniques as problem solving and coping skills training, whereas behavioural therapies use classical conditioning and operant techniques to modify habits. However, cognitive and behavioural procedures are not easily separated in theory or research but, instead, are intermingled almost always in actual clinical practice,[16,17] including the adaptation of CBT to pain management.[18,19] In essence, CBT is an organized set of psychotherapy procedures that emphasize the following:

- The importance of thought patterns and behavioural habits, as well as social influences on emotional functioning
- The necessity of learning, social skills and self-management in overcoming human difficulties
- Interactions between thoughts and feelings, mind and body, the person and their environment
- Scientific methods as the most legitimate ways to test our theories and treatment outcomes.

While much can be learned from other schools of thought in psychology, such as psychoanalytic theory or existential approaches to human growth, it remains fair to say that, so far, only cognitive–behavioural psychology has systematic methods of pain management than can be coherently integrated with medical care. Again, in a nutshell, the goals of CBT in this context are to reduce pain, or at least the emotional distress that goes with pain, help patients increase coping skills for managing chronic or recurrent symptoms more effectively, improve their health habits and rebuild meaningful lives. Cognitive behavioural treatment has traditionally been conducted most often in outpatient psychology clinics, which patients usually attend weekly for 1-hour sessions, over the course of 8 to 16 weeks. Often, this provides adequate psychological care to enable individuals to move forward on their own; but sometimes longer-term treatment is required, or other formats need to be considered.

## Psychotherapies in marital and family formats

When dysfunctional relationships are part and parcel of the emotional problems, when an individual lacks the resources to make effective changes alone, and/or when the difficulties impact a partner or children, then it makes sense to treat the couple or the family together in psychological treatment.

## Multidisciplinary pain management and rehabilitation programmes

When patients are emotionally distressed about their pain and in need of physical rehabilitation, and they cannot maintain coping skills or reasonable physical activities on their own, then it is wise to consider referral to a structured pain management programme (PMP). At the very least, a good PMP should have dedicated professional staff from clinical psychology, medicine and physical therapy. Larger or more established PMPs will typically have occupational therapy and nursing staff, along with administrative support staff, and more than one medical specialty on the pain team. Generally, the outcome goals of PMPs are similar to the CBT approach described above. For this reason, clinical psychologists tend to serve as leadership roles for the pain team, often as programme director or co-director, usually with a physician as medical director of the PMP. Guidelines about the desirable characteristics of PMPs are available elsewhere,[20] and multidisciplinary programmes are described in further detail in Chapter 33.

# Coordinated care between physician and psychologist

Every pain clinic physician will see some patients whose disability levels are strikingly more severe than might be expected from their injuries. Examples include the patient with a mechanical back sprain, or minor disc prolapse, who spends his days at home on disability benefit, or the patient with painful wrists diagnosed as repetitive strain injury, who believes she should never work again, or the patient who had minor knee surgery years ago and has remained in a wheelchair since then, and now wants a morphine pump. None of these complex biopsychosocial problems are likely to be solved with any type of medicine or surgery. These are the patients who may benefit most from referral to an inpatient or residential multidisciplinary rehabilitation PMP.

However, some patients who need such intensive multidisciplinary treatment will not be suitable for the group format of a PMP. On the one hand are those whose emotional disturbance or personality problems would disrupt or undermine group treatment. These individuals often carry a psychiatric diagnosis along with their painful medical condition. As such, they may do better with a combination of outpatient care that is coordinated between the General Practitioner (GP; in UK) or Primary Care Physician (PCP; in USA) and the pain physician working with a pain psychologist, and perhaps a psychiatrist, family therapist or community social worker. On the other hand are people whose good psychological functioning will make treatment in a group PMP seem too elementary. Such persons are likely to still be working, or involved in suitable social and leisure activities, but they could obtain better pain management or greater functioning with assistance of psychological intervention.

Over the course of caring for patients in a pain clinic, one point at which physicians will want to consider adding psychological treatments is whenever they plan to repeat medical treatments or try experimental procedures. It may be helpful to remember that most of the sensible medical treatments are tried early in the course of care. Repeating medical treatments that have failed in the past, or trying procedures that are clearly experimental, are both good indicators that psychological interventions may be warranted.

# References

1. Chapman CR, Turner JA, Psychologic and psychosocial aspects of acute pain. In: Bonica JJ, Loeser JD, Chapman CR, Fordyce WE, eds. *The Management of Pain*, 2nd ed. London: Lea & Febiger, 1990, pp. 122–132
2. Bonica JJ, General considerations of chronic pain. In: Bonica JJ, Loeser JD, Chapman CR, Fordyce WE, eds. *The Management of Pain*, 2nd ed. London: Lea & Febiger, 1990, pp. 180–196
3. Bromm B, Desmedt JE, eds. *Advances in Pain Research and Therapy: Pain and the Brain – From Nociception to Cognition*. New York: Raven Press, 1995
4. Wall, PD, Introduction. In: Wall PD, Melzack R, eds. *Textbook of Pain, 3rd ed*. Edinburgh: Churchill Livingstone, 1994
5. Price DD. *Psychological and Neural Mechanisms of Pain*. New York: Raven Press, 1988
6. Wade JB, Price DD. Nonpathological factors in chronic pain: Implications for assessment and treatment. In: Gatchel RJ, Weisberg JN, eds. *Personality Characteristics of Patients with Pain*. Washingtion DC: American Psychological Association, 2000, pp. 89–107
7. Fishbain DA, Cutler R, Rosomoff HL, Rosomoff RS. Chronic pain associated depression: Antecedent or consequence of chronic pain? A review. *Clin J Pain* **13**: 116–137, 1997
8. Sullivan MJL, Reesor S, Mikail R, Risher R. The treatment of depression in chronic low back pain: Review and recommendations. *Pain* **50**: 5–13, 1992
9. Wickramasekera I. *Biofeedback, Behavior Therapy and Hypnosis*. Chicago: Nelson-Hall, 1976
10. Lehrer PM, Woolfolk RL, eds. *Principles and Practice of Stress Management, 2nd ed*. New York: Guilford Press, 1993

11. Fredericks LE, *The Use of Hypnosis in Surgery and Anesthesiology.* Springfield, Illinois: Charles C Thomas, 2001
12. Hilgard ER, Hilgard JR. *Hypnosis in the Relief of Pain, 1st, 2nd & 3rd eds.* New York: Brunner/Mazel, 1975, 1983, 1994
13. Barber J, *Hypnosis and Suggestion in the Treatment of Pain: A Clinical Guide.* New York: WW Norton, 1996
14. Tarrier N, Commentary: Yes, cognitive behaviour therapy may well be all you need. *Br Med* **324:** 291–292, 2002
15. Green J. Psychological therapies in pain management. In: Dolin S, Padfield N, Pateman J, eds. *Pain Clinic Manual.* Oxford: Reed, 1996.
16. Jacobson NS, ed. *Psychotherapists in Clinical Practice: Cognitive and Behavioral Perspectives.* New York: Guilford Press, 1987
17. Mahoney MJ. *Cognition and Behavior Modification.* Cambridge, Massachusetts: Ballinger Books, 1974
18. Turk DC, Meichenbaum D, Genest M. *Pain and Behavioral Medicine: A Cognitive Behavioral Perspective.* New York: Guilford Press, 1983.
19. Gatchel RJ, Turk DC, eds. *Psychological Approaches to Pain Management: A Practitioner's Handbook.* New York: Guilford Press, 1996.
20. Sears K, Williams AC, Richardson P, Collett B, Main CJ. *Desirable Criteria for Pain Management Programmes.* Report of a Working Party of The Pain Society, 1996.

Note: Preference in this chapter has gone to references of books, and book chapters, as these can provide the interested reader with a more thorough background than isolated journal articles. However, the obsessive reader may also find these books and chapters contain extensive bibliographies and references to the primary journal articles.

# 33 Pain Management Programmes

## Jane M Green

The prevalence of chronic pain within the community is very high. However, many people with chronic pain continue to function effectively and enjoy a good quality of life in spite of the pain and with no external help, and so never become patients. A large number of those who do present to physicians may be helped effectively by intermittent interventions and support from their general practitioners. Where this proves insufficient, referral to a pain clinic may be necessary. Many of those referred may be helped successfully with single types of procedures or combined physical and psychological approaches within the pain clinic. These may improve the patient's quality of life to the point where they no longer seek further help. For some patients, however, these interventions will not be enough to enable them to achieve an acceptable quality of life. These patients may have had pain for many years and, over time, have functioned less and less effectively in a variety of areas of their lives. Others may be functioning at a reasonably high level, on objective assessment, but feel distressed that they cannot do more. Attending a pain management programme (PMP) may help such patients to regain control over their lives and cope adequately with pain.

## Type of patient

The criteria that determine which people with chronic pain are referred to a pain clinic include: the level to which the pain interferes with the person's life, their ability to learn coping strategies, the degree of support they have from family and friends, their pre-morbid personality, and the characteristics of the pain. Patients treated in the pain clinic fall into three categories:

- Treatments employed are successful and reduce pain or improve function.
- Treatments fail to reduce pain, but the patient continues to function well.
- Treatments fail and the patient also functions poorly.

This last group of patients is that for whom referral to a PMP is usually appropriate. It is important that the patient has had all the appropriate physical investigations and treatments before referral to a PMP, and is being helped to understand that there is nothing more to be gained from a constant search for a diagnosis and cure for their pain. If litigation is active, this can severely adversely affect the patient's ability to benefit from attending a PMP and so, ideally, referral should wait until the litigation has been completed. Because this may well be a lengthy process, it may sometimes be necessary to refer a patient whose litigation is still active, and the likely effects of this will need to be considered as part of the assessment procedure.

Signs of failing function include inappropriate drug usage, crumbling family support, with either antagonism or overprotection, general reduction of physical abilities and inappropriate expectations of the future. When a patient develops into a sick role within the family unit, secondary gains may become established for the other members of the family as well as for the patient, and these become entrenched over time. The influence of the patient's family can be fundamental and, ideally, patient selection would involve the patient's close relations, who may be involved in the treatment programme. Appropriate support from family or a significant other is a significant factor for a good outcome. Over reliance on drugs reduces performance, clouding cognitive faculties and reducing physical activity. Poor functional ability may further decrease as chronic inactivity, pathological interpersonal relationships and dependence on others for physical, emotional and often financial support become established. If no intervention is made, these patients will often continue to seek a definitive diagnosis and treatment for their condition, undergoing more and more invasive interventions, with the risk of further morbidity, as well as reinforcement of the sick role. This pattern may be well established by the time of referral to a PMP, and have contributed to the failure of single-modality treatments.

A patient who is referred to a PMP is typically someone who:

- Is disabled in multiple areas of their life
- Is physically inactive
- May be passive in relationships with their immediate family
- Is isolated from other contacts
- Is usually not in employment
- May be taking multiple drug treatments
- May have a poor understanding of the nature of their condition.

# Structure and content of pain management programmes

Pain management programmes are multidisciplinary psychoeducational cognitive behavioural group programmes aimed at helping patients to improve the quality of their lives despite having pain. They are not designed to remove or necessarily reduce the pain, but to equip people to manage the pain and minimize the effect of it on their lives. Patients, although frequently apprehensive at the prospect of joining a group, usually find being part of a group of people suffering from the same kind of condition one of the most helpful aspects of the programme. They find it reassuring that they are not alone in their suffering. They can learn practical coping skills from one another, and derive considerable emotional support from the other members of the group. Most importantly, other members of the group can help individuals keep to their targets and can provide reinforcements for their achievements.

The psychological input to the PMP is based on cognitive behavioural principals, described in Chapter 32, and includes other psychotherapeutic techniques as appropriate. The cognitive and behavioural[1] aspects of the therapy are integrated with each other and with other aspects of the programme. It is important that all members of the team involved in the PMP understand the theoretical basis of the cognitive behavioural approach and work within its structure, thus giving patients and their significant others a consistent view of the nature and management of chronic pain.

## The multi-disciplinary team

In 1995, a working party of the Pain Society[2] listed the minimal interventions constituting a PMP as:

- Physical reconditioning
- Posture and body mechanics training
- Applied relaxation techniques
- Information and education about pain and pain management
- Medication review and advice

- Psychological assessment and intervention
- Graded return to activities of daily living.

Optimal interventions would include also:

- Work with families/significant others
- Vocational and educational guidance
- Welfare advice
- Liaison with other agencies as necessary.

Essential members of the PMP multi-disciplinary team are:

- The psychologist
- The physiotherapist
- The occupational therapist.[3]

Other contributors include:

- A pain medical consultant
- A pain nurse
- A pharmacist
- A dietitian.

## The timetable

Whilst all incorporate the above features, PMPs vary in their structure and timetable. Some run as inpatient programmes, typically Monday to Friday for 4 weeks. In these, the patients may be accommodated in a hostel-type environment or, less often, in a ward setting. As far as possible, patients are encouraged to manage their own activities of daily living during the programme. More programmes are run on an outpatient basis. Patients will normally attend for the equivalent of 12 half-day sessions over a period of 6 weeks. Follow-up sessions may take place after 1, 3 and 6 months and at 1 year.[4]

## The content

The PMP provides patients with input of three main types: education about the nature of pain; practical measures and behavioural coping strategies; and cognitive and emotional coping strategies.

### Education about the nature of pain
- Understanding the nature of chronic pain[5,6] and that it differs from acute pain in that it does not signify ongoing damage. In an acutely painful condition, the purpose of the pain is to warn the individual of damage and to encourage rest of the affected part, preventing further damage and increasing healing. However, in a chronic pain condition, periods of absolute rest further increase pain when activity does occur, decrease fitness so that pain actually spreads to neighbouring parts and lead to see-sawing levels of activity with both under- and over-activity, known as 'activity cycling'.
- A basic understanding of the physiology of pain perception, and an understanding of the gate control theory of pain.[7] When patients are told that no cause can be found for their pain, they tend to interpret this as being told that it is 'all in their mind' and, therefore, that they are being regarded as malingerers or 'mad'. It is often useful to explain to patients the phenomenon of phantom limb pain to help them realize that the experience of pain in the absence of a local cause is a common one, albeit not one susceptible to physical treatment.

**291**

- Learning about the vicious circle of stress and pain and how to break it by using relaxation, exercise and effective problem-solving strategies (Figure 33.1). Pain is interpreted by the brain as a warning. This leads to the build up of the 'fight or flight' stress response. In the stress response, breathing becomes faster, which may lead to hyperventilation, the heart rate is increased, which may cause the person to imagine they are having a heart attack, blood is diverted to the major muscles, often causing intestinal disturbances, and the major muscles become tense and tight, ready for action. In the absence of any appropriate fight or flight action to be taken, this muscle tightness remains and itself leads to pain. Thus a vicious circle of pain and muscle tension ensues. Long-term muscle tension will also lead to fatigue and to stiffness and immobility. It may also lead to cramp or spasm, which may cause a major flare-up of pain. Learning to breathe efficiently, using the diaphragm, and learning to recognize and relax muscle tension when it first begins will break this circle. Regular stretching and exercise will contribute to this and counteract stiffness and immobility. External stress in the form of everyday worries will lead to a build-up of muscle tension through the stress response, and even people not suffering from chronic pain may experience headaches or other pains in response to this. Patients with chronic pain will experience an increase of pain in response to everyday worries and so need to evolve effective ways of recognizing and solving their problems.
- Learning about the range of investigations and treatments used in the management of pain and their limitations. Many patients feel cheated that they are not being offered ever more medical treatments or high tech investigations such as computed tomography (CT) or magnetic resonance imaging (MRI). It is important for them to understand why the clinicians have ceased looking for a diagnosis or cure for their pain. Only when they understand fully that there is no treatment currently available to rid them of their pain will they be able to accept the necessity of adopting new behavioural strategies for living with it.
- Dietitic advice to address such problems as increased weight following decreased activity and constipation resulting from the use of opiate medication.
- Education on the use of medication and understanding the reasons for taking analgesia on a time- and not a pain-contingent basis. Most patients will believe intuitively that they should take analgesics in response to pain. By taking their medication in this way, they have to monitor their level of pain constantly, thus keeping the pain gates open all the

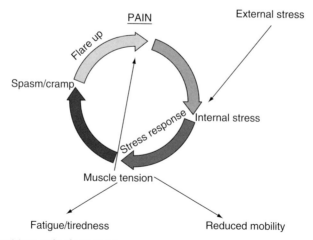

**Figure 33.1**   The vicious circle of pain and stress

time. They will also fail to maintain therapeutically adequate levels of the analgesic in their blood. By taking their regular medication on a time-contingent basis they will usually find their overall use of the analgesics is reduced, that the beneficial effect of the medication is increased and that they are able to stop monitoring their pain level constantly, so allowing the pain gates to close and thus experiencing less pain. They may benefit from taking additional medication in anticipation of an activity that would be likely to increase their pain. In that situation, they should take the additional medication in advance of the activity and not wait for the increase in pain.

### Practical measures and behavioural coping strategies
- Overcoming the fear-avoidance[8] of exercise by doing gentle stretches and exercise during the sessions and working out an appropriate exercise plan with the physiotherapist to be continued after the programme ends. The fear of pain causes most patients to avoid exercise and so become physically greatly de-conditioned. Patients need to gain an understanding of the value of taking optimal amounts of exercise to keep fit, prevent the build up of stiffness and encourage the production of endorphins, the body's naturally occurring opioids.
- With the occupational therapist, learning how to analyse tasks and look at new ways of tackling activities of daily living, set priorities, plan and pace activities and achieve a balance between chores and leisure activities. Pain patients typically adopt a pattern of 'activity-cycling'. When their pain is less they become very active in an attempt to 'make hay while the sun shines'. This will lead to an increase in pain and a subsequent major reduction in activity. Over time the level of activity during even the active periods is reduced. Patients become demoralized and fearful of any activity. Patients are taught to break down their activities into small components and to pace these activities according to what they are able to do even when their pain level is high. They are then able to maintain a constant level of activity, regardless of their level of pain, paced by measures other than pain, thus helping to keep the pain gates closed. Most patients will have given up a variety of activities. Often they continue with chores but cease taking part in recreational activities. They benefit from reviewing their priorities and achieving a balanced lifestyle.
- Setting specific, measurable, achievable, realistic, time-limited, interesting, enjoyable and satisfying goals –'SMARTIES'. Patients will have had the experience of setting themselves unrealistic goals, failing to achieve them and becoming demotivated as a result. Learning to work out realistic goals and experiencing success will restore motivation.
- Relaxation training to avoid the build up of unnecessary muscle tension, which leads to an increase in pain, fatigue and immobility, and which can provoke flare-ups of pain. Relaxation will also encourage the production of endorphins, the body's naturally occurring opioids.[9]

### Cognitive and emotional coping strategies
- Cognitive therapy aimed at helping patients to recognize, challenge and replace unhelpful thoughts which may be preventing them from adopting more effective coping strategies
- Training in appropriate assertive behaviour
- Training in mental relaxation and distraction
- Training in recognizing emotional problems and learning strategies for solving them
- Patients with chronic pain need to go through a process of bereavement. If they can successfully mourn and come to terms with the loss of their previously healthy selves, they are more able to adjust their lives appropriately to the nature and degree of their disability and so achieve a better quality of life. Thus, modified bereavement therapy is incorporated into the group sessions.

- Usually patients experience considerable anger, both about their chronic pain and its cause and about the treatment they have received to date. They often feel that their pain has not been taken seriously and that they have been dismissed as malingerers or written off as psychologically disturbed. Frequently, they believe that some medical cure is being withheld until they prove themselves as 'worthy' of receiving it. Those working in the PMP need to be aware of these feelings and beliefs and be prepared to help patients resolve their anger in ways that enable them to make the best use of the programme.

## Outcome

Many patients attending a PMP have had multiple therapeutic attempts to reduce pain, which may have failed. The primary goal of the PMP is to improve quality of life[10] rather than to attempt to reduce pain. Improvement can be measured as rates of return to work, achievement of goals, reduction in illness behaviour, changes in medication usage, rates of presentation to physicians and ratings of mood and depression. However, given the heterogeneous nature of the pain population,[11] it is easy to see that factors such as rates of return to work depend on much more than the success or failure of the treatment programme[12] and can vary widely between programmes depending on such factors as their geographical location. A body of evidence indicates that PMPs have an important role to play in helping the chronic pain patient.[13] A systematic review of PMPs for patients with chronic low back pain by Guzman *et al.* in 2001[14] concluded: 'The reviewed trials provide evidence that intensive multidisciplinary biopsychosocial rehabilitation with functional restoration reduces pain and improves function in patients with chronic low back pain. Less intensive interventions did not show improvements in clinical relevant outcomes.'

## Resources

- A video demonstrating a PMP in action called 'No Illusions' is available from: The Pain Management Unit, Royal Cornwall Hospital (City), TRURO, Cornwall TR1 2HZ
- 'Pain Management Manual' is available from: The Pain Management Centre, Gloucestershire Royal Hospital, Great Western Road, Gloucester GL1 3NN. Tel: 01452–394151, fax: 01452–394448
- Patients can be put in touch with self help organizations such as: Pain Concern: *www.painconcern.org.uk*; The Chronic Pain Organisation: *www.chronicpain.org.uk*; Pain Support: *www.painsupport.co.uk*

## References

1. Fordyce WE, Behavioural science and chronic pain. *Postgrad Med J* 60: 865–868, 1984
2. Seers K, Williams A, Richardson P, Collett B, Main CJ. Desirable criteria for pain management programmes – Report of a working party of the pain society, 1995. 1996
3. Aylwin L. Minimum requirements for an occupational therapist working in pain management. *Newsletter Pain Soc* 1: 7–11 2001
4. Gloucester Pain Management. "*Pain Management Programme Training Manual*" 2nd ed. 1999 (available from: The Pain Management Centre, Gloucestershire Royal Hospital, Great Western Road, Gloucester GL1 3NN.)
5. May CR, Rose MJ, Johnstone FC. How patients account for non-specific low back pain. *J Psychosom Res* 49: 223–225, 2000

6. Klaber Moffet JA, Newbronner E, Waddell G, et al. Public perceptions about low back pain and its management: a gap between expectations and reality. *Health Expect* **3**: 161–168, 2000
7. Melzack R, Wall PD Pain mechanisms: a new theory. *Science* **150**: 971–979, 1965
8. Waddell G, Newton M, Henderson I, Somerville D, Main CJ. A fear-avoidance beliefs questionnaire and the role of fear-avoidance beliefs in chronic low back pain and disability. *Pain* **52**: 157–168, 1993
9. Payne, RA. *Relaxation Techniques – A Practical Handbook for the Health Care Professional.* Edinburgh: Churchill-Livingstone, 1995
10. Skevington, SM, Carse, S, Williams, AC. Validation of the WHOQOL–100: Pain management improves quality of life for chronic pain patients. *Clin J Pain* **17**: 264–275, 2001
11. Gatchel, RJ, Noe CE, Pulliam C, et al. A preliminary study of multidimensional pain inventory differences in predicting treatment outcomes in a heterogeneous cohort of patients with chronic pain. *Clin J Pain* **18**: 139–143, 2002
12. Marhold C, Linton SJ, Melin L. A cognitive-behavioural return-to-work program: effects on pain patients with a history of long-term versus short-term sick leave. *Pain* **91**: 155–163, 2001
13. Turk, Dennis C. Combining somatic and psychosocial treatment for chronic pain: perhaps 1+1 does = 3. *Clin J Pain* **17**: 281–283, 2001
14. Guzman J, Esmail R, Karjalainen K, Malmivaara A, Irvin E, Bombardier C. Multidisciplinary rehabilitation for chronic low back pain: systematic review. *Br Med J* **322**: 1511–1516, 2001

# 34 Interventional Pain Procedures

*Simon J Dolin and Nicholas L Padfield*

This chapter will illustrate a sample of interventional techniques in common currency amongst interventional pain specialists. The list is not exhaustive but is here to illustrate the range of techniques available. For details on less commonly performed local anaesthetic/neurolytic blocks the reader is advised to look in a large textbook specifically on regional block techniques.

## Cervical epidural

There are three positions in which a cervical epidural can be done, and individual patient circumstances will dictate which approach is the most appropriate. As with all epidurals, it is mandatory to establish intravenous access and have appropriate physiological monitoring and resuscitation facilities immediately available. The patient should also spend the subsequent 20 minutes in a properly staffed recovery immediately after the procedure.

### Prone

With the patient lying prone, arms by their sides with a pillow under the chest and the brow resting on a head-ring so that respiration is unhindered, the back of the neck is prepped with cleaning solution and the spine of C7 palpated. The next easily palpable interspace, moving cranially, is identified and the skin infiltrated with 1% lignocaine. A 22 gauge spinal needle is then inserted in the midline and the trajectory checked with anterior–posterior (AP) imaging to correct any deviation from the midline. The needle is then advanced a few centimetres until it is held by the tissues. Lateral imaging is then checked to determine the advancement of the needle tip towards the line formed by the anterior edge of the vertebral spines.

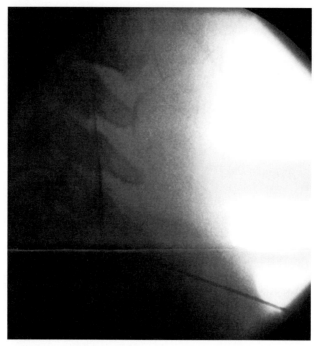

**Figure 34.1**    Cervical epidural (lateral radiograph)

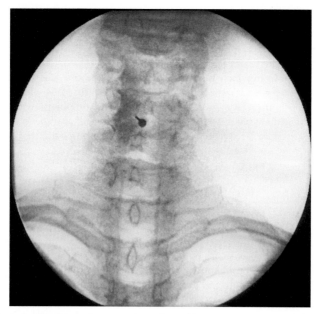

**Figure 34.2**    Cervical epidural (anterior–posterior radiograph)

Note that, in the cervical spine, the epidural space lies behind the facet pillars in the lateral projection. The need for altering the angulation of the needle cranially or caudally to avoid impingement on the spines will be also apparent. When the needle tip is near this line, an intravenous giving set connected to a paediatric burette containing normal saline is connected. The drip chamber is then inspected as the tip of the needle is slowly advanced. As the epidural space – only 1.5 mm deep in the cervical spine – is entered, the drip will start to run giving a clear end point. The intravenous giving set is then disconnected and about 0.5 ml Isovist 240 (iotrolan at iodine equivalent, 240 mg/ml) contrast is then injected and the spread of the contrast checked on both AP and lateral images. It should look like a straight line running just in front of the vertebral spines with well defined edges (Figures 34.1 & 34.2). Triamcinolone 40 mg mixed with 20 mg lignocaine and normal saline to make a total volume of 5 ml is then slowly injected. In the unlikely event that there is severe pain on injection, it should be stopped immediately and, if possible, imaging undertaken to ascertain the problem.

## Lateral

With the patient lying on their most comfortable side, pillows are placed so that the line of the ENTIRE vertebral column is straight and parallel to the floor. The patient should also be lying at 90° to the floor. Careful positioning at this point will prevent difficulties in obtaining the correct trajectory of the needle. The rest of the procedure is then undertaken in a similar manner as described above, however, the imaging will be reversed.

## Sitting

This is rather more controversial. The patient sits on a stool with their arms comfortably resting on a pillow on the imaging table. The C-arm is then positioned from the end of the table and swung round 90° so that the AP and lateral images are both parallel to the floor. This has advantages for nervous or arthritic patients, as the positioning for them is much simpler as less claustrophobic. However, if there is any predictable likelihood that the patient may faint then it is best avoided. Otherwise make sure there is plenty of strong-armed help available. Even so, with experience, this position can make a potentially scary procedure much easier for patient and clinician.

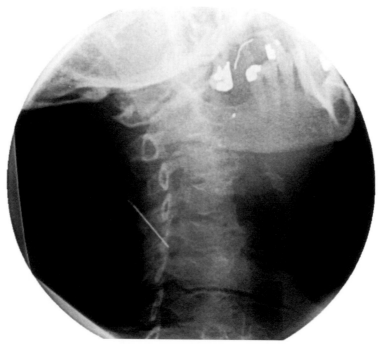

**Figure 34.3**   Cervical nerve root injection (lateral radiograph)

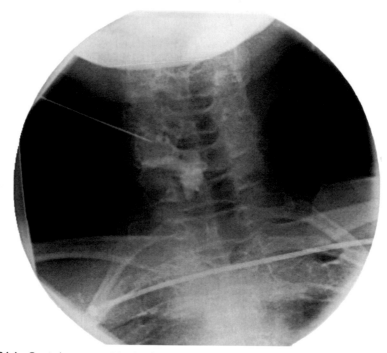

**Figure 34.4**   Cervical nerve root injection (anterior–posterior radiograph)

# Cervical nerve root injection

Patients are positioned supine for these blocks. The imaging table must allow for angled views as well as the classic AP and lateral views. The C-arm is angled 30° up from the lateral position to demonstrate the intervertebral foramina. Remember the first foramen to be seen is between C2 and C3 and contains the C3 root (the majority of the innervation to the lesser occipital nerve). The skin entry point is located over the selected level with a sponge holding forceps under fluoroscopy and is then infiltrated with local anaesthetic. The chosen needle is then inserted, aiming for the upper margin of the facetal pillar so that it can be 'walked' off anteriorly to lie at the apex of the intervertebral foramen. Anterior–posterior views should confirm that the tip of the needle is lying halfway between the outer edge of the transverse process and the outer edge of the vertebral body. The 50 mm 23 gauge POLE stimulating needle is ideal, as direct stimulation once the radiological position is optimal will confirm the correct level and distribution as well as giving an indication of the proximity of the needle tip to the root (Figures 34.3 & 34.4). It is possible to place a 22 gauge spinal needle with the use of contrast to confirm positioning, but the author favours a stimulation–location technique. 1.5–2 ml solution containing 20–40 mg depot methylprednisolone and local anaesthetic are then injected slowly. Severe pain indicates an intraneural or a seriously compressing injection that would jeopardize the blood supply to the cord at that level and must be stopped immediately.

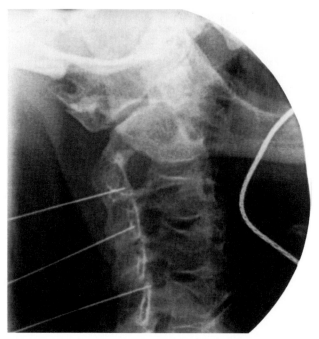

**Figure 34.5**  Cervical facet joint radiofrequency denervation (45° angle radiograph)

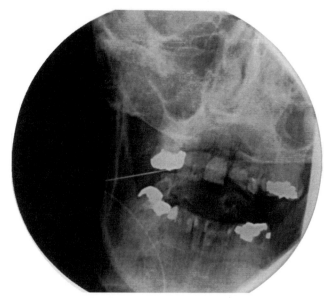

**Figure 34.6**  Cervical facet joint radiofrequency denervation (anterior–posterior radiograph)

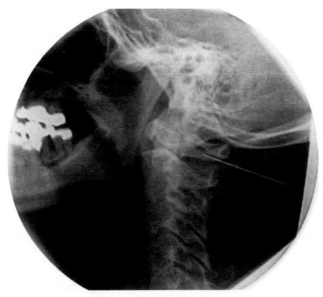

**Figure 34.7**   Pulse radiofrequency dorsal root ganglion (lateral radiograph)

## Radiofrequency cervical facet joint denervation

A line demonstrating the posterior border of the sternocleidomastoid is marked, as this is the line from which the skin is entered. With a 45° angle from the lateral the facet pillars and the intervertebral foramina are demonstrated. The tip of 50 mm SMK needle is advanced until it hits the facet pillar at the same level as the apex of the intervertebral foramen. The tip of the needle is then advanced until the tip lies just behind the posterior margin of the intervertebral foramen. The AP view is then checked, and the proximity of the needle tip to the facet pillar can be checked (Figures 34.5–34.7). Most facet pillars are 'waisted', and the ideal position is anywhere from the top to the middle of the waist. A current is then passed down to the exposed needle tip via the electrode from the radiofrequency (RF) lesion generator, and the voltage threshold for paraesthesia sought. Ideally, it should be between 0.3 and 0.5 V and should be felt in the neck and *nowhere else*. Because the median branches of the posterior primary rami divide and course in a variety of positions, it is often necessary to make several lesions up and down the facet pillars at each selected level. Lesions are made after local anaesthetic infiltration for 60 seconds at 80°C.

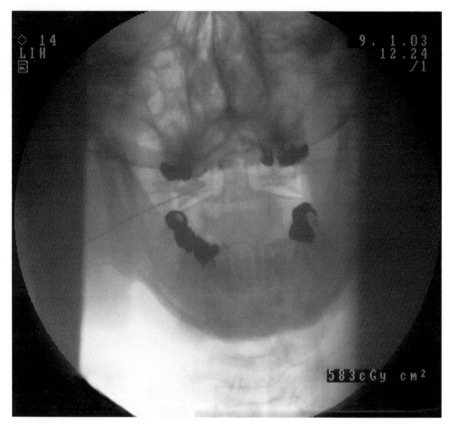

**Figure 34.8** Pulsed radiofrequency cervical dorsal root ganglion (anterior–posterior radiograph)

## Pulsed radiofrequency cervical dorsal root ganglion

Patients are positioned supine for these blocks. The imaging table must allow for angled views as well as the classic AP and lateral views (Figures 34.8). The C-arm is angled 30° up from the lateral position to demonstrate the intervertebral foramina. Remember, the first foramen to be seen is between C2 and C3 and contains the C3 root (the majority of the innervation to the lesser occipital nerve). If pulsed RF treatment to the C2 root is required to treat the greater occipital nerve, the posterior intervertebral foramen needs to be imaged, which requires a 'jaw up' position and angling of the image intensifier to show this level clear of double shadows from the mandible.

A 50 mm 23 gauge SMK needle is then directed to lateral aspect of the foramen avoiding entry into the dural sac. For the lower levels down to C7, the skin entry point is located over the selected level with a sponge holding forceps under fluoroscopy and is then infiltrated with local anaesthetic. The needle is then inserted aiming for the upper margin of the facetal pillar so that it can be 'walked' off anteriorly to lie at the apex of the intervertebral foramen. Anterior–posterior views should confirm that the tip of the needle is lying halfway between the outer edge of the transverse process and the outer edge of the vertebral body. Once the radiological position is optimal the current is passed through the tip of the needle and paraesthesia elicited to confirm the correct level and site of the stimulation. The output of the pulsed RF treatment needs to be titrated so that it is just felt, and then continued for 8 minutes at each level. At the end of treatment, patients will volunteer that prior pain has been replaced by pleasant feelings, variously described as tingling, light and warm.

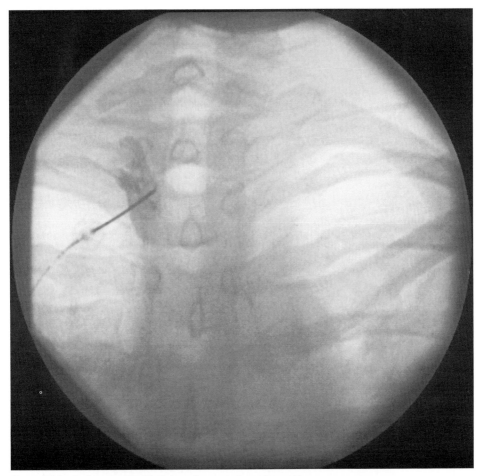

**Figure 34.9**  Stellate ganglion block (anterior–posterior radiograph)

## Stellate ganglion block

The stellate ganglion is formed by the coalescence of the superior thoracic and cervical sympathetic ganglia. Consequently, the spread of agent needs to cover several vertebral levels. The patient is positioned supine, and the cricoid cartilage palpated, which indicates the level of the transverse process of C6. The groove between the carotid pulsation and the trachea is located, and a 22 gauge spinal needle inserted at right angles to the skin directly posteriorly until the tip of the needle finds bone. 0.5 ml Isovist 240 contrast is injected, and the spread checked in AP and lateral images to confirm sharp edges as the contrast lies in front of the prevertebral fascia (Figures 34.9). For a diagnostic block, 6 ml 0.5% bupivacaine and 40 mg methyl prednisolone are injected, and the patient is then sat up. A Horner's syndrome should then develop over the next 5 minutes, confirming successful spread and placement of the local anaesthetic solution. For a neurolytic block, the patient must understand and accept the possibility of a permanent ptosis, although unlikely, and even then the author would only use 2–3 ml 6% aqueous phenol.

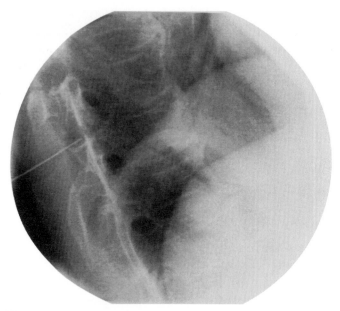

**Figure 34.10**   Thoracic epidural (lateral radiograph)

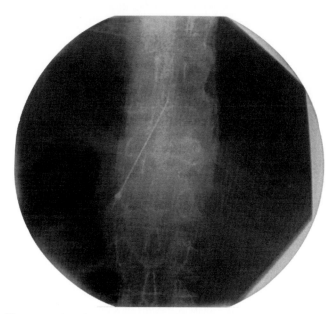

**Figure 34.11**   Thoracic epidural (anterior–posterior radiograph)

# Thoracic epidural

Ideally, the patient should be sat on a table at a height that will permit easy access of the C-arm to image AP and lateral views. After screening to determine the selected interspinous space, the skin over it is infiltrated with 1% lignocaine and a 22 gauge spinal needle, Quincke ended, is inserted and then advanced, screened in both planes to ensure the optimal trajectory to avoid impingement on the angled thoracic vertebral spines (Figures 34.10 & 34.11). As the tip of the needle approaches the epidural space, an intravenous giving set attached to a paediatric burette is attached and opened. The tip is then gently advanced whilst observing the drip chamber. As the epidural space is entered, the saline will start to drip, giving a clear end point. 0.5 ml Isovist 240 contrast is then injected and the spread checked to confirm correct intraepidural placement, then 1 ml 1% lignocaine and 20 mg depot methylprednisolone injected per vertebral level to be treated. Patients should then have physiological monitoring in a suitable environment for at lest the next 20 minutes.

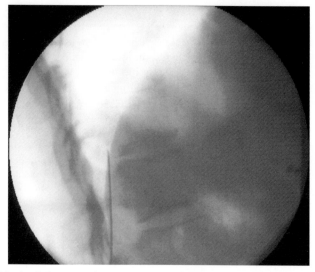

**Figure 34.12**   Pulsed radiofrequency thoracic dorsal root ganglion (lateral radiograph)

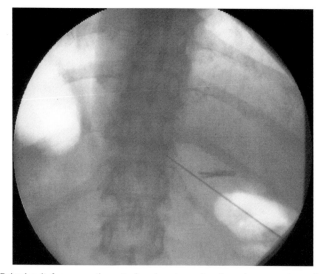

**Figure 34.13**   Pulsed radiofrequency thoracic dorsal root ganglion (anterior–posterior radiograph)

# Pulsed radiofrequency thoracic dorsal root ganglion

The dorsal root ganglia in the thoracic region lie behind the facet pillars, and they are the most difficult to reach with the tip of the SMK needle. To guarantee needle placement at the dorsal root ganglion, a hole needs to be drilled through the transverse process, which makes the procedure far more invasive and greatly increases the potential morbidity. The lateral approach is technically difficult, as the rib lies at the same level as the intervetebral foramen; therefore, to avoid the rib and to get access to the foramen, the trajectory will almost certainly pass very close to the segmental neurovascular bundle, and the likelihood of nerve damage or vessel damage is high. However, it may be the only possible approach, and the patient should be warned of the risks accordingly. The use of curved SMK needles will increase the chance of success as they are easier to manoeuvre around the bony obstacles.

Alternatively, an interspinous approach may be worth trying if fluoroscopy indicates a generous interspinous space and a likely success of placing the tip of the needle laterally within the epidural space. It is important to note that the longitudinal ligaments may well be needled by this technique, which can lead to a variety of pains from the occiput to the low back.

When the needle tip is positioned as optimally as circumstances will allow (Figures 34.12 & 34.13), the threshold voltage for paraesthesia is sought as it will give an indication of the proximity of the dorsal root ganglion to the needle tip (and, therefore, the likelihood of success). If paraesthesia can be elicited at 0.5–1 V then it is worth proceeding, if the threshold is much higher, it is probably not going to be effective, in the author's experience. The output should be adjusted on the pulsed RF mode until the pulses are just felt but not uncomfortable. The treatment needs to be continued for 8 minutes in each segment. If the pain has subsided at the end of the procedure, the outcome is likely to be favourable.

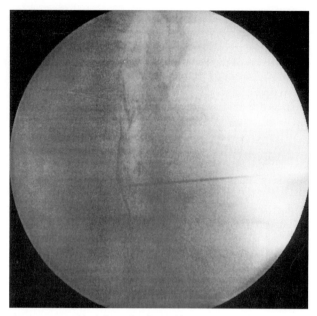

**Figure 34.14**  Lumbar nerve root block (lateral radiograph)

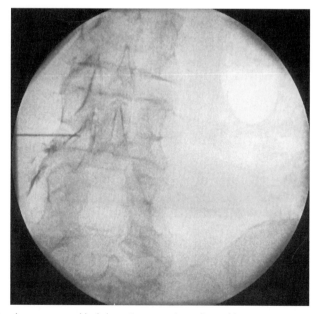

**Figure 34.15**  Lumbar nerve root block (anterior–posterior radiograph)

## Lumbar nerve root blocks

The intervertebral foramina are easiest to visualize fluoroscopically in the lumbar region. The patient is positioned prone on the screening table and the image intensifier is turned to 45%, so that the top of the pedicle and the anterior aspect of the facet is easily seen. A 22 gauge spinal needle is then inserted along this trajectory, 'looking-down-the-needle' until bone is encountered. As long as the tip of the needle is kept up to lie just underneath the pedicle, it is unlikely that the nerve root will be encountered. Lateral imaging should confirm that the needle is touching the posterior surface of the vertebral body and that the tip is lying at the apex, superiorly, of the lateral foramen (Figure 34.14). Anterior–posterior views should confirm that the needle tip is lying at the medial border of the facet joint (Figure 34.15).

0.5 ml Isovist contrast is injected, which should outline the nerve sheath and produce an anterior epidurogram. 2–3 ml of a mixture of 40 mg depot methylprednisolone and 0.5% marcain is then injected.

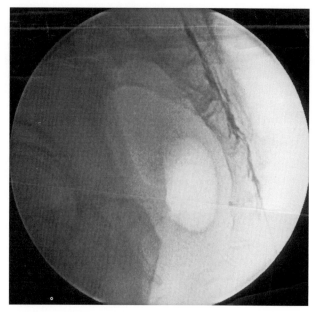

**Figure 34.16**   Sacral epidural (anterior–posterior radiograph)

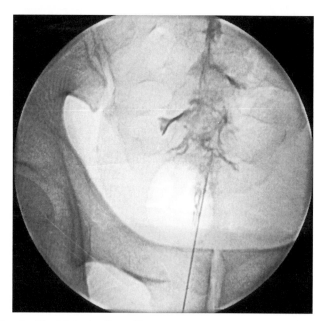

**Figure 34.17**   Sacral epidural (lateral radiograph)

# Sacral epidural

The patient is positioned prone on the imaging table and lateral fluoroscopy performed to demonstrate the sacral hiatus at the entrance to the caudal epidural canal. The skin over the midline at this level is then infiltrated with 1% lignocaine and a 22 gauge spinal needle inserted at an angle of 45° in the sagittal plane. The tip is advanced until it touches bone, and then angled more cranially until it enters the sacral hiatus with the characteristic 'give'. This should be apparent on lateral imaging (Figure 34.16) and, to confirm epidural placement of the tip, 0.5 ml Isovist 240 contrast is injected (Figure 34.17). This should outline the epidural space, lying posteriorly within the canal, and should show the branches of the nerve roots in the typical 'Christmas tree' pattern. 4–6 ml 40 mg depot methylprednisolone and 0.5% marcain mixture are then injected and the needle withdrawn.

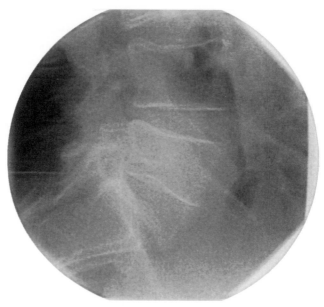

**Figure 34.18**   Lumbar epidural (anterior–posterior radiograph)

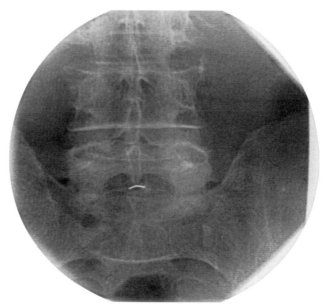

**Figure 34.19**   Lumbar epidural (anterior–posterior radiograph)

# Lumbar epidural

With the patient in the prone position a 22 gauge spinal needle is inserted under direct fluoroscopy through the interspinous space. Once the needle is gripped by the interspinous ligaments, the trajectory is confirmed (Figures 34.18 & 34.19). It is possible to perform one-sided epidurals when the pain is predominantly one sided by steering the needle tip towards the lateral canal. The proximity to the epidural space is then checked by lateral fluoroscopy and penetration of the epidural space confirmed, initially, by loss of resistance to the injection of saline or by connecting to an intravenous giving set and watching the drip chamber. As the epidural space is entered the saline will start to drip; a useful technique for difficult spines, but probably not necessary in unremarkable spines. The volume of solution injected depends on the number of vertebral levels to be treated, and whether the block is unilateral or bilateral. The author uses 10 mg triamcinolone per vertebral level mixed with 1 ml 0.5% lignocaine and makes a slight reduction of the total volume if a unilateral approach is employed.

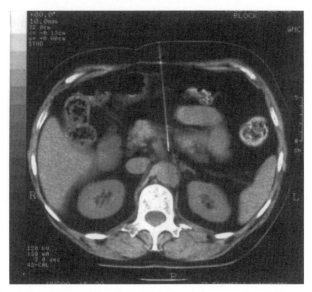

**Figure 34.20** Coeliac plexus block (CT-guided axial view)

# Coeliac plexus block

This was classically performed with patient in the prone position, relying on gravity to reach the plexus. Large volumes were injected on either side and, not surprisingly, there have been several reports of serious permanent neurological sequelae arising from this route. It will be described for the sake of completeness, but, in the author's view, should not be employed when other equally effective and much safer techniques exist. In all cases, intravenous access and fluids along with full physiological monitoring are mandatory.

## Prone

The patient is positioned prone on the screening table, and the area from the lower thoracic vertebral spines to the top of the sacrum cleaned with prep solution. The body of the first lumbar vertebral is located and the skin marked with a pen. The lower border of the 12th rib is located and the area below, about 7 cm from the midline, is infiltrated with 1% lignocaine The fluoroscope is then angled 45° in the coronal plane and then angled and screened in the sagittal plane until the body and the facet of L1 are clearly defined without interference from the rib. The 22 gauge 150 mm needle is then advanced so that it passes anterior to the facet joints and the tip ends up at the level of the anterior surface of the vertebral body. The needle tip position is then checked in AP and lateral views without sagittal angulation.

To confirm its position just anterior to the vertebral body and medial to the lateral edge of the body, Isovist 240 contrast is then injected, and the spread checked to confirm the flow anteriorly up and down in front of the body of L1, well away from the segmental nerves emerging from the intervertebral foramina. For a diagnostic block, 10 ml 0.5% bupivacaine and 40 mg depot methylprednisolone is injected each side. For a neurolytic block, 20 ml 50% alcohol is injected. It is often necessary to give analgesia as the intense initial burning sensation after the injection of the alcohol can be excruciating. Patients should be nursed prone for a further 40 minutes to minimize the risk of spread/tracking of the alcohol back towards the segmental nerves.

## Supine

This approach is best achieved in the computed CT scanner. The origin of the superior mesenteric artery as it leaves the aorta anteriorly is located by scanning at the level of the bodies of L1–L2. It is sometimes necessary to angle the CT scanner up to 10° in the sagittal plane. The axial views allow accurate visualization of the plexus, which lies anterior to the aorta and the pancreas (Figure 34.20). The depth from the skin surface and the trajectory necessary to reach the ganglia, which can usually be seen discretely with this technique, can then be calculated. The spread of contrast (which must be diluted to third normal strength) will localize the ganglia of the plexus and confirm the site of the spread of agent. 8–10 ml aqueous phenol 6% is then injected, and the spread monitored by further scanning. At this stage, it may be evident whether a further injection needs to be made, changing the trajectory of the needle to the other side of the midline to treat both sides of the plexus, or whether the single injection has reached both sides satisfactorily. As with the alcohol injection, analgesia should be given as the injection of phenol is followed initially by an intense burning feeling. In the case of repeat procedures, scarring from the previous neurolytic injections may distort the anatomy making, in the author's opinion, a CT-guided approach preferable to the 'blind' posterior approach.

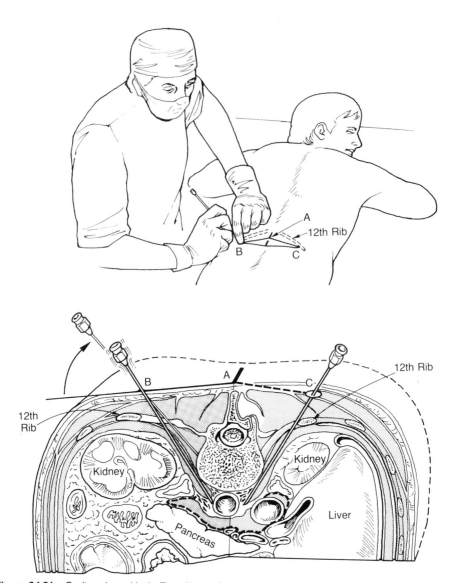

**Figure 34.21** Coeliac plexus block. Top: skin markings, position of patient and initial insertion of needle. Note: Triangle formed by skin marks on lower border of 12th ribs (B and C) in line with inferior border of L1 spinous process and joined to inferior border of T12 (A). Bottom: needle insertion and deep anatomy. Skin markings and triangle (A, B, C) are still shown. Needle initially directed in the plane of the line BA or CA, and at 45° to the horizontal axis of the body, to contact the lateral aspect of L1 vertebral body. It passes inferior to the 12th rib and medial to the kidney. The angle of insertion of the horizontal axis of the body is then increased until the needle slips past the lateral aspect of the vertebral body, still in line BA or CA to reach to the antero-lateral aspect. On the left side the aortic pulsations will be deleted at the needle hub before puncturing the artery.

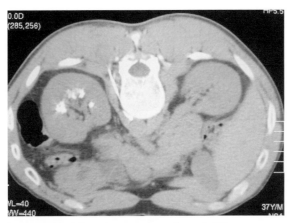

**Figure 34.22**   Spanchnic nerve block (anterior–posterior radiograph CT)

## Splanchnic nerve block

The splanchnic nerves arise as the greater, lesser and least splanchnic nerves from the coalescence of the lowest thoracic sympathetic ganglia. They pass anteriorly through the crura of the
diaphragm to form the coeliac plexus anteriorly to the aorta and pancreas. They can be
blocked retrocrurally with a much smaller volume of agent than the coeliac plexus, and the
technique is associated with a far lower incidence of adverse side-effects and permanent neurological sequelae. In all cases, intravenous access and fluids along with full physiological monitoring are mandatory.

The skin about 7 cm from the midline, just inferior to the lower edge of the 12th rib, is
infiltrated with 1% lignocaine, and the spine of the 11th thoracic vertebra identified. The trajectory of the 22 gauge 150 mm needle is such that the tip of the needle will lie alongside the
body of the T11. This can be confirmed by fluoroscopy in AP views. Skewed views in the
sagittal plane are generally unhelpful as the ribs make interpretation difficult. CT gives much
more precise localization where the axial images scan the bodies of T10–T11 and the nerves
can be seen in relation to the crura of the diaphragm. 0.5 ml Isovist 240 contrast is injected
after satisfactory needle tip placement by fluoroscopy and the same volume of third strength
contrast after localization by CT scanning (Figure 34.21 & 34.22). The contrast should not
move on respiration, and it should spread up and down the vertebral body. It should not pass
into the lung parenchyma, the pleura or retrogradely towards the segmental intercostals
nerves. Inadvertent neurolytic block of the intercostals nerves is frequently accompanied by
severe neuropathic pain, which can be refractory to treatment. 8 ml 0.5% bupivacaine with 40
mg depot methylprednisolone are injected for a prognostic block, and 8 ml 6% aqueous phenol injected for a neurolytic block. As intense burning pain is initially experienced with the
neurolytic block, analgesia needs to be administered first.

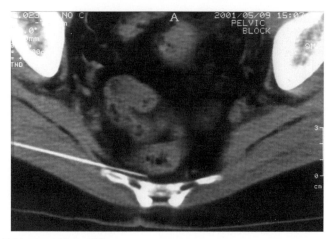

**Figure 34.23** Pelvic plexus block (CT)

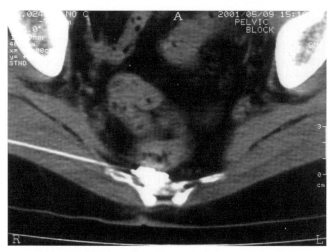

**Figure 34.24** Pelvic plexus block (CT with contrast)

## Pelvic plexus block

The pelvic plexus can be reached as it lies anterior to the sacrum by passing a 22 gauge 150 mm needle over the iliac crests underneath the lamina of L5, so that the needle tip lies in front of the sacrum on lateral views and towards the midline on AP views (Figure 34.23). 1 ml Isovist 240 contrast is injected and the spread should confirm the spread just anterior to the presacral fascia (Figure 34.24). 6–10 ml 0.5% bupivacaine and 40 mg depot methylprednisolone should inject easily. For a neurolytic block, 6–8 ml 6% phenol is injected. This will affect the neurogenic control of the bladder and anal sphincters.

## Presacral neurolytic block for relief of pain from pelvic cancer: description and use of a CT-guided lateral approach

Oral contrast is administered 2 hours prior to the procedure to highlight the small bowel. The patient lies supine on the CT (Sytec) couch and routine monitoring of pulse and blood pressure is applied. Preliminary axial scans of the pelvis (10 mm thickness every 10 mm) are taken to identify the greater sciatic notch and the presacral fat plane, which lies just anterior to the vertebral bodies of the sacrum at the level of S3 and S4. The pelvic pain fibres, in close association with the pelvic sympathetic nerve supply, lie close to this fat plane. Measurements are taken from the fat plane to the skin of the buttock. The point on the skin is highlighted by a laser light from the CT scanner and marked accordingly. Using an aseptic technique, a 22 gauge needle is passed from the buttock, perpendicular to the skin, posterior to the hip joint and through the greater sciatic notch into the pelvic cavity. Under CT guidance, the needle is directed towards the presacral fat plane in the midline. Once a satisfactory position is reached, correct placement is confirmed with 1 ml contrast (Isovist 240 diluted 2-fold). Correct placement occurs when the contrast runs freely in the presacral area and when intravascular injection does not occur. Following correct positioning of the needle, either local anaesthetic (5 ml 0.5% bupivacaine) is injected to perform a diagnostic block or 5 ml 6% phenol in water is injected to perform a neurolytic block. The sciatic nerve and major blood vessels are clearly observable and easily avoided by guiding the needle posterior to them.

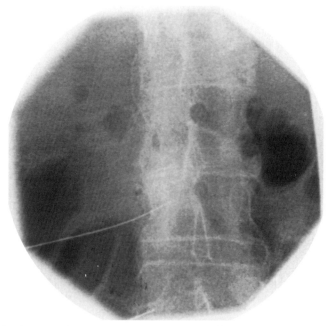

**Figure 34.25** Lumbar sympathectomy antero-posterior radiograph

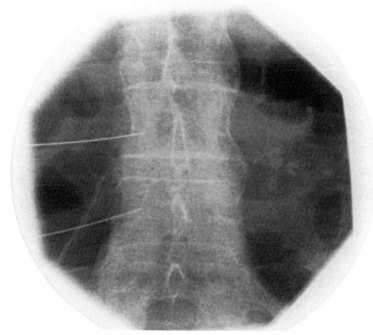

**Figure 34.26** Lumbar sympathectomy (anterior–posterior radiograph)

# Lumbar sympathectomy

The patient is positioned prone and the spine of L3 identified. The skin 7 cms lateral is infiltrated with 1% lignocaine and then the fluoroscope is angled 45° in the coronal plane. A 22 gauge 150 mm needle is then introduced, aiming for the anterior border of the vertebral body passing anterior to the facet joint. When it has been advanced sufficiently to hold it firmly, lateral and anterior views are checked as the needle continues to be advanced until the tip lies at the anterior border of the vertebral body on the lateral view and is tucked inside by the medial border of the zygoapophyseal joint (Figure 34.25 & 34.26). 1 ml Isovist 240 contrast is injected and the spread is checked to ensure it lies anteriorly to the body without moving on respiration and not demonstrating the fibres of psoas major. Anterior view should confirm spread anteriorly to the vertebral body, and not lateral spread outlining psoas major. For a diagnostic block, 10 ml 0.5% bupivacaine with 40 mg depot methylprednisolone is injected. For a neurolytic block, 6–8 ml 6% aqueous phenol is injected, warning the patient that they will feel a transient burning feeling, which may leave an area of hyperaesthesia in the flanks. This is usually only temporary, rarely lasting longer than 3 weeks.

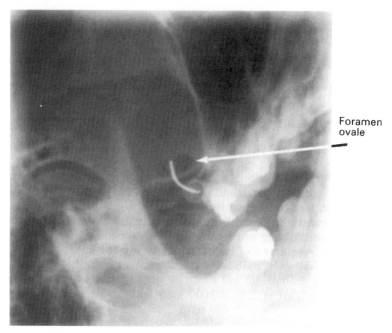

**Figure 34.27** View of foremen ovale with needle *in situ*. The foramen can be readily seen by extending the patient's neck and adjusting the angle of the image intensifier to 10° rotation and approximately 30° skew from the anteroposterior.

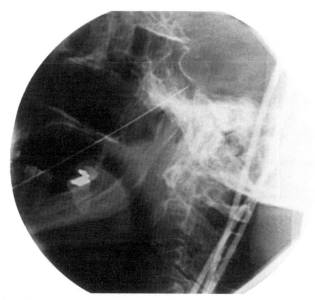

**Figure 34.28** Radiofrequency trigeminal ganglion thermocoagulation (lateral radiograph)

# Radiofrequency trigeminal ganglion thermocoagulation

With patient lying prone, a 100 mm RF insulated needle, with a 5 mm active tip, is inserted 2–3 cm lateral to angle of mouth. The midpoint of the ipsilateral pupil can be used as a rough guide to correct alignment in the sagittal plane (Figure 34.27). Keeping away from the angle of the mouth avoids the needle entering the oral cavity. The foramen ovale is visualized by fluoroscopy: with neck extended angle the beam approximately 10° rotation away from the midline towards the side of the needle, and 20–30° of skew in a caudad direction. The foramen will appear as an oval shaped structure between the maxilla (medial) and mandible (lateral). The needle can be advanced using 'tunnel vision' directly into the foramen. As it enters the operator has a sense of the tissues giving way (see Figure 34.27). Change to lateral view: the needle should be caudad to sella turcica and between foramen and clivus (Figure 34.28). Using a wake-up technique for sedation or anaesthesia the correct trigeminal division can be located by sensory stimulation 50–100 Hz (threshold 0.2–0.3 V). The third, second and first divisions will be stimulated in succession the closer to the clival line the needle tip is. Sedation/anaesthesia is increased and RF lesion (75–80°C; 1–2 minutes) is performed.

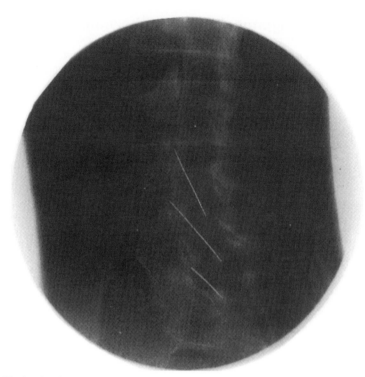

**Figure 34.29** Lumbar facet joint injection (anterior–posterior radiograph)

## Lumbar facet joint injection

With patient lying prone the fluoroscope C-arm is rotated 25–35°. The lumbar facet joints are usually clearly visible, although there are anatomical variations in facet joint angles, and the angle may need to be adjusted to give the best view. A 22 gauge 9 cm (3.5-inch) needle is introduced percutaneously, and advanced into the joint using 'tunnel vision' (Figure 34.29). The operator can usually feel the needle enter the joint, where it takes a slightly medial course. Contrast material can be introduced to perform an arthrogram, prior to injection. The volume of the joint is small and will only tolerate injection of 0.5–1 ml local anaesthetic and methylprednisolone. Various numbers of joints can be injected at the same time.

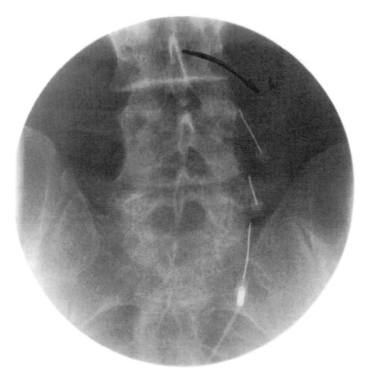

**Figure 34.30** Lumbar radiofrequency facet joint rhizolysis (anteroposterior view).

## Radiofrequency lumbar facet denervation

With patient lying prone, the true AP is established by fluoroscopy. For lumbar vertebrae L1–L4, rotation 15° on side of the lesion for initial needle placement. A metal pointer is placed over the junction of the transverse process and inferior articular facet process. A 100 mm RF insulated needle, with a 5 mm active tip, is introduced percutaneously, and advanced to touch bone at this junction, using 'tunnel vision'. The needle is rotated with bevel facing medial and slipped slightly off the junction of bone. Change to AP, to check needle is snuggled in close to the facet joint and just cephalad to transverse process. Change to 45° rotation on side of needle. Needle tip should be lying across the base of a triangle of bone made up of the inferior articular process of the facet joint. It should not project beyond this triangle (Figure 34.30).

For L5 needle placement, use 10° rotation and 10° skew in a cephalad direction. This is needed to clear the iliac crest, especially in men. Otherwise, AP and 45° views as above.

S1 level can be lesioned as well. The needle can be placed in the posterior part of the S1 foramen using an AP view and 'tunnel vision', although some cephalad skew may be needed in some patients. The operator will feel the needle enter the S1 foramen. A lateral view should show the needle at the junction of S1 and S2 vertebrae. The needle should be advanced to about the midline of the spinal canal, but no further, in the lateral view. Stimulation of 50–100 Hz (threshold 0.3–0.4 V) should give stimulation in the back or buttock, but not in the leg. Once correct position has been located, RF current is increased to give 75°C for 60 seconds.

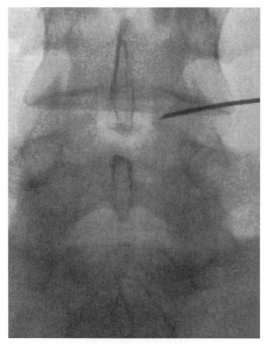

**Figure 34.31**   Lumbar discography (anterior–posterior radiograph)

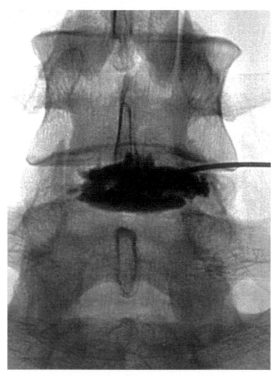

**Figure 34.32**   Lumbar discography (lateral radiograph)

# Lumbar discography

With patient lying prone, C-arm is rotated to one side about 30°, so that facet joints lie approximately in the middle of the vertebral body. The C-arm will need to be skewed in either a cephalad or caudad direction to line up the vertebral end-plates, which opens up the best view of the disc. A metal pointer is placed at the junction of the transverse process and inferior facet pillar. A 22 gauge 12.5 cm (5-inch) needle is introduced percutaneously and advanced under 'tunnel vision' onto the junction. The needle is then advanced beyond the junction and introduced into the intervertebral disc. Keeping close in to this junction will avoid needle contact with the anterior nerve root. Move to an AP view: needle should be in the centre of the disc (Figure 34.31). Move to a lateral view: needle should be in centre of disc (Figure 34.32). A 10 ml syringe containing 8 ml Isovist 240 mg/ml and 2 ml gentamicin (80 mg) is connected to rigid extension tubing and then to the needle hub. Under direct fluoroscopy the disc is injected. A healthy disc will take a volume of 2 ml, without producing pain and without contrast leakage. A degenerated disc will take greater volume and may have some contrast leakage, in a posterior direction into the epidural space. Discography is positive when the patient experiences their typical pain, perhaps at its most severe for a few seconds during injection; there is often accompanying leakage from the disc. Intravenous antibiotic cover is often given as well, to prevent discitis, which is a rare complication.

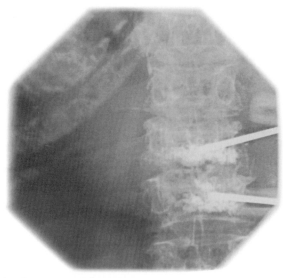

**Figure 34.33** Vertebroplasty anteroposterior view.

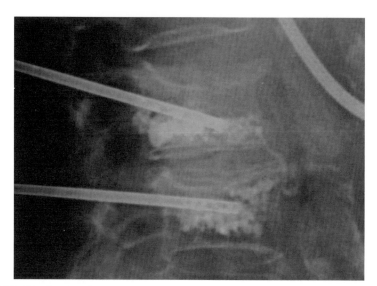

**Figure 34.34** Vertebroplasty lateral view.

# Vertebroplasty

The patient is positioned prone (Figures 34.33 & 34.34). For vertebral fractures from the mid-thoracic to the lumbar region an 11 gauge needle is used, for fractures above that level a 15 gauge needle is used. Fluoroscopy initially should entail an oblique view of 10–15°; the pedicle should appear as an oval-shaped structure, and the needle should be introduced through the skin to contact the pedicle in its lateral position using this view. A degree of angulation in the cephalad/caudad plane may be needed to ensure the needle follows the pedicle; this can be verified in the lateral view. The needle is then introduced through the bone and, under gentle pressure, is advanced down the pedicle and into the body of the vertebra. A bone hammer may be useful to give small, controlled increments of pressure. Some clinicians use an approach just lateral to the pedicle and enter the bone in the vertebral body itself. Either approach is designed to avoid the nerve roots as they exit the foramina above and below. The needle is advanced to the anterior one-third of the vertebral body in the lateral plane and, ideally, into the middle of the vertebral body in the AP view. When the needle is in place, attempts should be made to aspirate blood, if so, a venogram can be performed with some contrast, and if this shows spread into the epidural or anterior veins then the needle should be moved slightly until this effect disappears. Bone cement (Vertebroplastic, Osteopal) is then mixed and can be introduced into the needle directly via a syringe, although many clinicians now prefer the use of a hand held injector, which enables small increments of cement to be injected.

Injection should only occur during continuous fluoroscopy in the lateral view, with care taken to make sure the cement does not enter the epidural canal nor the intervertebral disc nor the adjacent blood vessels. The bone cements used have added contrast, so are easily visible using fluoroscopy. The usual volumes of injection are 2–3 ml in the thoracic area and up to 5 ml in the lumbar area. The needle is then withdrawn using a rotational movement. The patient should lie still for about half an hour, which should provide sufficient time for the bone cement to set. Antibiotic cover is recommended.

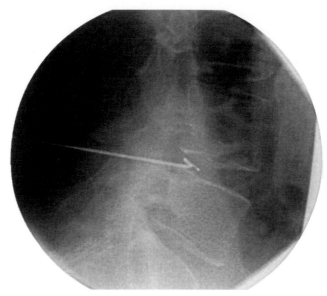

**Figure 34.35** Annuloplasty (lateral radiograph)

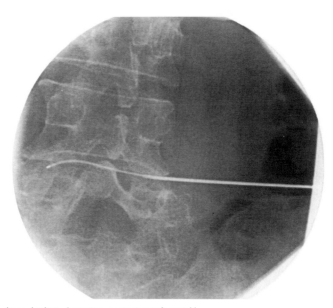

**Figure 34.36** Annnuloplasty (anterior–posterior radiograph)

# Anuloplasty

With the patient lying prone an oblique view is obtained at about 35°. Under fluoroscopy, the vertebral end plates of the appropriate disc are lined up by adding skew in either a cephalad or caudad direction. The facet joint should appear approximately mid-way across the disc with the end plates lined up. An introducer (Radionics) is inserted percutaneously, this may require a small skin incision to aid skin entry. The introducer is then passed down lateral to the facet joint, and then advanced into the intervertebral disc; continuous impedance monitoring is recommended – once the introducer enters the disc the impedance falls to under 300 Ohms. There is a distinct feeling of resistance as the introducer enters the disc. The RF disctrode (Radionics) is then introduced through the curved introducer in a medial direction and passes across the back of the anulus; this should be confirmed in the anterior and lateral planes (Figures 34.35 & 34.36). A thermocouple is then introduced into the disc on the other side, using an insulated needle. The RF current is then applied as follows: 2 minutes at 45°C; 2 minutes at 50°C; 2 minutes at 60°C; and 4 minutes at 65°C. The current is adjusted to maintain the temperature in the thermocouple at or below 48°C. The full lesion time is 10 minutes. Antibiotic cover is recommended.

# Invasive Procedures: Technical Details

*Simon J Dolin and Nicholas L Padfield*

Pain management has developed in many different directions. Those trained in this sub-specialty who wish to embrace all branches of pain medicine will need to be aware of invasive techniques for pain relief. This chapter will deal with four key areas:

- Implantable drug delivery systems.
- Cryo analgesia.
- Radiofrequency thermocoagulation.
- Electrical stimulation analgesia (including transcutaneous nerve stimulation or TENS).

# APPENDIX I

## Implantable intrathecal drug delivery systems

### Indications

It is difficult to give specific indications for implanted drug delivery systems. They are confined to patients whose pain is opioid sensitive but whose pain has proved difficult to control with oral opioids alone because of escalating dosages or increasing side-effects of oral or transdermal opioid administration.

It is used in a mixed range of cases, including pain of malignant origin, failed back syndrome, complex regional pain syndromes and even phantom limb pain, although the literature is confined to a series of case reports and there have been no randomized controlled studies in this area. Intrathecal drug administration is also considered for patients with painful spasticity.

Prior to implantation most investigators would consider a trial of intrathecal drug administration, which is usually done by inserting a temporary intrathecal catheter and running a continuous infusion of the drug over one to several days. Some investigators may even consider sending the patient home with a trial infusion for one or more weeks with a portable pump. There are, however, some investigators who feel that a single shot of the drug is a sufficient trial. There is no universal agreement on this, although common sense would dictate that the longer the trial lasts and the more the patient is able to simulate day-to-day conditions in their life, the more the trial will predict success of the final technique.

## Drugs used for intrathecal administration

- Opioid – morphine is the most commonly used drug because of its longer stability in solution. Diamorphine is available in the UK, but it has a relatively short stability time. Morphine is known to be stable for in excess of 70 days, which is the usual time between pump refills. Morphine is available commercially at 30 and 40 mg/ml; in the USA, 50 mg/ml is available. While doses in the range of 0.3 mg per day are usually sufficient for postoperative analgesia, daily requirements for patients with cancer pain or chronic non-malignant pain are in a range of 2–20 mg per day. Most patients run at under 10 mg per day. The dose needs to be gradually increased, but there can be periods of long stability for many months, or even years, between dose increases.

- Clonidine can be used either alone or in combination with morphine. Intrathecal doses range from 30–120 µg per 24 hours.
- Bupivacaine has also been used by intrathecal administration, particularly in patients with cancer pain, usually in combination with morphine. Doses range from 30–300 mg per 24 hours.
- Baclofen is used primarily for treating painful spasticity in patients with multiple sclerosis, given in doses of 50–800 µg per 24 hours.
- Other drugs have been tried including ketamine, midazolam and ketorolac, but their use is not widespread.

# Equipment

Pumps are placed on the anterior abdominal wall muscles in a surgically created pocket and securely anchored by sutures to stay points. All implanted pumps have a central port for easy refilling and a separate port for aspiration or bolus of the intrathecal catheter. The ports are accessed percutaneously under sterile conditions; there is a hand-held template, which marks the refill entry point. Purpose-made refill kits are required

- Fully programmable lithium battery pumps – the main one on the market is the Medtronic SynchroMed with a reservoir of 18 ml (Figure A.1). This is fully programmable, using an external radio transmitter attached to a laptop computer. The operator is able to programme the rate, and it can run simple, continuous or complex infusions including varying rates at different times of the day and bolus injections with continuous background infusions. The advantage of this pump is that it gives great flexibility when the intrathecal medication is first commenced. This is particularly useful for patients with cancer pain, who may have rapidly escalating analgesic requirements. The lithium battery has a life of approximately 7 years, although this may be less depending on the rate at which the pump runs. This is generally the pump of first choice, at least for the initial pump.
- Mechanical pumps – these are gas driven, using either Freon or n-butane, or have a spring mechanism. The principal of these is that the spring or gas is compressed by filling the reservoir and the reservoir is emptied against a fixed constriction, which is a long constricted tube or a ceramic chip, designed to give a fixed flow rate over many weeks. These pumps lack flexibility for dose adjustments, as the rate is fixed and dose changes necessitate emptying and refilling the pump with a different concentration of drug.
- Single bolus ports can be implanted under the skin and can be accessed directly, so the patients or their carers can administer bolus doses. These systems, such as Portacath, are used almost entirely for treating cancer pain. They are less satisfactory because the bolus dose technique has the intrinsic disadvantages of higher dose-related side-effects, as well as repeated access to the implanted system with the increased risk of infection.
- Patient-activated systems are also available. This involves the patient emptying some of the main reservoir into a secondary reservoir and then emptying that as a bolus dose intrathecally. While these are less expensive, they are generally less widely used than the programmable intrathecal pumps.

While the fully programmable pump is the preferred first choice; the fact that it needs replacing every 5–7 years, as determined by battery life, does commit the patient to a number of

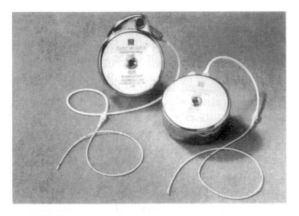

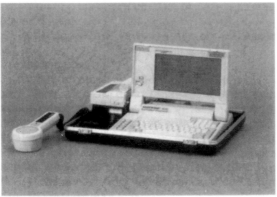

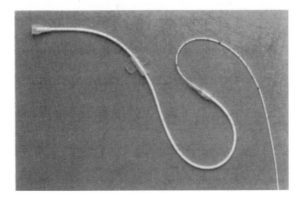

**Figure A.1** Medtronic Synchromed pump, fully implantable.

operations throughout their lives, especially if the pumps are put in when they are relatively young. Some investigators prefer mechanical pumps as the replacement pump, as this, in theory, means that only two pumps are required for the patient's lifetime.

## Complications

• Infection remains the major risk; if these pumps get infected the patient develops meningitis and can be seriously ill. Scrupulous attention to aseptic techniques and use of laminar flow facilities for drug preparation are advised. By careful attention to detail, it is possible to run these pumps for many years without this complication.

- Catheter migration – intrathecal catheters do on occasion migrate out of the intrathecal space and, sometimes, right out of the spine to come to lie subcutaneously. This is most likely to happen in the initial stages before the whole system has settled in. One patient who gave us particular problems with this had an amputated leg and, because of her prosthesis, walked with a marked limp; the movement of the spine appeared to encourage the catheter to migrate out of the intrathecal space.
- Catheter disconnections and kinking and breakages – intrathecal catheters are made of silicone, and the newer generation of catheters should be very robust in terms of not being able to kink or break. Small tears on inserting the catheter in the needle may, at a later stage, lead to catheter fracture. Catheters have also been known to become disconnected from the pump. Any thought that there may be a catheter problem can be checked by X-raying the system intact, as all catheters are radio-opaque, and it will be clear if the catheter is in the wrong position; by putting contrast through the bolus access port, it is possible to identify leakages.
- Intrathecal pumps have been known to come loose from the anchor points where they are sutured into the anterior abdominal wall. In that case, the pumps have been known to turn over so that the access port is facing posteriorly; this will require surgical revision.
- Drug side-effects – morphine and clonidine are both potentially sedative drugs and excessive dose will result in somnolence, as well as other opioid side-effects including nausea and vomiting. Baclofen overdose can cause drowsiness and hypotension. Bupivacaine can result in neurological disturbances such as paraesthesia and gait disturbances.

Intrathecal pumps require great commitment from a well-organized team. They require help with surgical implantation; while some pain clinicians may want to put their own pumps in, many will prefer to work with a surgical colleague, especially for creating the pocket and securing the catheter and pump. Refilling can be done by a clinical nurse specialist, who will require additional training and facilities for refilling. The use of aseptic facilities and support from the local pharmacy is essential. These patients become the responsibility of the pain clinic for the life of the patient, and back up needs to be provided when the pain clinician is on leave.

# APPENDIX 2

## Radiofrequency thermocoagulation

Radiofrequency thermocoagulation was first introduced in 1974 by Shealy for facet joint denervation of the lumbar spine.

### Procedures for which radiofrequency is used.

- Lumbar facet denervation
- Thoracic facet denervation
- Cervical facet denervation
- Root ganglion lesioning (pulsed radiofrequency)
- Trigeminal thermocoagulation
- Sympathectomy
- Cordotomy
- Peripheral nerve lesions
- Lumbar anuloplasty.

## Equipment needed for radiofrequency

The needles used are Teflon coated, and they are available at 5, 10 and 15 cm, with exposed tips from 1–10 mm, depending on requirements. A probe is inserted down the needle. The probe contains 3 wires: one wire carries radio-frequency current from the radio-frequency lesion generator to the tip of the probe; a second wire completes the circuit to the earth plate, which is attached to one of the patient's extremities; the third wire runs from a thermistor at the tip of the probe to a temperature display on the radio-frequency machine. Once the earth plate is attached and the needle and probe are in place, the circuit can be judged to be intact when the temperature display is at body temperature (37–38°C). Both resistance and current can also be displayed and all radio-frequency machines will also have a timer, which can be operated manually or pre-set. Radio-frequency machines will also have the ability to stimulate using a sensory (50–100 Hz) or motor (1–2 Hz) frequencies.

Once the nerve that requires lesioning is located, there are two forms of radio-frequency lesioning; the most commonly used one is to increase the power output from the radio-frequency lesion generator to produce a temperature display of 60–80°C for 60 seconds (Fig A.2). Radio-frequency current does not heat the probe or needle as such, but heats the surrounding tissue in the same way as a microwave does. This causes heating without tissue destruction, although thermocoagulation of the nerve will occur as nerves are more temperature sensitive than other tissues. However, the nerve itself remains intact as simply the peripheral process of the axon that is affected. The nerve architecture is preserved and the nerve is thought to regenerate down this with the passage of time. Because of this concern about nerve injury and the possibility of subsequent neuropathic pain (although this appears to be a rare occurrence with this technique), there has been more recent interest in the use of pulsed radiofrequency. The aim of this is to produce pulses of radiofrequency (300 KHz for 30 milliseconds out of a 1 second cycle with the output adjusted so the temperature reaches no more than 42°C). This technique is still under evaluation, although is becoming increasingly widely used.

(a)

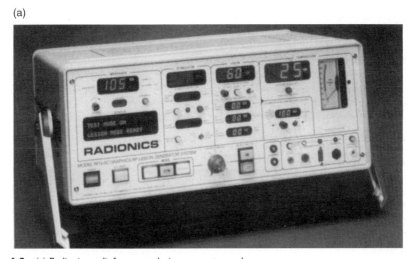

**Figure A.2**  (a) Radionics radiofrequency lesion generator and

*Continued*

(b)

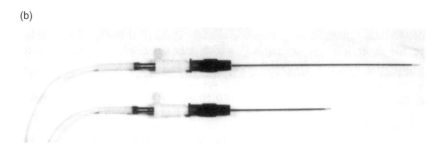

**Figure A.2 cont'd**   (b) Sluyter-Mehta needles.

# APPENDIX 3

## Transcutaneous electrical nerve stimulation

Transcutaneous electrical nerve stimulation (TENS) appears to alleviate the appreciation of pain in certain circumstances where there is a peripheral nociceptive component (Figure A.3). Conversely, it does not help in central pain states and psychological pain problems.

### Indications

- Myofascial syndromes
- Peripheral nerve injuries
- Phantom limb
- Stump pains
- Possible in some mechanical back, neck and joint pains.

A variety of electrodes, some of which are self-adhesive, are available. They need to be of adequate size, (at least 4 cm²). They are placed in order, surrounding the painful area. Good electrical contact is essential, and may necessitate plenty of electrode gel to ensure this. The patient is instructed to control the amplitude and frequency of the output from a small light portable stimulator.

There are numerous designs of TENS machines on the market at differing prices. The choice is up to the individual. Differences lie in the design of the controls, knobs versus electronic, number of pads (2 or 4) and shape of the casing.

The main advantages of the technique are that it has virtually no side-effects and it moves the locus of the control of pain back to the individual. Even if it does not afford complete relief, it can often be very helpful in combination with physiotherapy and analgesics.

Caution has to be exercised in patients with implanted cardiac pace-makers. Although most recent makes of these are relatively proof against electrical interference, it is probably wise to avoid their employment unless the manufacturers endorse their product as safe for use with TENS.

Skin care can be a problem in some patients whose skin is sensitive to adhesives. It can, therefore, be wise to rotate types of paddle, gel and adhesive tape.

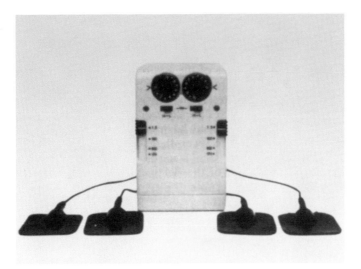

**Figure A.3**  Transcutaneous nerve stimulator and pads.

# APPENDIX 4

## Cryoanalgesia

Pain relief can be achieved by freezing nerves directly. While histological studies show that epineural and endoneural circulation is disrupted, leading to severe odema with diapedesis of polymorphonuclear cells through the vessel walls, there is a low incidence of long-term deafferentation problems since the nerve sheaths are not disrupted. Thus, the nerve axons can regenerate down the old neural tubes without scarring. Analgesia can be expected to last between 12 days and a few months and, interestingly, the analgesia can outlast the return of sensation.

It is useful therefore in self-limiting conditions or in order to give the patient a 'pain holiday' for a special event (e.g. a wedding). Cryoprobes are electrically insulated up to the tip and thus the target nerves can be stimulated at 2 and 100 Hz for confirmation of accurate placement before the tip is cooled to $-60°C$ by the adiabatic expansion of nitrous oxide or carbon dioxide. The ice ball that forms after 60 s is 2–4 mm in diameter depending on the vascularity of the tissue. It can be performed with the help of local anaesthesia; in fact patients will often tell you how soothing the actual cryotherapy is! As a form of treatment it has its advocates and its detractors.

### Indications

- Neuromas
- Fractured ribs (intercostal nerves)
- Postherapetic neuralgia (sometimes)
- Facet joint pain
- Coccydynia
- Scar pain.

**341**

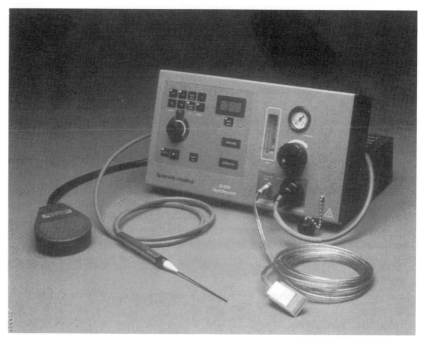

**Figure A.4**   Lloyd Neurostat and probe for cryotherapy.

## Use of cryoprobe (Figure A.4)

- Infiltration of skin surface with 1% lignocaine
- Insertion of cryoprobe under image intensification
- Stimulation to 100 Hz to 2 Hz for sensory confirmation and motor fibre exclusion
- Injection of 1% lignocaine at site for lesion
- Lesion at −60°c for 120 s
- Injection of 0.5 ml of bupivacaine/Depo-Medrone mixture (10 ml 0.5% plain bupivacaine + 40 mg Depo-Medrone).

# APPENDIX 5

## Spinal cord stimulation

Stimulation of the spinal cord has been performed since the 1960s by direct placement of the electrodes on the surface of the dura mater overlying the target level of the cord at open laminectomy. The technique then fell in relative disrepute, as the scientific basis for its action was then unexplained.

From animal work, it is now quite clear that spinal cord stimulation (SCS) works by neuromodulation; mobilizing γ-amino-butyric acid (GABA) and adenosine, restoring depleted GABA levels in certain neuropathic pain states, antidromic inhibition of spinothalamic afferent activity and direct neuronal effects resulting in the altered expression of C-fos. Undoubtedly, there will be more basic science discoveries with time. It is, however, usual for the stimulation-induced analgesia to significantly outlast the period of stimulation.

Thousands of patients worldwide now attest to its benefit. It is rarely 100% pain relieving in the highly selected and complex refractory pain problems for which it is employed, but then what is?

Developments in leads, electrode arrays, materials and batteries have enormously improved the SCS systems available to patients. Stimulation patterns are more focussed, and efficacy continues to improve, as our knowledge of best-suited systems and electrode arrays expands.

## Patient selection

Before considering the expensive form of treatment the following criteria should be satisfied:

- There is a physical basis for the complaint.
- All forms of alternative therapy have been tried.
- Psychiatric assessment has confirmed motivation and long-term commitment without major issues of secondary gain (compensation, litigation).
- The underlying pathology and topography are suitable for stimulation by the appropriate electrode system.

## Indications

After initial over-enthusiasm for this form of treatment, collected wisdom would suggest rather fewer conditions than indicated in the first edition of this book respond well to this expensive treatment. Since, in these cost conscious times, such expense has to be justified, most responsible implanters of SCS systems have been refining their patient-selection criteria with the resulting improvement in outcome. Within the groups mentioned here, the results are now much better than the global results often previously quoted as 50% pain relief at 2 years in 50% of patients. It must also be remembered that conditions change within patients over time, and that patient compliance with coincident functional restoration programs, for example, will be relevant to overall outcomes.

The best indications at present are:

- Intractable angina unsuitable for further revascularization procedures
- Complex regional pain syndromes, where all other treatment modalities have been tried
- Intractable sciatica from arachnoiditis, 'failed back surgery syndrome'.

Other less clear-cut indications, but where a trial of SCS should be considered if all other treatment modalities have failed:

- Neuropathic, including diabetes, and deafferentation pain
- Peripheral vascular disease and its sequelae-stump and phantom pain.

## Implantable systems

There are two types of system currently in use:

- Those where there is an implanted impulse generator powered by a lithium battery, which has to be replaced – the interval for which depends on the amount of use and the size of the system (vide infra) implanted.
- Those where the implanted receiver is activated by a radiofrequency signal from an antenna placed on the overlying skin.

Since the last edition of this book, the differences between the systems are reduced to the following:

- Implantable battery-driven impulse generators that can stimulate one or two electrode arrays, either vertically or horizontally, whose battery life dictates the size of the implant. Thus ®Synergy, which has a battery life of 7–10 years depending on stimulator usage is the largest, with the ®Itrel 3 and the ®Genesis impulse generators being smaller (Figure A.5). Externally driven radiofrequency receivers driven by antennae placed on the overlying skin, where the radiofrequency signal is then converted to square-wave direct current by the receiver to stimulate the electrodes. The antenna is connected to the pulse generator powered by a replaceable 9 V battery.
- All the parameters that can be programmed are accessible to the patient with the radiofrequency system, whereas only limited parameters, (amplitude, frequency and pulse width), can be changed by the patient with the implanted impulse generators.
- The implanted impulse generators are easy to activate, do not have any external attachments, which may limit activity, and do not have the problems of skin sensitivity to the adhesives commonly used to keep the antenna in place in the radiofrequency systems.
- The radiofrequency systems, once implanted and working satisfactorily should not require further surgery, and therefore cost!

## Which leads should be selected?

Selection of leads depends on which arrangement will give the best paraesthesia coverage to the painful area.

At present up to sixteen electrodes can be stimulated by one system. Thus a patient could have two octrodes, which could be placed parallel to each other or at two different vertical sites. Alternatively, four quatrodes could be inserted to cover two different sites bilaterally or up to four sites vertically.

## Which level?

The representation of the dermatomal level in the dorsal columns of the spinal cord is much higher than the corresponding vertebral level, thus, for example, the 'sweet spot' for sciatic pain, (dermatomal levels L5 and S1) is around T10. These levels have been mapped out by G-C Barolat and J Holsheimer in 1998 and show the likelihood of obtaining paraesthesia coverage for different parts of the body at different vertebral levels.

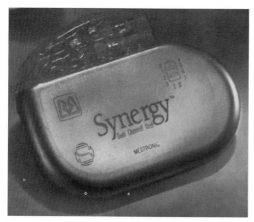
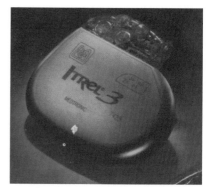

**Figure A.5**   Illustration of (a) ®Synergy and (b) ®Itrel 3 impulse generators.

This is complicated by the fact that the posterior cerebrospinal fluid (CSF) space varies up and down the spinal cord, which in turn affects the distance between the electrode, placed epidurally, and the dorsal columns. When this distance is large, the stimulation amplitude required to stimulate the dorsal column fibres stimulates the dorsal root fibres, which, although more distant, have lower electrical stimulation thresholds. This can result in painful segmental stimulation rather than soothing paraesthesia. Different electrode configurations have been tried to overcome this and include:

- Close parallel arrays sited as close to the physiological midline as possible (one radiographic study showed that the physiological midline was up to 2 mm right of the anatomical midline).
- 'Guarded cathode' or positive–negative–positive electrodes vertically or, in some cases, transversely where three electrodes are placed parallel to each other.
- Inter-electrode spacing of 2 mm rather than 4 mm.

## Ante-operative care

Antibiotic prophylaxis is controversial. All are agreed that a 'loading' dose of a broad-spectrum antibiotic intravenously prior to skin incision is mandatory. In our institution, all patients are swabbed to screen for methicillin-resistant *Staphylococcus aureus* (MRSA) 1 week prior to surgery. If positive, they are treated with nasal mupirocin ointment. Otherwise, 1200 mg of augmentin (or equivalent if the patient is allergic to penicillin) is given intravenously at the start of the procedure before skin infiltration with local anaesthetic.

## Placement of the electrodes

Electrodes can be introduced into the epidural space either directly at laminotomy or through a needle whose tip has entered the epidural space.

Surgically placed electrodes can be 'paddle-type', which are flatter and broader, or parallel arrays of slimmer electrodes. This approach is often necessary because adhesions, epidural fibrosis or anatomical variations prohibit the passage cranially of percutaneously introduced electrodes.

Figure A.6 illustrates ®Resume and ®Lamitrode electrodes.

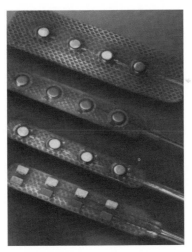

**Figure A.6**   Illustration of ®Resume electrodes.

It is important to radiologically confirm the desired level. On-table confirmation of satisfactory paraesthesia coverage of the painful area is rarely undertaken since the patients will be anaesthetised, at least for the laminotomy. Even if they are then allowed to waken half-way through the procedure, they can be notoriously unreliable in confirming appropriate paraesthesia coverage.

The percutaneous placement of electrodes has been facilitated by the development of ®Epimed cannulas which slide over the modified Tuohy needles used to locate the space. The use of guide-wires, introde cannulas and curved or straight stylets in addition give the pain specialist much more flexibility in how to achieve successful electrode placement (Figure A.7).

Since the patients are awake for this, electrodes can be placed with the patient prone, in the lateral position or sitting up. Each position has advantages and disadvantages in terms of access, manoeuvrability or vaso-vagal episodes. All these factors have to weighed by the pain specialist and a plan made individually for each patient. Whichever position is decided upon, the author always uses a loss-of-resistance to saline technique monitored by a paediatric burette drip chamber. As the epidural space is entered the saline starts to drip in a definite manner giving a clear end-point.

The electrode then needs to be inserted into the epidural space aiming for the desired vertebral level. Once this has been achieved, on-table stimulation is then undertaken to confirm appropriate paraesthesia coverage and further manoeuvring of the electrodes or the decision to place a second parallel electrode made.

Once paraesthesia coverage is satisfactory, the electrode(s) is/are anchored to the interspinous ligaments with ®Ethibond braided sutures. These have the advantage of being brightly coloured so that, should it be necessary to re-explore the site at a later date, they can be easily identified.

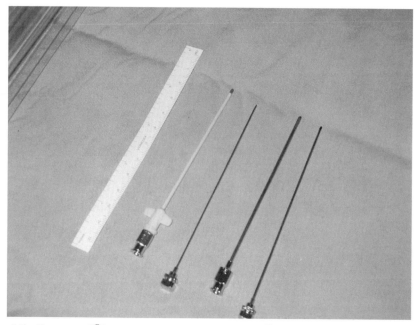

**Figure A.7**    Illustration of ®Epimed, guide-wire, Tuohy needle and ®Introde.

## Which settings?

- The cathode is about thirty times stronger than the anode in stimulating the dorsal column fibres. Therefore, the 'sweet spots' are usually located by stimulating the cathodes.
- Ideally it should be in the middle of the electrode, so any migration up or down of the electrode within the epidural space can be compensated for electronically by moving the site of the cathode.
- The pulse width determines the field of fibres that are stimulated, therefore a wider pulse width will increase the field and the patient experiences a broader area of paraesthesia.
- The frequency will be felt individually and, as such, is an individual preference. Some patients like a low frequency 'beating' sensation whereas others prefer a high frequency 'buzzing'. Anything goes!
- The threshold amplitude that paraesthesiae are felt depends on a number of factors. Previous epidural scarring, posterior CSF space and changes to the dorsal column fibres from trauma or other intrinsic conditions like diabetic neuropathy. Ideally paraesthesiae should be felt between 2–4 V. Much higher than this will rapidly drain the battery of an implanted impulse generator, which will then require replacement much sooner than it normally should, thus adding to the cost. Similarly with a radiofrequency system the 9 V batteries require replacement more often than usual, again adding to the cost. It may be an indication for a surgically placed electrode if it is likely to be due to epidural scar tissue that could be removed at subsequent operation.

## Implantation

After successful on-table stimulation, the pain specialist then has to decide whether to proceed there and then to implant the whole chosen system or connect the electrodes to temporary leads, which are then externalized for a trial period before the decision is made to implant or not. At the author's institution, practice has been changed. If on-table stimulation produces satisfactory paraesthesia coverage, the rest of the system is implanted immediately. We have found this reduces the incidence of infection and reduces the cost of hospitalization by avoiding two separate admissions, two episodes in the operating theatre and reduplication of drugs. Because of very stringent screening and selection criteria we have had very few 'unnecessary' implants. Looking back through our old patients records, the late failures had all had trials first. Most patients want to believe it will work and extremely few would choose not to have the implantation, since this effectively prolongs the trial period.

To complete the implantation, the electrodes are connected to barrel-shaped connectors at the proximal end of the extension cables, and the electrode contacts are tightened gently; they are then covered by a silicon sheath in one manufacturer's system or are already encased in a self-sealing silicon case in another's. A subcutaneous pocket is created in the hypochondrium or iliac fossa on the side chosen by the patient, and the proximal end of the cable tunnelled subcutaneously. The distal end of the extension cable is then attached to the chosen impulse generator or radiofrequency receiver and the skin of the pocket closed.

## Postoperative care

The selected intravenous antibiotics are continued for a further three doses then discontinued.

Patients are urged to avoid excessive bending and stretching for the first 24 hours, but otherwise mobilization is encouraged. They are usually ready to go home 48 hours or so after the procedure. There will always be exceptions when patients want to stay longer because they

**347**

need a lot of analgesia. The procedure is painful in its own right, and patients will experience considerable acute nociceptive pain, which must be treated accordingly and appropriately. For example, if a patient is already on 60 mg MST (slow release morphine) twice per day prior to the procedure it is illogical to prescribe a mere 10 mg morphine 4 hourly as required for post-operative analgesia as this won't touch their postoperative pain.

The author favours subcuticular monocryl sutures for skin closure, buttressed with ®Steristrips. A ®mepore dressing is applied as the initial dressing and then this is changed on the second postoperative day to a clear bio-occlusive dressing, so that the patient can go into the shower if desired. The wounds are usually healed and sealed in 10 days.

## Complications

The following have been reported:

- Infection localized and immediate or delayed – even sinus formation
- Transient paraplegia, which took 3 months to resolve
- Postoperative allodynia, which can necessitate change in the implant site
- Seroma and local tenderness over the anchor site, dorsally, or the implant site in the abdomen
- CSF leakage as a result of dural puncture – more likely at laminotomy when there has been considerable epidural fibrosis or scarring
- Postdural puncture headache – particularly severe because of the calibre of the needle used if following attempted percutaneous insertion
- Electrode migration – usually as a result of a trip or a fall
- Electrode failure – disconnection of the electrode/extension/implant electrical contacts or separation because of seepage of blood or serous fluid
- Receiver failure
- Expanding epidural haematoma causing ascending paralysis.

# APPENDIX 6

## Deep brain stimulation

In rare cases deep brain stimulation may be the last resort.

## Indications

- Certain head and neck pains
- Thalamic pain
- Neural injury
- Complex regional pain syndrome (CRPS)
- Failed back surgery syndrome
- Pains whose topography is not amenable to dorsal column stimulation
- Underlying lesion has caused loss of dorsal columns
- Failure of SCS.

As with SCS the patient must have a suitable psychological profile.

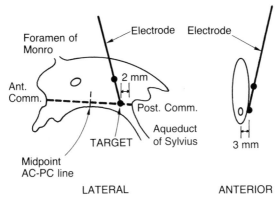

**Figure A.8** Electrode placement in reference to an outline of the third ventricle and aqueduct (Schaltenbrand-Bailey coordinates FP-10, HT-0, LT-4)

## Sites

- Sensory thalamus
- Periaqueductal grey nucleus (Figure A.8).

There are other sites targeted as well, but this lies in the realms of extremely specialized neurosurgery and is outside the scope of this publication.

## Complications

- Incidence of haemorrhage – 3%
- Diplopia (when periaqueductal grey nucleus is the target)
- Transient paraesthesias when the ventral basal thalamus is the target
- Incidence of infection – 3%, not usually in the central nervous system
- Malfunction of the equipment – 10%
- Development of tolerance, especially when the periaqueductal grey nucleus is the target.

# Index

'vs' indicates differential diagnosis.